OXFORD MEDICAL PUBLICATIONS

Phase I Cancer Clinical Trials

Oxford University Press makes no representation, express or implied, that the drug dosages in this book are correct. Readers must therefore always check the product information and clinical procedures with the most up to date published product information and data sheets provided by the manufacturers and the most recent codes of conduct and safety regulations. The authors and the publishers do not accept responsibility or legal liability for any errors in the text or for the misuse or misapplication of material in this work.

Phase I Cancer Clinical Trials
A Practical Guide

Elizabeth A Eisenhauer MD, FRCPC
Director, Investigational New Drug Program,
NCIC Clinical Trials Group
and
Professor of Oncology,
Queen's University, Kingston, Ontario, Canada

Chris Twelves B Med Sci, MB ChB, MD, FRCP
Professor of Clinical Cancer Pharmacology
University of Leeds and Bradford Hospitals
NHS Trust, Yorkshire, United Kingdom

Marc Buyse ScD
Executive Director,
International Drug Development Institute,
Brussels, Belgium
and
Director, Institut National du Cancer
Department of Clinical Research and Biostatistics,
Paris, France

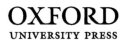

OXFORD
UNIVERSITY PRESS

OXFORD
UNIVERSITY PRESS

Great Clarendon Street, Oxford OX2 6DP

Oxford University Press is a department of the University of Oxford.
It furthers the University's objective of excellence in research, scholarship,
and education by publishing worldwide in

Oxford New York

Auckland Cape Town Dar es Salaam Hong Kong Karachi
Kuala Lumpur Madrid Melbourne Mexico City Nairobi
New Delhi Shanghai Taipei Toronto

With offices in

Argentina Austria Brazil Chile Czech Republic France Greece
Guatemala Hungary Italy Japan South Korea Poland Portugal
Singapore Switzerland Thailand Turkey Ukraine Vietnam

Oxford is a registered trade mark of Oxford University Press
in the UK and in certain other countries

Published in the United States
by Oxford University Press Inc., New York

Library of Congress Cataloging in Publication Data
Eisenhauer, Elizabeth A.
   Phase 1 cancer clinical trials: a practical guide / Elizabeth A. Eisenhauer, Christopher Twelves,
Marc Buyse. – 1st ed.
   p.; cm.
   Includes bibliographical references and index.
1. Cancer–Treatment. 2. Clinical trials. I. Twelves, Christopher. II. Buyse, Marc E. III. Title.
   [DNLM: 1. Neoplasms–therapy. 2. Clinical Trials, Phase 1–methods. QZ 266 E36 2006]
   RC270.8.E37 2006
   616.99'406–dc22
                                        2006014770
Typeset by SPI Publisher Services, Pondicherry, India
Printed in Great Britain
on acid-free paper by Biddles Ltd., King's Lynn

ISBN 0–19–856719–7 (Pbk.:alk.paper)   978–0–19–856719–6 (Pbk.)

10 9 8 7 6 5 4 3 2 1

Foreword

The phenomenal expansion in our knowledge on the molecular biology of cancer, as witnessed over the last decade, has very important implications for the performance of our clinical trials in Oncology Drug Development.

This is particularly so for phase I clinical studies. Most of the 'druggable' targets identified by molecular biology research require a continuous exposure to drug for an effective suppression of cancer growth. As a consequence we will increasingly witness chronic dosing of agents, which, in turn, will result in different definitions of dose-limiting toxicities. A side-effect that may be acceptable for a short while may not be at all acceptable when experienced daily and continuously. In addition we will be moving to different dosing regimens. Beside the consequences of newly identified targets, the changes in dosing regimens will also have implications from the regulatory perspective. Different pre-clinical data will be needed as study requirements and phase I study designs will also change. Finally outcome measures of phase I studies are changing as well. The continuous debate on surrogate markers of effect is ongoing and it can be anticipated that the importance of phase I clinical studies will only increase over the next few years, while the relative importance of phase II studies will decrease.

Given all of the above, it is of crucial importance to have an appropriate guideline for designing, writing, and performing clinical phase I trials. Such a guideline was missing up to now. *Phase I Cancer Clinical Trials: a practical guide* provides this guidance. The editors have succeeded in providing a very complete and comprehensive overview of all of the topics that are of importance for the clinical investigator. This book is an indispensable tool for all of those interested in and participating in phase I clinical trials in oncology.

Professor Jaap Verweij, MD, PhD
Medical Oncologist
Erasmus University Medical Center Rotterdam
The Netherlands

Acknowledgements

There are many individuals and organizations that deserve special thanks for their assistance in completing this book.

Joseph Pater and Lesley Seymour of the National Cancer Institute of Canada Clinical Trials Group (NCIC CTG) reviewed and commented on several sections, provided permission to use certain NCIC CTG documents which, with some modification, were added to the Appendices, and covered my duties at the CTG while I was on sabbatical from Queen's University to complete this project.

Jaap Verweij (Rotterdam Cancer Institute), Janet Dancey (Cancer Therapy Evaluation Program, Bethesda), Lillian Siu (Princess Margaret Hospital, Toronto), Steven Hirschfeld (US Food and Drug Administration), and Melanie Walker (NCIC CTG) all contributed their wisdom in reviewing draft versions of some chapters.

Janet Manzo and colleagues at the Ontario Cancer Research Network provided permission to use some of their clinical trials tools as appendices and offered valuable feedback on issues related to study start-up.

Colleagues at FECS, ASCO, and AACR granted me permission to modify and use the Phase I Generic protocol used at the workshop they co-sponsor on Methods in Clinical Cancer Research (details on how to apply for this course and other similar workshops are found in Appendix IV).

-Elizabeth Eisenhauer

Abbreviations commonly used in this book

ALT	alanine aminotransferase
AST	aspartate aminotransferase
AUC	area under the curve
BA	biological activity
BSA	body surface area
CRF	case report form
CRM	continual reassessment method
CT	computerized tomography
CTA	Clinical Trial Authorisation (Europe) or Clinical Trial Application (Canada)
CTC	common toxicity criteria
CTCAE	Common terminology criteria for adverse events
DCE	dynamic contrast enhanced
DLT	dose-limiting toxicity
EGFR	epidermal growth factor receptor
EMEA	European Medicines Agency
EWOC	Escalation With Overdose Control
FDA	Food and Drug Administration (US)
FDG	fluorodeoxyglucose
GCP	Good Clinical Practice (a guideline from ICH)
GFR	glomerular filtration rate
GLP	Good Laboratory Practice
GMP	Good Manufacturing Practice
ICH	International Conference on Harmonization
IC_{50}	concentration needed to inhibit 50% activity
IEC	Institutional Ethics Committee or Independent Ethics Committee
IRB	Institutional Review Board
IND	Investigational New Drug Application
LD_{10}	lethal dose in 10% of animals
MAD	maximum administered dose
MBAD	minimum biologically active dose

$MELD_{10}$ mouse equivalent LD_{10}

MTD   maximum tolerated dose (or maximum tolerable dose)

MRI   magnetic resonance imaging

NCI   National Cancer Institute

NOAEL   no observed adverse effect level

OBAD   optimum biologically active dose

PBMC   peripheral blood mononuclear cell

PET   positron emission tomography

PIS   patient information sheet

PK   pharmacokinetic

PD   pharmacodynamic

REB   Research Ethics Board

RECIST   Response Evaluation Criteria In Solid Tumours

RD   recommended (phase II) dose

SAE   serious adverse event

SUADR   serious unexpected adverse drug reaction

SOP   standard operating procedure

VEGF(R)   vascular endothelial growth factor (receptor)

WHO   World Health Organization

Contents

Appendices:

Chapter 1

Introduction

Elizabeth A. Eisenhauer

1.1 Drug development in cancer

The development of new agents for cancer therapy is an orderly and systematic process. Beginning with preclinical evidence for efficacy, as well as data on toxicology and mechanism of action, the classical clinical development of a new agent proceeds through three steps or phases. These steps have as their major goals: (a) establishment of a recommended dose and schedule; (b) discovery of whether the drug shows any preliminary evidence of activity in specific tumour types (or subtypes); and, finally (c) determination of whether the new agent alone, or in combination, has a meaningful impact on survival or other measures of efficacy in cancer patients. In all phases of investigation, compilation of drug safety and other data also takes place. Table 1.1 outlines these steps and highlights the types of questions, trial design, and endpoints that are typically associated with each in cancer drug development.

1.1.1 Cytotoxic chemotherapy development

Historically, the process of clinical development arose in the era of cytotoxic chemotherapy in the 1960s. As summarized in a recent historical review by Chabner and Roberts [1], early research into the relationship between dose and cell kill by Schabel and Skipper [2,3] provided the foundation for the strategy of giving the highest tolerable dose in clinical studies, and in fact laid the foundations for research in high-dose chemotherapy with stem cell support that occupied a great deal of clinical research activity in the 1980s and 1990s. Thus, phase I trials employing dose escalation to achieve levels of the 'maximum tolerated dose' of the cancer agent became the norm [4,5], not

Table 1.1 Cancer trial goals, designs, and endpoints

Phase	Goal	Question(s)	Design	Usual outcome measure(s) (primary endpoint)	Issues for 'non-cytotoxic' agents
I	Determine recommended dose for further evaluation	What maximum dose that can be administered? What is pharmacokinetic behaviour?	Non-randomized Dose escalation	Toxic effects using standard criteria	Is dosing to toxicity appropriate or necessary? Can direct measures of target effect be utilized to determine dose?
II	Determine if sufficient evidence of biologic effect to continue drug development	What is the response rate of the drug in a defined population? Does it surpass a pre-set minimum?	Non-randomized (some phase II trials may be randomized) Multistage enrolment to allow early stopping	Objective response	Is phase II necessary? If tumour regression is not anticipated, what endpoints are appropriate for non-randomized trials screening for efficacy? Should population be restricted to those expressing target? How should biomarker for efficacy be defined and identified?
III	Determine relative efficacy of new versus standard treatment	Does the treatment incorporating the new drug produce improved survival or freedom from relapse? Is the new treatment superior in terms of quality of life?	Randomized Early stopping rules for extreme differences allowed	Survival Relapse-free survival Quality of life measures	Should population be enriched for expression of relevant biomarker or target? How to combine/sequence with other agents? Should early stopping for futility be used?

only because of the preclinical science but also because the toxic effects that limited dose, usually myelosuppression, provided evidence of the biological effects that were desired of the new agent on the tumour.

Following completion of phase I trials, phase II evaluation, designed to screen new drugs for signals of antitumour activity meriting further investigation, utilized tumour regression, defined by objective standard measures, as the primary endpoint [6,7].

Finally, phase III trials in which the new agent was evaluated (alone or incorporated into combination) in comparison with standard treatment, provided a mechanism for unbiased assessment of the impact of the new drug in randomized designs that utilized clinically meaningful endpoints of relapse-free or overall survival.

1.1.2 Non-cytotoxic drug development

Some decades later, although many new cytotoxic drugs and other agents identified by empirical screening and other means continue to enter clinical trials, the landscape of new anticancer agents has changed. Therapeutic agents entering the clinic that are rationally designed or selected to affect specific intracellular and extracellular targets thought to be relevant to malignant transformation are commonplace. In this new era of 'molecular targeted therapy', questions have been posed about the appropriateness of applying the same clinical development paradigm and utilizing the same endpoints as are employed for cytotoxic drugs. Agents that are targeted to molecular aberrations in cellular and extracellular pathways may be devoid of traditional toxic effects, may not cause tumour regression, and may have effects only in molecularly defined subpopulations. Although it is generally agreed that phase III trials utilizing clinical endpoints are the final vital step in the development of newer agents, special attention needs to be paid to how the early clinical evaluation of such novel agents should most rationally proceed. Some of the questions that face targeted therapies are highlighted in the final column of Table 1.1.

1.2 Special role of phase I trials: finding the dose and schedule

Regardless of the debate about the endpoints and design of trials testing different types of cancer agents, it remains the case that phase I cancer trials are a critical first step in cancer drug development [8]. They are small sample size, non-randomized, dose escalation studies that define the recommended dose for subsequent study of a new drug in each schedule tested; they also produce early observations about the drug's safety, pharmacokinetic behaviour, and preliminary evidence of antitumour activity. The recommended dose is based on observations of toxic effects, pharmacokinetic outcomes or other measures as this book will describe. A wealth of preclinical information is utilized to inform phase I trial starting dose and design. Furthermore, statistical and other research has been undertaken to address issues of safety, ethics, and efficiency in the trial conduct and dose escalation methodologies.

As the subsequent development path for a drug is heavily dependent on the dose and schedule recommended from phase I trials, it is critically important to assure that the design, conduct, and analysis of these trials are rigorous. Rushing to finish phase I trials, inclusion of patients very different from those who will be treated in later studies, or taking a poorly justified decision at the end of phase I (e.g. choosing a schedule based only on convenience rather than supported by other data) may paradoxically *increase* the overall time of subsequent drug development or jeopardize the drug's future altogether.

The stories of gemcitabine and marimastat provide examples of some of these problems, albeit in diverging directions.

When the phase I trials of gemcitabine were originally conducted, it was recognized early on that schedule played a very prominent role in the dose of drug that could be delivered and in its toxic effects: the daily$\times$5 schedule was fraught with significant flu-like effects and only relatively small doses could be administered [9]. When the dose was given as a 30-minute infusion for 3 of 4 weeks, more drug could be delivered per cycle and myelosuppression, particularly thrombocytopenia, was dose-limiting. The latter schedule was thus selected for further development and the recommended phase II dose was 790 mg/m^2 (rounded to 800 mg/m^2 in initial phase II trials) [10]. However, as is often the case in phase I trials, heavily pretreated patients made up the population enrolled, and dose escalation was very conservative, resulting in a large number of patients treated at low doses without any toxicity, and very few patients treated near the recommended dose. When gemcitabine began its phase II evaluation at the recommended dose, little in the way of toxic effects were seen, and doses were first escalated to 1000 mg/m^2 then to 1250 mg/m^2 [11–14]. In the end, the phase I trial was repeated in non-small cell lung cancer patients who were treatment naïve: a dose of 2200 mg/m^2 was recommended [15], although many continued to use single agent doses in the range of 1000 mg/m^2 (the dose that was in fact approved for use in pancreatic carcinoma in the USA in 1996). In the same interval, exploration of increasing dose by giving a fixed dose rate infusion for increasingly long periods of time was undertaken [16]. This new approach was based on the knowledge gained through early trials that there was a fixed rate at which gemcitabine could be converted into its active phosphorylated form by deoxycytidine kinase. Recently, a randomized phase II trial in pancreatic cancer compared the maximal doses of gemcitabine delivered by the two methods: $1500 \, mg/m^2$ as a $10 \, mg/m^2$ per min infusion and $2200 \, mg/m^2$ as a 30-minute bolus [17]. In that trial, although there was no observed impact on the primary endpoint of time to treatment failure, there was an observed survival advantage (5 vs. 8 months) for the fixed dose rate arm, suggesting that that approach in drug delivery merited further evaluation. This example illustrates two things: first, that the initial choice of starting dose in the weekly schedule proved too low because the patients enrolled in the original phase I trial were not representative of those enrolled in the phase II setting; secondly that the knowledge about the best schedule is still emerging. Both these factors added time to the development process for the drug.

The second example is that of marimastat. This agent was one of the earliest drugs developed to inhibit matrix metalloproteinases (MMPs), which have a critical role in angiogenesis and metastasis by degrading extracellular matrix in response to appropriate signals. MMPs are therefore an attractive target for experimental cancer therapeutics. Initial phase I trials of marimastat in healthy volunteers indicated that doses of 50–200 mg p.o. at 12-hourly intervals were well tolerated and could produce steady-state trough levels of free drug sufficient to inhibit metalloproteinases. On the basis of these data, a dose of 100 mg p.o. twice daily was selected for the initial clinical trials in cancer patients. However, it was soon recognized that this dose exceeded tolerable levels when dose-limiting myalgia and arthritis appeared [18,19]. Subsequent studies demonstrated that, in cancer patients, the plasma levels of the drug were much higher, dose for dose, than in the normal volunteer population. For example, at a dose of 50 mg p.o. twice daily, the mean trough plasma level was $59.4 \, \mu g/1$ in healthy volunteers and $286.2 \, \mu g/1$ in a population of colorectal cancer patients [20,21]. There was considerable time spent after trials began in redefining the tolerable dose for the cancer population.

It is possible that if phase I trials were undertaken today with both gemcitabine and marimastat the same issues could arise; citing these experiences is *not* intended to fault the decisions taken at the time, which were carefully considered. However, these historical examples serve to highlight how important it is that the phase I trials that determine the dose for future studies be designed to include appropriate numbers and types of subjects in order to limit the risk of making inaccurate recommendations. Otherwise, considerable time and effort will need to be invested when the drug is undergoing phase II investigation to refine dosing, leading to potential delays in the overall drug development process.

1.3 Differences between cancer and other therapeutic areas

Unlike most other therapeutic areas, studies of cancer therapeutics usually are conducted first in *patients with the disease* rather than in normal healthy volunteers. The major reason for this is that anticancer agents often cause substantial toxic effects, or may need to be given in doses producing such effects, which are thought to be inappropriate for healthy subjects. Furthermore, the pharmacological behaviour of drugs may differ between patients and healthy subjects, as was illustrated in the case of marimastat referred to above. Thus, even if a cancer drug is first studied in a dose-seeking design in healthy subjects, it must eventually undergo a similar study in cancer patients to assure that dosing and pharmacology are similar in that population.

The study of cancer patients in a phase I setting poses unique ethical issues. Patients who have disease for which no active therapy remains who are offered participation in phase I trials may see this as an opportunity to help future patients but more often are hopeful that this treatment may prove effective in controlling their disease. While this may indeed be possible, it is not the goal of the phase I trial to establish efficacy but rather dosing and safety information. This and other ethical issues associated with phase I trials in an advanced disease population oblige investigators, institutions, and sponsors to address these through appropriate review of the study protocol and development of a process of trial conduct and consent that is rigorous, balanced, and in compliance with internationally accepted standards.

1.4 What this book will do

This book will describe the process of phase I development for cancer agents from the preclinical information required before a new agent is given to humans for the first time, through to generation of the final phase I study report. Agents that have direct effects on cancer and its tissue environment will be the major focus of the book; immunological therapies will not be emphasized, though many of the principles in their study are similar. Regulatory, ethical, and practical issues will be covered. Chapters 2–6 offer theoretical considerations in phase I trial design and conduct. Chapters 7–11 give practical information and examples covering protocol development, trial conduct, pharmacokinetic and pharmacodynamic assay development, and how to report the study. Finally, numerous appendices will offer useful resources for the clinician or investigator interested in studying new therapies or combinations of agents in a first-in-man assessment.

References

1. Chabner BA, Roberts RG Jr. (2005). Timeline: chemotherapy and the war on cancer. *Nat Rev Cancer* 5: 65–72.

2. Skipper HE, Schabel FM Jr, Wilcox WS (1964). Experimental evaluation of potential anticancer agents. XIII. On the criteria and kinetics associated with 'curability' of experimental leukaemia. *Cancer Chemother Rep* 35: 1–111.

3. Skipper HE, Griswold DP (1984). Frank Schabel 1918–1983. *Cancer Res* 44: 871–2.

4. Carter SK (1977). Clinical trials in cancer chemotherapy. *Cancer* 40 (Suppl. 1): 544–7.

5. EORTC New Drug Development Committee (1985). EORTC Guidelines for phase I trials with single agents in adults. *Eur J Cancer Clin Oncol* 21: 1005–7.

6. Miller AB, Hoogstraten B, Staquet M, Winkler A (1981). Reporting results of cancer treatment. *Cancer* 47: 207–14.

7. Therasse P, Arbuck SG, Eisenhauer EA, *et al.* (2000). New guidelines to evaluate the response to treatment in solid tumors (RECIST Guidelines). *J Natl Cancer Inst* 92: 205–16.

8. (1997) Critical role of phase I clinical trials in cancer treatment. *J Clin Oncol* 15: 853–9.

9. O'Rourke TJ, Brown TD, Havlin K, *et al.* (1994). Phase I clinical trial of gemcitabine given as intravenous bolus on 5 consecutive days. *Eur J Cancer*, 30A: 417–18.

10. Abbruzzese JL, Grunewald R, Weeks EA, *et al.* (1991). A phase I clinical, plasma, and cellular pharmacology study of gemcitabine. *J Clin Oncol* 9: 491–8.

11. Cormier Y, Eisenhauer E, Muldal A, *et al.* (1994). Gemcitabine is an active new agent in previously untreated small cell lung cancer (SCLC). A study of the National Cancer Institute of Canada Clinical Trials Group. *Ann Oncol* 5: 283–5.

12. Mertens WC, Eisenhauer EA, Moore M, *et al.* (1993). Gemcitabine in advanced renal cell carcinoma. A phase II study of the National Cancer Institute of Canada Clinical Trials Group. *Ann Oncol* 4: 331–2.

13. Anderson H, Lund B, Bach F, Thatcher N, Walling J, Hansen HH (1994). Single-agent activity of weekly gemcitabine in advanced non-small cell lung cancer: a phase II study. *J Clin Oncol* 12: 1821–6.

14. Catimel G, Vermorken JB, Clavel M, *et al.* (1994). A phase II study of gemcitabine (LY 188011) in patients with advanced squamous cell carcinoma of the head and neck. EORTC Early Clinical Trials Group. *Ann Oncol* 5: 543–7.

15. Fosella FV, Lippman SM, Shin DM, *et al.* (1997). Maximum-tolerated dose defined for single-agent gemcitabine: a phase I dose-escalation study in chemotherapy-naïve patients with advanced non-small cell lung cancer. *J Clin Oncol* 15: 310–16.

16. Brand R, Capadano M, Tempero M (1997). A phase I trial of weekly gemcitabine administered as a prolonged infusion in patients with pancreatic cancer and other solid tumors. *Invest New Drugs* 15: 331–41.

17. Tempero M, Plunkett W, Ruiz van Haperen V, *et al.* (2003). Randomized phase II comparisons of dose-intense gemcitabine: thirty-minute infusion and fixed dose rate infusion in patients with pancreatic adenocarcinoma. *J Clin Oncol* 21: 3402–8.

18. Hidalgo M, Eckhardt SG (2001). Development of matrix metalloproteinase inhibitors in cancer therapy. *J Natl Cancer Inst* 93: 178–93.

19. Quirt I, Bodurtha A, Lohmann R, *et al.* (2002). Phase II study of marimastat (BB-2516) in malignant melanoma: a clinical and tumor biopsy study of the National Cancer Institute of Canada Clinical Trials Group. *Invest New Drugs* **20**: 431–7.

20. Millar AW, Brown PD, Moore J, *et al.* (1998). Results of single and repeat dose studies of the oral matrix metalloproteinase inhibitor marimastat in healthy male volunteers. *Br J Clin Pharmacol* **45**: 21–6.

21. Primrose JN, Bleiburg H, Daniel F, *et al.* (1999). Marimastat in recurrent colorectal cancer: exploratory evaluation of biological activity by measurement of carcinoembryonic antigen. *Br J Cancer* **79**: 509–14.

Chapter 2

Preclinical data and requirements
Elizabeth A. Eisenhauer

2.1 Introduction

This chapter is intended to guide investigators through some basic principles of preclinical evaluation. It is not expected that it will provide recipes for the conduct of preclinical studies or offer instructions for assembling the documentation necessary to have a new drug submission made to government authorities. Rather, this chapter will offer investigators advice regarding the critical evaluation of preclinical studies on new agents that they may be asked to consider studying in a phase I trial. The following questions will be addressed:

- What scientific and other data are needed before studying a new agent in cancer patients?
- What aspects of preclinical evaluation are subject to government regulation?

In particular, this section is geared to examining the data needed before the first human trials of a new agent may take place, although the preclinical studies described are also of importance to later combination phase I studies as they may facilitate decisions about drug combinations and study design.

2.2 General comments

Before considering the study of any new anticancer therapy in humans, the body of preclinical (also referred to as non-clinical) data must provide substantial evidence to support the initiation of clinical studies. The issues that should be addressed are: the *biological plausibility* of the agent having activity in cancer; the *expectation of benefit for patients; a reasonable expectation of safety;* and sufficient information on which to base a *starting dose* [1]. Although this framework was proposed in the context of phase I paediatric studies, it is more generally applicable to all first-in-man cancer trials.

In effect, the subsequent sections of this chapter will focus on the experimental studies and other information that, together, provides the compilation of evidence required to satisfy these general conditions.

2.3 The agent: its target and chemistry

The reward of decades of research aimed at understanding the biological basis of cancer is an ever-increasing list of molecular changes believed responsible for instigating or maintaining the malignant behaviour of tumours. This list is also viewed as one of potential therapeutic targets for drug development. Thus the starting point for review of a 'package' of information for a new therapeutic begins with the question: *What is its target?*

For most new agents the target is known (or believed to be known) largely because the drug in question has been *designed* to affect a particular molecular target. This is not always the case, however; drugs discovered through empirical screening of natural products are also brought into clinical trial. Although the decision to evaluate empirically discovered agents in the clinic may be based on efficacy in animal models, considerable effort goes into defining the molecular targets of these drugs before first-in-man studies commence. None the less, this work may be incomplete when clinical trials are initiated.

Assuming that most new agents have a putative target and thus a mechanism of action defined in preclinical experiments, an important question to consider as part of the evaluation of a phase I study proposal is *how important* the drug's target is likely to be for cancer therapy. Most investigator brochures and protocols contain relevant background information on the drug target to assist in making a judgement: it is wise to supplement these overviews with additional readings, unless the target is well known to the investigator as one of probable relevance. Evidence of the validity of a target for cancer therapy comes from a variety of experimental sources: (a) the association of its expression with prognosis or its impact on a signalling pathway of documented relevance in cancer; (b) the consequences of its amplification or inhibition in laboratory test systems; (c) its relevance in carcinogenesis experiments; (d) the frequency or pattern of its expression in a variety of tumour types; and (e) the efficacy of agents already in the clinic affecting the same target. The sum of such information provides the 'validation' that the target of a new agent is of relevance in cancer biology and, by extension, drugs affecting valid targets are interesting to study.

Beyond target validation, the identification of the drug target creates a burden to show, in preclinical experiments, that the drug has the desired effect on its target. For agents designed to inhibit the action of a specific protein, such as a kinase, this should include demonstration of protein inhibition *in vitro* and *in vivo* and also documentation that antitumour effects are accompanied by (and, by inference, due to) inhibition of the target kinase. More on this follows in subsequent sections.

Another key aspect of compound review relates to its *chemistry*. This does not mean one must understand the chemical synthetic process for the agent in question, but knowledge of the general chemical class and structure can point to a set of data that ought to be considered. What chemical class does the new agent belong to [small molecule, antibody, anti-sense oligodeoxynucleotides (ODN)]? Is it of novel structure? A natural product? An analogue? Answers to these questions will have implications for what to look for elsewhere in the preclinical data package. Examples include the following:

- Hydrophobic natural products may carry with them special challenges for formulation and, by consequence, administration.
- Agents that are of a particular chemical structure: e.g. antibodies, anti-sense ODNs or HLA class restricted peptides, may have species specificity that can render preclinical animal efficacy and toxicology studies challenging. Furthermore, agents such as these may have toxicological effects related to their chemical structure rather than effects on their target. ODNs are a case in point: The propensity for large anionic compounds such as ODNs to cause complement activation mandates specific toxicology tests to determine the critical levels at which this may happen.
- Finally, agents that are analogues of marketed cancer therapeutics are of greater interest if their preclinical evaluation distinguishes them sufficiently from their parent compound. Generally, this means they should be either less toxic (for example, carboplatin's great appeal lay in its relative renal-sparing toxicological profile compared with the parent cisplatin), or more effective in either the range of tumour types sensitive to the drug or in overcoming mechanisms of acquired or *de novo* resistance.

Thus the nature of the agent, its target and chemistry, provide the *plausibility* that the drug may be effective in treating cancer. This knowledge creates expectations for the content of the preclinical evaluation package. Understanding what to look for gives the investigator some direction and may also lead to pertinent questions to ask of the new drug's sponsor, if the anticipated experiments have not been done.

2.4 Preclinical efficacy data (non-clinical pharmacology)

If the previous section discussed, in general terms, the requirement for *plausibility* of the new drug having an impact in cancer, this section deals with another important topic: the *expectation for benefit*.

Although it is not reasonable to expect a new drug to show substantial antitumour effects in phase I trials where the goal is to identify its recommended dose, there should be a reasonable expectation, based on preclinical data, that the drug will have efficacy in later clinical development. This expectation is primarily based on the results of *in vitro* and *in vivo* efficacy experiments.

There is little prescribed by regulatory agencies vis-à-vis the laboratory models that are to be used to address efficacy. In fact, the International Conference of Harmonization (ICH), a project devoted to the development of standard international recommendations for non-clinical and clinical assessment of pharmaceuticals, is largely silent on this aspect of (cancer) drug evaluation. The ICH guideline on *General Considerations for Clinical Trials* mentions only that non-clinical pharmacological studies should include 'mechanism of action, dose-response ... relationships, and studies of the potential clinical routes of administration' [2].

The Committee for Medicinal Products for Human Use (CHMP—formerly the Committee for Proprietary Medicinal Products—CPMP) of the European Medicines Agency (EMEA) has provided a more specific guidance on preclinical evaluation of anticancer medicinal products [3]. This document suggests a variety of *in vitro* and *in vivo* studies to consider in the preclinical testing of an anticancer agent. Table 2.1 lists the tests that are described in the CHMP Guidance document. As can be seen, the recommendations are very general, and do not include any reference to which preclinical models are advised, or which methods are advised to assess the impact of the drug's effect on its molecular target within efficacy models.

United States Food and Drug Administration regulations are listed in Title 21 of the Code of Federal Regulations in section 312.23(a)8. No particular species tests are mandated, but the record keeping and reporting requirements are summarized in the regulations and described in an FDA Guidance

Table 2.1 Suggested Pre-clinical Studies of Antitumour activity: from the CPMP (CHMP) Note for Guidance

Nature of study	Detailed description	Comment in guideline
In vitro	Drug activity: In appropriately selected cell panel Identify IC_{50} for each line to develop drug-specific activity profile If drug has specific target, activity can be determined in cell lines expressing different target levels	Cell line panels that are well characterized, such as the US National Cancer Institute cell line panel may be used.
	Mechanisms of resistance: In parallel with above studies, develop profile with respect to possible mechanism of resistance	e.g. overexpression of P-glycoprotein, multidrug resistance protein, changes in topoisomerase I or II as appropriate to mechanism
	Exposure time and cell-cycle dependency	
	Disease specific activity	Further profile may be obtained using fresh human tumour samples
In vivo	Tumour-bearing animals Route of administration and dosing regimen (schedule)—should mimic planned human testing Efficacy criteria can include: tumour growth measures, survival time, and degree of remission or cure	Both xenograft or allograft models are possible

document 'Content and Format of Investigational New Drug Applications (INDs) for Phase 1 studies of drugs including well-characterized, therapeutic, biotechnology-derived products' [4].

The absence of required minimal preclinical efficacy standards means it is left to the judgement of those developing the agent, potential clinical investigators and review committees (including those in government review agencies) to judge if a given agent has demonstrated sufficient preclinical efficacy to justify human clinical trials. The studies described in the following section therefore represent, in our view, an ideal (not a mandatory) list of preclinical efficacy studies. These are studies that both academics and those with commercial interests ought to consider in evaluation of a new agent, particularly for a new agent that represents a novel class of therapeutic or one that has a novel target. Any individual drug must be assessed on the basis of the *totality* of preclinical information available supporting its human testing: efficacy models are but one aspect of that data set.

Table 2.2, which summarizes published *in vitro* and *in vivo* data on ZD6474, a compound with vascular endothelial growth factor receptor 2 (VEGFR–2) inhibiting activity, will be referenced throughout the next sections as an example of the output in a variety of preclinical efficacy studies [5].

2.4.1 Evidence of target effect

As noted earlier, agents that are developed specifically to affect a molecular system or target, should be evaluated with respect to that effect in preclinical development.

As many drugs affect aberrant proteins and enzyme systems found in malignancies and are intended to inhibit gain of function behaviour, the usual assessment begins with determination of the concentration of drug needed to inhibit its target enzyme. Results are expressed in terms of the IC50 (the inhibitory concentration of the drug needed to inhibit 50% of enzyme activity). This evaluation should include not only the putative drug target, but also other molecules in the same class or family in order to determine the spectrum of inhibition and the relative potency of the drug. Table 2.2 provides the data obtained for a small molecule inhibitor of VEGFR–2, ZD6474. As can be seen in this example, the agent not only inhibits the target tyrosine kinase enzyme, but also other kinases with varying degrees of potency. The degree to which high levels of specificity is desirable depends on the drug and its intended target, and also the prevailing views of the time. It was argued a decade ago that highly specific inhibitors were ideal; the views have now shifted with the successes seen with several small molecules such as BAY 43–9006 (sorafenib), which has multiple targets relevant to malignancy [6].

Target inhibition should also be assessed in cellular and in *in vivo* systems (see later sections of this chapter). These experiments may be somewhat more challenging. Generally, for kinase inhibitors, demonstration that the drug changes phosphorylation or changes measures of downstream signalling are the types of assays used. Other approaches include assessment of the agent's ability to inhibit the consequences of signalling stimulation [for example, see the vascular endothelial growth factor stimulated human umbilical vein endothelial cell (HUVEC) experiment in Table 2.2]. When dealing with agents such as ODNs, target inhibition is assessed by measuring levels of target protein or mRNA before and after treatment in controlled conditions.

Extremely useful experiments are those that show target inhibition in implanted tumours and relate the degree of inhibition to the dose administered, the measured antitumour effects (growth delay or survival for example),

Table 2.2 Example of preclinical *in vitro* and *in vivo* mechanistic and efficacy data: ZD 6474[*]

Assay	Assay type	Goal (s)	Results	Interpretation
Kinase inhibition	*In vitro* Non-cellular	To determine the IC$_{50}$ of ZD6474 in inhibiting target enzyme activity: VEGF receptor-2 tyrosine kinase. To assess selectivity against other kinases	IC$_{50}$(μM): VEGFR2: 0.04 PDGFR 1.1 Flt-4: 0.11 MEK >10 Flt-1: 1.6 CDK2 >10 EGFR 0.5 AKT >100	ZD6474 inhibits kinase activity of VEGFR2 (KDR) in submicromolar concentrations. It is relatively specific but also has micromolar inhibitory activity on EGFR, PDGFB, FLT-4, and Flt-1
HUVEC inhibition	*In vitro* Cellular Non-cancer cell line	To determine if ZD6474 can inhibit the *in vitro* growth of VEGF-stimulated endothelial cell line HUVEC	IC$_{50}$(μM): 0.06	ZD6474 inhibits VEGF stimulated endothelial cell growth in submicromolar concentrations as assessed by [³H]thymidine incorporation
Tumour cell growth	*In vitro* Cellular Cancer cell lines	To determine if ZD6474 can inhibit the *in vitro* growth of human and murine cancer cell lines	IC$_{50}$(μM): 2.7–13.5	ZD6474 inhibits *in vitro* tumour cell growth in micromolar concentrations as measured by [³H]thymidine incorporation Concentrations required to inhibit *in vitro* cell growth are 45–225-fold greater than those required to inhibit HUVEC growth
Inhibition of VEGF Signalling responses *in vivo*	*In vivo* Non-tumour-bearing rat model	To determine if ZD6474 can affect VEGF-stimulated hypotension and VEGF-dependent growth plate morphology in a rat model compared with control	2.5 mg/kg i.v. produces a 63% inhibition of VEGF-induced hypotension 50 mg/kg p.o. × 14 days: 57% increase growth plate 100 mg/kg p.o. × 14 days: 75% increase growth plate	Oral ZD6474 caused a partial reversal of VEGF-induced hypotension *in vivo*; it also produced a dose-dependent hypertrophy of the growth plate in young rats. Both observations support an *in vivo* effect on VEGF signalling

(Continued)

Table 2.2 *Continued*

Assay	Assay type	Goal (s)	Results	Interpretation
Intradermal tumour angiogenesis	*In vivo* Tumour-bearing animal	To determine the effect of ZD6474 on tumour vascularization in an intradermal model compared with control	ZD6474 administered daily × 5 days: 50 mg/kg: 63% inhibition of new tumour blood vessels 100 mg/kg: 79% inhibition of new tumour blood vessels	Oral ZD6474 cased inhibition of tumour-induced new vessel formation in an intradermal murine tumour model
Tumour growth inhibition	*In vivo* Tumour-bearing animal	To determine the effect of daily oral chronic administration of ZD6474 on *in vivo* tumour growth in a variety of subcutaneous human xenograft models compared with control. Tumours grown to 0.15 – 0.47 cm^3 before treatment	At 12.5 mg/kg/day p.o. × 3 weeks: 5/7 xenografts had significant growth delay At 25 mg/kg/day p.o. × 3 weeks: 7/7 xenografts had significant growth delay (46–89% growth inhibition) At 100 mg/kg/day p.o. × 3 weeks: 7/7 xenografts had significant growth delay (79–100% inhibition)	Dose-dependent growth inhibition. Maximal effects seen at 75 or 100 mg p.o. daily in most models
Tumour growth inhibition	*In vivo* Tumour-bearing animal	As above, except in established xenografts (0.65 – 1.4 cm^3 before treatment)	At 100 mg/kg/day p.o.: ZD6474 caused regression of established PC-3 xenografts and growth delay of Calu-6 xenografts	ZD6474 has activity in well established tumours

EGFR, epidermal growth factor receptor. *Data abstracted from Wedge *et al.* (2002) *Cancer Res* **62**: 4645–55.

and if possible, plasma levels of drug. This type of experiment, though complex, neatly links four critical parameters for phase I trial design: (a) the *dose*; (b) the *plasma level*; (c) the maximal *efficacy*; and (d) the *degree of target inhibition*. Unfortunately, experiments evaluating all of these elements are not often performed: there may be correlation between dose and target inhibition or antitumour effects and target inhibition, but rarely are all four elements dissected in a single set of experiments. Increasing preclinical investment in assessing pharmacokinetic (PK)–PD effects will facilitate intelligent phase I trial conduct and design.

2.4.2 Single agent *in vitro* studies

In vitro assessment is the usual starting point for the efficacy evaluation of a potential new cancer agent.

In vitro cellular assays may examine mechanistic questions, for example as in Table 2.2 where the vascular endothelial growth factor receptor targeted drug ZD6474 was tested for growth inhibition of human umbilical vein endothelial cells, an endothelial cell line whose growth is dependent on vascular endothelial growth factor signalling. Other *in vitro* assays have been developed to evaluate antitumour effects in malignant cell lines or fresh tumour samples.

Antitumour *in vitro* assays include several types. For example, *antiprolifera-tive* assays use incorporation of [^{3}H]thymidine or colony formation as end-points. Others assess *viability or growth* using colorimetric assessment. The latter type of assay measure is the basis of the *in vitro* screen of the NCI Developmental Therapeutics Program. Using a 60-cell line system, patterns of dose–response can be identified and sorted using a computer algorithm. This has led to the development of a web-based tool known as 'COMPARE' where the patterns of activity are sorted to allow investigation of the mechanism of action of new compounds and assessment of a variety of other attributes, including comparison with other active cancer agents, tumour type specificity and more [7].

It is reasonable to expect that most new cancer agents that are likely to be effective in clinical testing will have demonstrated antiproliferative and/or cytotoxic effects in a number of *in vitro* assay systems, including cell lines. Exceptions to this are agents that have mechanisms of action that require engagement of a secondary biological system (e.g. biological response modifiers, angiogenesis inhibitors) or those whose activity derives solely from modulating the activity of other cancer drugs (e.g. chemotherapy resistance modulators). Under these circumstances, appropriate *in vivo* (for biologically activated agents) or combination *in vitro* studies (in the case of modulating agents) are needed.

2.4.3 Single agent *in vivo* efficacy studies

Much has been written about the value of *in vivo* tumour model systems as a method of predicting clinical activity. In short, there is no single system generally agreed to have reliable positive predictive value in human tumours. Some have argued, therefore, that *in vivo* data are unnecessary before proceeding into clinical trials in humans. This is, however, a minority view. Furthermore, there are no anticancer agents in use today that did not have preclinical *in vivo* efficacy testing. It is not clear what the merits would be in skipping this step as it provides at least some evidence that the drug to be evaluated has biological effects of the type considered relevant in intact animals. For many therefore, this is a critical 'test' of a new agent's mettle, which cannot be foregone. While positive *in vivo* results cannot guarantee clinical success, they offer additional favourable evidence that the agent can *reasonably be expected to provide benefit.* Furthermore, *in vivo* studies afford opportunities to assess the relative impact of route and schedule of administration on antitumour effects as well as on pharmacodynamic (PD) effects of the agent on its molecular target. These observations help guide the clinical development of the drug.

2.4.3.1 Choice of model system

The choice and number of *in vivo* models used in preclinical studies is somewhat arbitrary. A sampling of the types of *in vivo* models available and the major variables associated with tumour model studies are shown in Table 2.3. When the technology to evaluate human tumour xenografts in murine hosts became available and largely supplanted the use of murine tumour allograft models for new drug testing, this was widely hailed as an important means of determining more precisely if a new drug would indeed have activity in human cancers, and as well in which histological tumour types it was likely to have the greatest effects. Although xenograft models have been modestly more successful than allograft models in predicting the activity of agents in the clinic, the results have not been striking [8,9]. In a review of preclinical efficacy experiments of 31 cytotoxic cancer agents, Voskoglou-Nomikos *et al.* [8] showed that activity of a compound in a panel of ovarian xenografts was significantly correlated with activity of that same agent in phase II trials in solid tumours (in general) as well as in ovarian malignancies (in particular). In their review of the literature, no 'threshold' to declare activity was prospectively defined; rather activity as measured by the relative growth of tumour in treated versus control animals was evaluated as a continuous variable and correlated with phase II response rates. Johnson *et al.* [9] concluded that, while no specific relationship between activity in xenografts of a particular histological type and

Table 2.3 *In vivo* murine model variables

Parameter	Variables
Murine host	Immune-competent mouse Immune-deficient mouse (nude mouse or SCID mouse) Transgenic mouse
Type of tumour	Allograft cell line Human xenograft cell line Spontaneous (e.g. in transgenic mouse)
Tumour profile	Characterized with respect to key targets Not characterized
Tumour location	Subcutaneous Intraperitoneal Orthotopic Subrenal capsule Hollow fibre
Drug route of administration	Oral Intravenous Intraperitoneal Intratumoral
Drug schedule	Continuous (daily) Single dose Intermittent (e.g. days 1, 5, 9) Repeat dose (e.g. days 1–5)
Drug dose	Single or multiple dose levels Include MTD for each schedule or other doses
Timing of drug administration	At same time as tumour implantation After implanted tumour is established/palpable After implanted tumour has micrometastases After implanted tumour has macrometastases After resection of implanted tumour ('adjuvant')
Measures of efficacy	Tumour regression Tumour growth delay (%T/C) Animal survival Animal cures (or proportion long-term survival)

clinical activity in that tumour type could be found, activity in more than one-third of xenograft models was correlated with positive results in at least some phase II clinical trials. In both these reviews, results from cytotoxic drugs were compiled and xenograft studies generally used subcutaneous or intraperitoneal tumour cell implantation. The merely modest success of the use of human xenografts models in predicting clinical activity has been disappointing to many in the field. Approaches to developing more predictive models have included the use of orthotopic transplantation (tumour implantation in the relevant organ) [10], the use of models of naturally occurring tumours [11], and the integration of pharmacology with *in vivo* models to enhance their positive predictive value [12]. Furthermore, with the advent of molecular targeted agents, there has been interest in using models driven by specific molecular aberrations as are found in transgenic models (spontaneous tumour development in genetically predisposed rodents) [11], or at the very least, in using models whose genetic abnormalities are carefully catalogued (reviewed in [13,14]). None of these approaches, while intellectually appealing, has generated sufficiently large data sets on multiple agents to ascertain their positive predictive value. Transgenic and orthotopic approaches are relatively labour intensive and require special expertise in the research laboratory, so their widespread use will depend upon their demonstrated utility in predicting accurately success and failure in clinical development. Prospective research using standardized methodology will help resolve these questions.

An assay which has been developed to help select compounds for xenograft studies is the hollow-fibre assay. Cultured cell lines are flushed into hollow fibres that are subsequently implanted in the subcutaneous and intraperitoneal cavities of nude mice. Following 4 days of intraperitoneal drug administration the fibres are removed and cell viability determined using a colorimetric assay. Compounds are identified as active with the use of a detailed scoring system. Activity in the hollow fibre assay correlates well with subsequent xenograft activity [9] so it offers a rapid 'pre-screen' to select agents for full testing in xenograft models, thus reducing the overall resource burden in preclinical testing. This technique also has the advantage of permitting molecular analysis of treated tumours to investigate preliminary PD endpoints.

Besides the choice of model, how many should be evaluated? Generally speaking, activity in multiple tumour models or panels of models is more predictive of clinical activity than activity in only a single model. As noted earlier, Johnson *et al.* found in a retrospective analysis that activity in more than one-third of xenograft models is positively correlated with activity in at least some phase II clinical trials [9]. Similarly, Voskoglou-Nomikos *et al.* identified that activity in a 'panel' of ovarian xenografts (a panel being two or more xenografts of the same tissue of origin) was predictive of eventual activity in phase II trials [8]. Phase II response rates, in turn, may predict activity in randomized trials where clinically meaningful endpoints of survival or freedom from relapse are used.

Further prospective and retrospective work is needed to determine the utility of various *in vivo* efficacy models in predicting the clinical activity of non-cytotoxic, molecular targeted therapy. Now that many such agents are undergoing clinical evaluation, reviews such as those performed on cytotoxic drugs would be timely.

2.4.3.2 Choice of design and endpoints

Controversy also exists regarding the design of *in vivo* experiments. As will be seen, there is no widely used, standard methodology for the design and evaluation of *in vivo* efficacy experiments. Tumour cells can be injected subcutaneously, intraperitoneally, or orthotopically (in the organ of origin). Treatment may begin immediately (same day as tumour cell administration), after establishment of primary tumour growth to a minimum size, after metastatic disease appears, or after surgical excision of an established primary (a quasi-adjuvant design). Most studies evaluate several doses of drug in comparison with vehicle controls and generally utilize only one schedule of administration, although some deliver the drug in a variety of both doses and schedules. Table 2.3 shows some of the many variables at play in animal tumour model experiments. Clearly, the outcome of the experiment using the same cell line and the same investigational treatment can be dramatically influenced by these variables. By way of an example, Kerbel showed that different outcomes of various treatment approaches were seen in a MDA-MB 231 breast xenograft model in SCID mice depending on whether the mice had micro- or macrometastatic disease [15]. He goes on to argue that if models that more closely approximated human metastatic disease had been utilized historically, it is likely we would have had a more realistic expectation of the true clinical behaviour of agents when they were taken into phase II clinical trials in patients. That is, mouse outcomes following treatment with an anticancer agent seem overly optimistic in predicting clinical outcome not because something is special about the mouse, but rather because of the design of the experiments: they have not generally used tumour burdens that mimic the clinical scenario.

A further important consideration in interpreting the results of *in vivo* experiments relates to measures of efficacy. Tumour growth delay (expressed often as the treated over control tumour volume ratio [%T/C], or the tumour volume growth inhibition ratio [%GI]), tumour regression, survival and cures are all reported as outcomes. The observation of dose-dependent efficacy is considered ideal. However, the use of multiple outcome measures renders comparisons between agents and between new drug dossiers challenging. What does it mean if one agent results in significantly prolonged survival and another in the same xenograft model leads to significant growth delay? Are they similar or is one likely to be better? Furthermore, there are varying *thresholds* applied to these measures to claim activity: 40% T/C is a cut-off often applied to define activity, but there has been little work to determine, based on *subsequent* clinical efficacy, what the threshold for activity in animal tumour models ought to be.

As well as exploration of a variety of doses to establish a dose–effect relationship, *in vivo* experiments offer the opportunity to evaluate a variety of routes and schedules of administration to guide clinical development. Often a single xenograft or allograft model is selected to define the schedule that has maximal efficacy and thereafter this schedule is evaluated in a wider array of models. For agents in which an oral formulation is available and planned for clinical development, experiments sometimes focus solely on oral administration or may compare oral and intravenous formulations of the agent to quantify outcomes and define doses by each route at which maximal effects are seen. *In vitro* work may suggest that certain schedules are more likely to be efficacious (e.g. continuous exposure *in vitro* may translate into chronic oral daily administration) but it is important to confirm this hypothesis and optimize the schedule in animal studies.

A final note of caution: the cell lines used in preclinical models differ in several respects from 'normal' human tumours, but one of considerable importance is that they are very rapidly growing (providing the convenience to the lab investigator to have palpable tumours established in a few days and thus the ability to detect differences between control and treated animals within a 30-day observation period). The ability to grow this quickly to palpable size means these tumour lines must be extremely efficient at inducing angiogenesis (and by inference, particularly sensitive to agents that might interfere with new vessel formation). This behaviour is at variance with most human tumours where doubling in size usually requires months, not days, of growth.

2.4.3.3 Effects on target and their relation to *in vivo* activity

For agents designed to affect a particular molecular target, *in vitro* assays as described above can determine if the molecular interaction is happening but that, of course, is not the same as knowing if that interaction is happening *in vivo* or if it is responsible for the observed antitumour effects. In reviewing a dossier on a new drug that is supposed to exert its anticancer effects by inhibition of a specific target, it is therefore useful to see if there is evidence provided that, in animal studies, the agent's level of activity is related to the putative mechanism of action of the drug. A variety of assays can be conducted to study this. Which ones are appropriate depends on the nature of the investigational agent and its target as follows:

◆ *For antibodies and small molecular inhibitors of signalling or other enzymes.* Assess downstream measures of effect in the pathways affected by the agent in normal or tumour tissue in animal models. To be convincing, there should be a parallel relationship observed between the degree of antitumour effect and the quantitative effects on downstream measures: the greater the antitumour effect seen, the lower the levels of downstream measures.

◆ *For ODNs.* Measures of mRNA and protein should fall in response to higher doses of drug and those changes should have an inverse relationship to the degree of antitumour effect.

Assessment of these effects as part of the *in vivo* efficacy assessment of a new drug can also provide support for the use of similar measures in the clinical trial(s) of the agent: often, as will be described in Chapter 3, there is an interest in demonstrating that the drug is having its desired molecular effect in human tissues as well. Assays developed to study this as part of animal testing can play an additional role by becoming a means to evaluate similar endpoints in the clinic.

It should be noted that not all agents have a known target when the decision is taken to place them in clinical development. Under these circumstances, preclinical data showing a target–antitumour effect relationship is not possible. Even when the agent is believed to have its mechanism of action and target sorted out before the clinical trials begin, it is not obligatory that 'proof' of *in vivo* antitumour effects by target inhibition be available prior to clinical trials. Such information can, however, increase the interest in studying a new drug.

2.4.3.4 Comparative data with other agents

As noted earlier, some new agents are designed to be new and improved variations of active cancer drugs. Some are true analogues (e.g. platinum compound series or anthracycline series) while others may be new chemical entities having the same target (e.g. a small molecule versus an antibody affecting the same cellular receptor). In either case, the preclinical evaluation should include a number of studies that pit the new agent against the parent or prototype to address questions of efficacy and toxicology. With respect to efficacy, key questions include potency, impact on schedule, range of activity across a spectrum of tumour types as well as activity in models resistant to the parent. Potency alone is not particularly interesting *except* when it facilitates greater ease of delivery (fewer or smaller volume infusions, smaller tablets) or is associated with a different therapeutic index (i.e. increased activity but not at the cost of a parallel increase in toxicity). In terms of schedule impact, here one seeks to find a drug that may need less frequent administration due to its chemistry. When it comes to efficacy, the new agent will be most interesting if it appears to be active across a broader spectrum of tumour types, including those with *de novo* or acquired resistance, so experimental models set up to address these questions are the most pertinent. In designing comparative studies it is important to administer all agents using their optimal dose and schedule to adequately interpret results. Finally, most laboratories involved in drug discovery also evaluate new agents against the 'best' drugs available (whether analogue or not) for treating particular xenografts in order to provide a benchmark for interpretation of *in vivo* results.

2.4.3.5 Combination efficacy data

For most anticancer agents there is no requirement to undertake combination *in vivo* studies before beginning phase I first-in-man trials, unless both agents are investigational. However, *in vivo* studies may provide insight into subsequent development steps and, thus, may have an impact on phase I design. For example, if it is intended to develop a drug for breast cancer, understanding its efficacy in combination with other active drugs such as taxanes or anthracyclines may contribute to the decision of the phase I schedule that is selected for study (i.e. a schedule that would fit well with the standard administration of the other drugs could be chosen). However in most cases, showing additive or supra-additive effects with other anticancer agents preclinically simply reinforces the interest in the development of the agent, provides added evidence that it may be effective in humans, and gives information that can help direct the future development plan.

An obvious exception to this argument is found with agents developed expressly to enhance the efficacy of other active drugs. Resistance modulating agents, for example, should be studied in combination both *in vitro* and *in vivo* with the relevant drugs in appropriate models to show they produce the desired effects on sensitization.

2.4.3.6 Summary of *in vivo* efficacy studies

As the foregoing indicates, there is no standard panel of *in vivo* efficacy testing that will be perfectly predictive of clinical efficacy. The following represents a synthesis of the studies that contribute positively to the decision to take an agent into phase I trials because of expectation of benefit, and linkage of that benefit to drug effects:

- *Multiple xenograft models.* Xenografts have greater predictive value than allografts and activity in multiple models is a reasonable indicator of clinical activity. Activity in a panel of ovarian xenografts is of interest. The independent value of orthotopic and transgenic models is uncertain but activity in those models clearly adds weight to the body of evidence that the drug may be active in humans. Studies in models that have been characterized vis-à-vis their molecular genetic changes may be particularly informative for targeted therapies.
- *Models that establish the tumour prior to treatment.* It seems intuitively reasonable that agents active in models that more closely resemble the clinical situation, whether overt metastases or adjuvant-like, are of highest interest to evaluate. Agents having activity *only* when administered at the same time as tumour cell injection are of little appeal.
- *Models that use intravenous or oral administration of drug.* Experiments in which drug is administered into a cavity or locally (especially if it is the same site as the tumour!) are not investigating a scenario likely to apply in humans so are not a good basis from which to infer efficacy.
- *Confirmation of target inhibition.* When the drug target is known, establishing its alteration in concert with dose/plasma level and in turn with efficacy outcomes is useful. These data provide further evidence that the putative mechanism of action is true and offers assistance in designing phase I PD studies. Research methods developed and standardized to study this in the animal model setting may be used in the clinic as well.

Table 2.2 shows a number of *in vivo* models that were studied in the evaluation of the example agent, ZD6474. All were established tumours at the time of initiation of therapy and many showed significant antitumour effects.

It is important to acknowledge that, given the large number of new targets and drugs being discovered as a result of the technological advances enabling discovery science and the rising cost of clinical development, there is an increasing urgency to utilize non-clinical studies to select active compounds with greater precision. This is not confined to cancer drug development: it is a movement spearheaded by the US FDA for application to the development of medicinal products in general. In a recent paper entitled 'Innovation or stagnation: challenge and opportunity on the critical path to new medical products' [16], the FDA calls for a better 'toolkit' to hasten development and limit the failure of new products once they reach clinical studies. For cancer, this means work in the development of better preclinical models and also in identifying useful surrogates for activity in both animal and human studies from which accurate predictions of efficacy can be made. Whether new types of *in vivo* or *in vitro* models are needed or new designs (e.g. using models having overt metastatic disease instead of barely palpable subcutaneous disease) is unclear: a first step in sorting this out will be a systematic review of data now in the hands of numerous pharmaceutical companies and academic laboratories, and the development of standard methodology to apply to design and measurement. A challenge to be sure.

2.5 Preclinical toxicology

As important as assessing the potential for benefit, is the determination of a *reasonable expectation of safety* based on toxicological data. The International Conference on Harmonization has developed guidelines for the non-clinical safety (toxicity) assessment of new agents prior to their study in humans. The following sections of this chapter are based on the content of several pertinent ICH guidelines (M3, S4A, S6, and S7A) and also refer to interpretive comments, when appropriate, from various regulatory agencies. Table 2.4 provides a general summary of required toxicology studies. In all cases, it is anticipated that toxicology studies be carried out using Good Laboratory Practice (GLP) standards or GLP-like quality [17,18].

2.5.1 Single dose toxicity studies

Using the formulation to be studied in humans, single dose studies should be conducted in two mammalian species. Dose escalation designs are used to establish the maximal dose compatible with survival (maximum tolerated dose [MTD] or LD10, lethal dose in 10% of animals). The CHMP in Europe has stated in its *Note for Guidance on Preclinical Evaluation of Anticancer Medicinal Products* that mice and rats can be the two species evaluated, unless the agent is of a class in which rodents are known to be poor predictors of human toxicity (e.g. antifolates) in which case a non-rodent should be the second species [3]. The US FDA guidance document PT 1 (not specifically for cancer drugs) recommends evaluation of a rodent and non-rodent species [19]. Specific details of requirements may vary therefore by jurisdiction.

Animals should be treated in dose groups of six to 10, including both males and females, and observations should continue for 2 weeks after dosing. Both the no-observed adverse effect level (NOAEL) and the MTD should be determined. The nature and extent of adverse effects are to be documented as well as their time of onset, reversibility, and duration. PK studies that accompany the toxicity evaluation will contribute to understanding the relationships between exposure and specific organ effects. For biological products (e.g.

Table 2.4 Required toxicology testing prior to phase I trials of anticancer agents*

Type of toxicology	Requirements	Comments
Single dose	Two mammalian species: rodent and non-rodent Clinical formulation Several doses studied Determine MTD and organ effects	Some jurisdictions will accept two rodent species under some circumstances For species-specific compounds such as monoclonal antibodies and ODNs, testing may need to be in a non-rodent that shares the same target, or may need to be conducted in the rodent with the rodent-equivalent homologue of the agent
Repeat dose	Two mammalian species: rodent and non-rodent Formulation, dose and schedule as is planned for the clinical study Several dose levels; animals of both sexes at each level Duration of treatment: same as planned treatment duration in clinic Determine highest doses that can be safely administered, organ effects, severity, and reversibility	Some jurisdictions will accept two rodent models in some circumstances For phase I trials, some jurisdictions require only 2–4 weeks or 1–2 cycles of repeat dose testing See note regarding species specific compounds above
Chronic toxicity (for clinical treatment planned to be >6 months)	Two mammalian species: rodent and non-rodent Formulation, dose, and schedule as is planned for the clinical study *Duration of treatment*: rodents: 6 months; non-rodents: 9 months Determine chronic or late effects of treatment and their severity, reversibility	Some variety in required duration of non-rodent testing in some situations in certain countries

(*Continued*)

Table 2.4 *Continued*

Type of toxicology	Requirements	Comments
Safety pharmacology	Evaluation for specific major organ effects Test system depends on organ system of concern or interest Basic battery includes cardiovascular, respiratory, CNS studies	Not required prior to phase I trials, unless drug is of class with known effects on major organs, target is likely to be relevant to a major organ, or findings of standard toxicology point to the need
Genotoxicity	*In vitro* tests for mutations and chromosomal damage from the experimental agent	Generally not required prior to initiation of phase I trials
Local toxicity	Assessment of local tolerance using routes relevant to method of administration	Generally performed as part of other toxicity studies

*Based on ICH guidelines S4, S4A, M3, S6, and S7A.

antibodies) or other agents with species specificity (e.g. anti-sense ODNs), care must be taken to include at least one species (preferably two, but this may not be possible) in which the test agent is pharmacologically active. This may require manufacture of the species-specific homologue of the agent if cross-reactivity with the human protein or nucleotide sequence is not achieved. This requirement also applies to repeat dose studies (below).

2.5.2   Repeat dose and chronic toxicity studies

The general approach for repeat dose toxicity studies is that they should be conducted in a rodent and non-rodent species using the *formulation* intended for clinical use, the *schedule* proposed for study in humans, and be of the same *duration* as the proposed clinical trial. For chronic (long-term) administration, ICH guidelines stipulate that the duration of rodent testing be 6 months and non-rodent be 9 months [20]. However, guidance documents from specific jurisdictions provide some modifications and exceptions to the above for phase I trials and/or for trials in life-threatening illness.

In the European CHMP guidance on anticancer products [3], it states that two rodent species may be evaluated, unless the product is of a novel mechanism of action in which case rodent and non-rodent testing is required. Further, it is specified that the equivalent of only 2–4 weeks or one to two cycles of treatment need be evaluated in toxicology studies prior to beginning phase I cancer trials. For phase II and III trials, 6-month toxicology studies in rodent and non-rodents are required. The requirement for use of a rodent and non-rodent species for novel compounds has been challenged by Cancer Research UK. A recent review of their database of preclinical and clinical studies showed that all but one of 39 agents (an antifolate) had a safe starting dose predicted using only rodent toxicology [21].

In the FDA guidance on this subject [22] some notes are added on the duration of chronic toxicity studies in non-rodents: 6-month or 12-month, rather than 9-month, studies may be indicated in particular circumstances. Six-month studies may be acceptable for 'drugs intended for indications for life-threatening disease for which substantial long-term clinical data are available, such as cancer chemotherapy in advanced disease'.

The FDA guidance is silent on the specific duration of toxicity studies required to commence phase I cancer trials: generally repeat dose studies representing one to three cycles of treatment have been sufficient. It is advised, however, that the sponsor of the trial seek guidance before the toxicology is well underway.

As for acute dose (single dose) toxicity studies, repeat and chronic dosing studies require multiple animals per group of each sex. Follow-up includes clinical observations, blood, and other laboratory tests and assessment of the nature, timing, and reversibility of any toxic effects. Observations from the repeat dose or chronic dose studies may lead to specific supplemental toxicity studies to evaluate particular organ effects in greater detail.

2.5.3 Special toxicology: safety pharmacology studies

In addition to the standard toxicology requirements detailed above, specific safety studies to investigate adverse pharmacological effects on major organ systems may be required in certain circumstances. Examples include the following: when the experimental agent is a member of a class known to cause renal, cardiac, neurological, or pulmonary damage; when *in vitro* or other data demonstrate it affects receptors or proteins of critical importance in a major organ; or when results of concern from standard toxicology studies mandate further investigation. Depending on the specific safety issue in mind various specialized *in vitro* or *in vivo* studies can be performed. The core battery of studies includes central nervous system, cardiovascular system, and respiratory system evaluation. Details of the studies required are found in the ICH Guideline S7A: Safety Pharmacology Studies for Human Pharmaceuticals [23]. For agents that have the potential to prolong QT interval, a special guideline (S7B) has been developed for recommended non-clinical electrophysiological studies [24]. This is a new guideline and is under review by regulatory authorities.

2.5.4 Toxicology for drug combinations

Phase I trials that combine two or more agents are not generally preceded by combination toxicology studies. Usually all the drugs will have undergone prior human evaluation to establish recommended single agent dosing, thus the combination trial will use this information to set safe starting doses (see Chapter 5). There are three exceptions to this approach: The first is when both agents are investigational. The second is when the experimental drug is designed to modulate the action of other agents, in which case preclinical toxicology (and PK evaluation) of the planned clinical combination is needed. For example, some classes of resistance modulators have caused PK and/or metabolic effects resulting in increased systemic exposure and toxicity of the combined chemotherapeutic agents. Here, knowledge of preclinical combination toxicology is important to determine safe starting doses. The third situation in which preclinical toxicology of combinations are needed is when the agents to be combined share significant organ toxicities. Under these circumstances knowledge of the combination preclinical MTD is useful to determine the safety of the planned combination.

2.5.5 Selecting the starting dose

One of the critical objectives of preclinical evaluation is to amass the data necessary to determine a safe *starting dose* for phase I trials. The calculation of the starting dose, also discussed in Chapter 3, is based on toxicology results obtained using the same formulation, route, and schedule planned for clinical trials. Usually the murine LD10 (or MTD) is converted from mg/kg to mg/m^2 using conversion factors (found in Chapter 3) and the human starting dose is 1/10th the mouse LD10 equivalent, unless the non-rodent species shows that this dose is excessively toxic. Under these circumstances 1/3 to 1/6 the lowest toxic dose equivalent in the more sensitive species becomes the starting dose for human trials. Other factors may play a role in determining the starting dose: clinical toxicity data from analogues of the experimental agent; data from *in vitro* studies comparing sensitivity of human and non-human cell lines; drug protein binding characteristics in human and rodent plasma, to name a few.

2.6 Animal pharmacokinetics

Information on drug distribution, absorption, and metabolism obtained from animal studies provide helpful data that can inform clinical development. For example, knowledge of the half life of a drug in animal studies will contribute to decisions regarding dosing intervals in animals for both efficacy and toxicology and thus have an impact on clinical trials design. Relationships between plasma drug levels and both toxicity and efficacy outcomes in animal models provide important linkage information that may contribute to phase I escalation decisions (e.g. pharmacologically guided dose escalation [25]) or to determination of recommended doses (see Chapters 3 and 6).

Knowledge of the major organs involved in excretion and/or metabolism such as liver or kidney will appropriately inform decisions about patient inclusion and exclusion criteria. Furthermore, if the agent is metabolized through a cytochrome P450 enzyme system, there may be a rationale to restrict co-medications to those not dependent on the same enzyme system in order to avoid adverse drug interactions, at least in the first-in-man trial of the experimental drug.

Studies on protein binding may be important if plasma drug levels or some measure of drug exposure will contribute to dose recommendations. In these circumstances knowledge of the binding in the test animal and in human plasma will allow appropriate calculations to be made to determine the projected effective level of free drug.

Finally, PK data should, whenever possible, be correlated with changes in measures of target effect in normal and tumour tissue in animal studies (PK–PD studies). These experiments can provide important information to link dose, exposure, and target inhibition and thus may contribute to rational dose selection in human clinical trials.

2.7 Correlative assays: preclinical assay development for use in human trials

It is increasingly common that early clinical studies of targeted agents will include some measure of effect on the putative target, whether as an endpoint for dose escalation or as a simple proof of principle that the agent is affecting the target as designed. All too often, the assays for such studies are first undertaken as part of the clinical trial itself. Ideally, the preclinical data set for such drugs should include assay development. The goal is to develop assays that can reproducibly and sensitively measure the key changes in the tissue(s) that will also be studied in the patient. Assay development ought to include measures in tumours or tissue resected from treated animals so that relationships between changes in target over time, as measured by the intended clinical assay, can be correlated with dose, PK, and antitumour effects. This means that tumour-bearing animals must be treated, and their blood and tissue sampled at several time points and dose levels. This type of study is not commonly undertaken prior to clinical development because of its complexity and cost but could certainly prove useful in early trial design, and may save time and money in the clinic by providing key information in advance of first-in-man exposure. Excised tumour tissue from patients, removed for diagnosis or treatment, is another source of material in which assay methods can be developed and tested. This may only be undertaken if appropriate consent from the patient has been obtained.

2.8 Chemistry, formulation, and manufacturing quality

Before any new pharmaceutical product is given to humans, it must meet government-defined quality control standards for its manufacturing and purity. While this topic is the purview of pharmaceutical manufacturers and government regulators, a few comments are relevant for this chapter.

'Good Manufacturing Practice' is a set of minimum standards for pharmaceutical manufacture that detail the equipment, processes, documentation and quality control procedures that are to be followed. Links for Good

Manufacturing Practice documents from the United States, European Union, and Canada are provided in Appendix I.

Intravenous drugs may present challenges for formulation. Excipients to aid in solubilizing or emulsifying the parent drug may be required (e.g. cremophor EL) as may substances that stabilize the drug. The importance of this is that these added agents may carry their own risk of toxicity and have special intravenous administration requirements. Cremophor EL is a case in point: it is a non-ionic surfactant derived from castor oil used to solubilize intravenous paclitaxel formulations, but it has its own toxic effects [26,27] and pharmacological effects (p-glycoprotein modulation) [28], which may contribute to the toxicity produced by paclitaxel and other drugs given concurrently. Furthermore, it cannot be given in standard polyvinyl chloride intravenous tubing as it can leach plasticizer from the tube. Thus knowledge of the specifics of the drug formulation can reveal additional issues for investigators to consider in the design and interpretation of first-in-man studies.

Biological agents and those derived from biotechnology are subject to special guidelines with respect to purity, manufacture, and potency testing. Depending on the source of the agent, special testing for viral contamination may be required, for example. At the International Conference for Harmonization website (http://www.ich.org) there are a number of specific guidance documents available on the quality and preclinical safety evaluation for these types of products. Individual countries may have additional regulations that apply over and above those listed.

2.9 Investigator's Brochure

The Investigator's Brochure (also called the Clinical Brochure; the Investigator Drug Brochure); is a summary document of the preclinical (and, if relevant, clinical) data available on the experimental drug. It includes information on the physical, chemical, and pharmaceutical properties of the new drug, summary data on preclinical studies (efficacy, toxicology, PK, and more) and on any clinical studies that have been conducted. For phase I first-in-man trials this latter section will be incomplete of course, but as clinical data emerges, the Investigator's Brochure is updated, often on an annual basis. This document thus provides an excellent overview of the evidence to support the initiation of human clinical trials with a new agent. Table 2.5 provides a list of the table of contents to be included in an Investigator's Brochure as defined by ICH.

Table 2.5 Investigator's Brochure: content

Major headings	Details/content
Title page	
Table of contents	
Summary	Brief summary of 1–2 pages highlighting significant physical, chemical pharmaceutical, pharmacological, toxicological, PK, and clinical information
Introduction	Summary of chemical name, active ingredients, pharmacological class of drug, rationale for performing research and likely indications. Include at the end a summary of the approach to the clinical evaluation
Physical, chemical, pharmaceutical properties and formulation	
Non-clinical studies	Pharmacology: includes efficacy models, receptor binding, or other mechanistic studies Other studies: *in vitro* and *in vivo* studies that support mechanism, establish IC_{50}, biomarker development (i.e. assays that may be used in clinical trials to establish proof of principle for drug's mechanism) PK and product metabolism: disposition, metabolism, and excretion in animal models. If oral, should include bioavailability studies. Relationship of PK to efficacy and toxicological findings Toxicology: At least two species (rodent and non-rodent). Single dose and, if multiple or repeat doses will be given in clinic, those schedules must be assessed as well. Genotoxicity and reproductive toxicology (may be waived for initial human trials of an anticancer agent in patients) Include species tested, number and sex of animals in each group, dose units, route of administration, dosing interval, duration of dosing, duration of postexposure follow-up and results. Results should include: nature, frequency and severity of toxic (or pharmacological) effects, time to onset, duration, and reversibility. Finally a summary regarding dose–response.
Effects in humans (if available)	*For phase I first-in-man studies, this section will usually be empty. If normal volunteer data are available, or if the drug was previously studied in a non-malignant condition, data should be summarized according to the following sections. For phase I combination trials, the information for the following sections will be available from studies in cancer patients* PK and product metabolism in humans Safety and efficacy: description of outcomes of phase I, II, and III studies, including recommended dose/schedule. In addition, a table summarizing overall safety experience Marketing experience
Summary of data	Guidance for the investigator
References	Publications Reports

Investigator Brochure content abstracted from ICH Good Clinical Practice Guideline (E6) found at http://www.ich.org

Table 2.6 Summary of preclinical evaluation: example for a targeted agent

Element	Assay	Study goals	Results/comments
Target effect	*In vitro*: non-cellular systems	Determine IC_{50} Comparison with other agents of similar structure or targeted intent Comparison with other targets in the same molecular family	Agents active at nanogram levels are more likely to achieve those levels *in vivo* than those that are active at microgram levels Non-specific compounds may still be of interest if other effects are on relevant targets.
	In vitro: cellular systems	Determine IC_{50} for effect on target protein Determine maximal suppression possible, concentration needed to achieve it, and time course for recovery Determine IC_{50} for growth inhibition in a few cell lines	Compare IC_{50} for cellular and non-cellular effects, for effects on target and on growth inhibition If IC_{50} is substantially dissimilar between target inhibition and growth inhibition, other mechanisms may be involved.
	In vivo: animal models	Determine dose and /or plasma concentration effects on measures of target effect in normal and/or tumour tissue (PK–PD studies)	Proof of principle in animals that the agent can affect the target Seek correlation between: dose–target effect–antitumour effect or PK parameter–target effect–antitumour effect (PK–PD efficacy) Refine assays for use in clinic
Efficacy	*In vitro*	Determine growth inhibitory concentrations across a range of malignant cell lines Assess activities in sensitive/resistant paired cell lines Assess activity by level of target expression (if possible)	Pattern of sensitivity may assist in confirming mechanism of action, similarity (or not) to other agents, clues to sensitive tumour types Activity based on concentration and level of target expression assist in confirming mechanism

(Continued)

Table 2.6 *Continued*

Element	Assay	Study goals	Results/comments
	In vivo	Assess activity in a range of xenograft models having, if possible, range of target expression levels	Look for agents with activity (dose-related) across a range of xenografts.
		Use models with established tumours, including some with large tumours or metastatic disease compare doses and schedules if formulation allows	Ovarian xenografts of particular interest
		Orthotopic models may be explored	Seek evidence of *in vivo* target inhibition and its magnitude and duration in reference to maximal antitumour effects and plasma drug levels
		Assess target level over time in tumour; add PK assessment to this experiment. If appropriate, determine efficacy in combination with other agents	How does the agent compare with other active drugs?
		Active and vehicle control groups	Look for evidence that schedule or route may play a role in efficacy
Toxicology	Single dose	Using clinical formulation, determine MTD in rodent and non-rodent species	Exceptions to requirement for non-rodent allowed in some jurisdictions
		6–10 animals per dose. Include both sexes. Observe 14 days after dosing.	Determine MTD (LD10), clinical signs, nature of organ and other toxicity
	Repeat dose/chronic	Using clinical formulation study rodent and non-rodents in schedule planned for clinical evaluation at several dose levels and in both sexes	Determine nature, severity, reversibility of toxicity
		Duration of treatment should be similar to planned human exposure	Determine MTD in mg/kg for rodent species in schedule planned for clinical study
		For planned chronic (long-term) treatment, rodent study is 6 months and non-rodent 9 months	Determine relationship between PK parameters and toxic effects
			Determine if need for special safety pharmacology studies
Animal PK		Assess PK with toxicology or separate study	Basic PK parameters
		Consider adding PK to some efficacy models (see above)	Organs/enzyme systems involved in excretion and metabolism
		Metabolism and excretion	

In reading the Investigator's Brochure for a new drug, reflect on the four items listed at the beginning of this chapter and evaluate the data provided to verify that the following are addressed: the *biological plausibility* of the agent having activity in cancer; the *expectation of benefit for patients; a reasonable expectation of safety;* and sufficient information on which to base a *starting dose.*

2.10 Summary

There is a large body of preclinical data required before a new agent can be investigated in its first human trials. While much of the data generated is in response to government regulation and guideline requirements, other aspects, particularly tests of efficacy and target inhibition, are not. Using the example of a novel targeted agent, Table 2.6 summarizes the elements of a preclinical data set that require careful review by the investigator before undertaking a phase I trial. The table describes the ideal list of information that should be available prior to initiation of human studies. Important in this list are not only standard toxicology and efficacy assays, but also data that provide linkages between dose or PK measures, target effect, and outcomes: whether efficacy or toxicity. These data will greatly assist in early clinical trial design.

References

1. Hirschfeld S. (2004). Clinical drug trials in children. In: Yaffe S, Aranda Y, ed. *Neonatal and Pediatric Pharmacology*, 3rd edn, pp. 69–91. Lippincott, Williams & Wilkins, Philadelphia, PA.
2. ICH Harmonised Tripartite Guidelines: General Considerations for Clinical Trials (E8) (quotation from p. 4) http://www.ich.org/MediaServer.jser?@_ID=484&@_MODE=GLB [last accessed August 2005]
3. CPMP Note for guidance on the pre-clinical evaluation of anticancer medicinal products. Found at: http://www.emea.eu.int/pdfs/human/swp/099796en.pdf [last accessed August 2005]
4. http://www.fda.gov/cder/guidance/clin2.pdf [last accessed August 2005]
5. Wedge SR, Ogilvie DJ, Dukes M, *et al.* (2002). ZD6474 inhibits vascular endothelial growth factor signaling, angiogenesis, and tumor growth following oral administration. *Cancer Res* 62: 4645–55.
6. Wilhelm S, Carter C, Tang LY, *et al.* (2003). BAY 43–9006 exhibits broad spectrum antitumour activity and targets Raf/MEK/ERK pathway and receptor tyrosine kinases involved in tumour progression and angiogenesis. *Clin Cancer Res* 9 (Suppl.): A78.
7. Zaharevitz DW, Holbeck SL, Bowerman C, Svetlik PA (2002). COMPARE: a web accessible tool for investigating mechanisms of cell growth inhibition. *J Mol Graph Model* 20: 297–303.

8. Voskoglou-Nomikos T, Pater JL, Seymour L (2003). Clinical predictive value of the *in vitro* cell line, human xenograft, and mouse allograft preclinical cancer models. *Clin Cancer Res* 9: 4227–39.

9. Johnson JI, Decker S, Zaharevitz D, *et al.* (2001). Relationships between drug activity in NCI preclinical *in vitro* and *in vivo* models and early clinical trials. *Br J Cancer* 84: 1424–31.

10. Bibby MC (2004). Orthotopic models of cancer for preclinical drug evaluation: advantages and disadvantages. *Eur J Cancer* 40: 852–7.

11. Hansen K, Khanna C (2004). Spontaneous and genetically engineered animal models; use in preclinical cancer drug development. *Eur J Cancer* 40: 858–80.

12. Peterson JK, Houghton PJ (2004). Integrating pharmacology and *in vivo* cancer models in preclinical and clinical drug development. *Eur J Cancer* 40: 837–44.

13. Suggitt M, Bibby MC (2005). 50 years of preclinical anticancer drug screening: empirical to target-driven approaches. *Clin Cancer Res* 11: 971–81.

14. Kelland LR (2004). 'Of mice and men': values and liabilities of the athymic nude mouse model in anticancer drug development. *Eur J Cancer* 40: 827–36.

15. Kerbel RS (2003). Human tumor xenografts as predictive preclinical models for anticancer drug activity in humans: better than commonly perceived—but they can be improved. *Cancer Biol Ther* 2(4, Suppl. 1): S134–9.

16. http://www.fda.gov/oc/initiatives/criticalpath/whitepaper.html [last accessed August 2005]

17. http://www.fda.gov/ora/compliance_ref/bimo/glp/78fr-glpfinalrule.pdf [last accessed August 2005]

18. http://europa.eu.int/comm/enterprise/chemicals/legislation/glp/index_en.htm [last accessed August 2005]

19. http://www.fda.gov/cder/guidance/pt1.pdf. Published in the US Federal Register August 26, 1996 (61 FR 43934). [last accessed August 2005]

20. ICH Harmonised Tripartite Guideline: Duration of Chronic Toxicity Testing in Animals (Rodent and Non-Rodent Toxicity Testing)(S4A). http://www.ich.org/MediaServer.jser?@_ID=497&@_MODE=GLB [last accessed August 2005]

21. Newell DR, Silvester J, McDowell C, Burtles SS (2004). The Cancer Research UK experience of pre-clinical toxicology studies to support early clinical trials with novel anti-cancer therapies. *Eur J Cancer* 40: 899–906.

22. US Federal Register Vol. 64 No. 122, June 25, 1999 (FR 99–16189) http://www.fda.gov/cder/guidance/62599.pdf [last accessed August 2005]

23. ICH Harmonised Tripartite Guideline: Safety Pharmacology Studies for Human Pharmaceuticals (S7A) http://www.ich.org/MediaServer.jser?@_ID=504&@_MODE=GLB [last accessed August 2005]

24. ICH Harmonised Tripartite Guideline: The Nonclinical Evaluation of the Potential for Delayed Ventricular Repolarization (QT Interval Prolongation) By Human Pharmaceuticals (S7B) http://www.ich.org/MediaServer.jser?@_ID=2192&@_MODE=GLB [last accessed August 2005]

25. Collins JM, Grieshaber CK, Chabner BA (1990). Pharmacologically guided phase I clinical trials based upon preclinical drug development. *J Natl Cancer Inst* 82: 1321–6.

26. Rowinsky EK, Donehower RC (1995). Paclitaxel (taxol). *N Engl J Med* 332: 1004–14.

27. Weiss RB, Donehower RC, Wiernik PH, *et al.* (1990). Hypersensitivity reactions from taxol. *J Clin Oncol* 8: 1263–8.

28. Webster L, Linsenmeyer M, Millward M, *et al.* (1993). Measurement of cremophor EL following taxol: plasma levels sufficient to reverse drug exclusion mediated by the multidrug-resistant phenotype. *J Natl Cancer Inst* 85: 1685–90.

Chapter 3

Basics of phase I design: first-in-man studies

Elizabeth A. Eisenhauer

This chapter will focus on the basics of design of phase I trials of agents that are entering the clinic for the first time. These trials are commonly referred to as 'first-in-man' (or occasionally 'first-in-human') studies and this terminology will also be utilized in this chapter. While combination phase I trials have many concepts in common with first-in-man studies, they are the subject of a more detailed description in Chapter 5, so will not be discussed here. Ethical considerations related to phase I trials are discussed in detail in Chapter 4.

3.1 Goals

The primary goal of first-in-man studies is to define the recommended dose of a new drug in the schedule(s) tested (see Table 3.1). Secondary goals of these trials are several and usually include at least those in Table 3.1 below.

Table 3.1 Goals of first-in-man phase I studies

Goals	
Primary	To determine recommended dose of the new agent for further study in the schedule under evaluation
Secondary	To describe the toxic effects produced by the new agent in the schedule under evaluation
	To determine the PK of the new agent
	To document any evidence of objective antitumour effect
	To describe any relationship between dose, or PK parameters, and effects on toxicity, or measures of molecular drug effect in tissues (PD effects)

PD effects are 'what the drug does to the body', so they can include things such as toxic effects, clinical antitumour effects, and also molecular and imaging changes in tissues. It is the latter two that are increasingly referred to as 'PD measures' in recent years. Not all phase I first-in-man studies include measures of PD, but increasingly in trials of targeted, non-cytotoxic agents, assays of normal or tumour tissues are undertaken to assess molecular effects of the new drug as will be described below.

3.2 Patient population

Normally the population enrolled in first-in-man phase I trials of new anticancer agents is cancer patients for whom no curative or standard therapy remains. The reason for this is that most anticancer agents, whether cytotoxic chemotherapies or other more targeted non-cytotoxic agents, commonly have toxic effects in normal tissues at doses that are likely to be effective. As is noted below, toxicity is often the primary endpoint of these studies and for that reason, initial testing is commonly conducted in cancer patients where doses are escalated to the maximum tolerated. Furthermore, this population affords the opportunity to document any hints of biological antitumour effects of a new agent that might contribute to further development decisions.

Despite the foregoing arguments, in some cases healthy volunteers are the subjects of first-in-man evaluation of an anticancer therapeutic. Examples include the first studies of hormonal agents, drugs with a known spectrum of toxicity, mechanism of assessing target effect (fall in hormone levels), and unlikely to be harmful in volunteers (for example, see [1]). Normal volunteers may also be enrolled in the first studies of some novel agents, which, in preclinical toxicology evaluation, appear to have limited adverse effects. Trials in this second setting often involve only limited dosing in volunteer subjects and their primary goal may not be to establish the highest safe dose but rather to understand the PK and absorption characteristics of a new agent, prior to finalizing the schedule for more protracted phase I trials cancer patient. Gefitinib (ZD1839), an oral inhibitor of the epidermal growth factor receptor (EGFR) tyrosine kinase, is an example of an agent for which the first human study was a normal volunteer trial designed to describe the drug's PK and its absorption with/without food. This study established that once daily dosing was appropriate [2]. Subsequent trials in the cancer population used once daily dosing continuously on the basis of the normal volunteer studies and determined a recommended dose based on toxic effects [3].

Although normal volunteer studies may offer some information relating to PK and safety, some caution is warranted in relying on these studies alone to determine recommended doses for phase II cancer trials. The experience with marimastat, a matrix metalloproteinase inhibitor, is a case in point. Normal volunteer studies of single and repeated twice daily dosing concluded that doses as high as 200 mg p.o. twice daily were well tolerated [4], but in cancer patient phase II trials, even 100 mg twice daily, the dose selected for initial phase II studies, proved unacceptably toxic. At this dose a syndrome of poly-arthralgia was seen, which was not identified in the phase I normal volunteer studies. A subsequent phase I trial [5] identified 100 mg twice daily to be above the dose that could be tolerated and phase II trials, which were started at the 100 mg b.i.d. dose were reduced to 25 or 10 mg b.i.d. midway through accrual [6,7]. The plasma levels in the cancer population were several times those of the healthy volunteer population given the same dose. No good explanation for this phenomenon has been found.

Thus while healthy volunteer studies may have a place in early cancer drug development, it is clear that they should not completely supplant careful study of a new agent in a population of cancer patients as a higher level of toxicity may be considered acceptable and PK may differ. Because the conduct of trials in a volunteer population may increase the overall time of drug development, it can be argued that their use should be limited to those situations where the information garnered will have a critical impact on the subsequent design of phase I studies in cancer patients.

The remainder of this section addresses entry criteria for the phase I evaluation of a new agent in a cancer population.

3.2.1 Patient entry criteria: general remarks

The patient population under study must be defined prospectively in the protocol. In general, the description of the eligible population is divided into several major areas as follows (see Table 3.2).

3.2.1.1 Disease characteristics

Tumour type   Most phase I trials are undertaken first in patients having a mixture of types of solid tumours. A second study in patients with haematological malignancies may follow this, or may supplant it, if the agent in question is destined solely for use in leukaemia or lymphoma, as were some recent monoclonal antibodies [8]. The separation of haematological from non-haematological malignancies in this way is an historical one. Myelosuppressive agents were often escalated to higher dose levels in haematological malignancies

Table 3.2 Patient entry criteria

Area	Specify	Comments
Disease characteristics	Solid tumours or haematological malignancy	Some protocols are even more restricted: e.g. to specific type(s) of tumour if drug is designed for use in only that population
	Disease extent	Most protocols specify no curative therapy available. Some may enrol better risk patients if justified
	Number of prior systemic therapies allowed	Most protocols allow extensive prior therapy. To assure phase I population is comparable with phase II, restriction in number of regimens is recommended at final stages of enrolment Restriction in total drug dose from prior therapy is appropriate for some agents (e.g. anthracyclines or platinum) if new agent is analogue or may have similar organ effects
	Prior surgery and radiation allowed	
Patient characteristics	Age	Generally restricted to adults, i.e. age ≥18 in most jurisdictions
	Performance status	Generally ECOG or WHO 0, 1, or 2
	Organ function: Haematology Biochemistry (liver, renal) Cardiac Neurological	First-in-man studies restrict to normal or, in case of biochemistry, modest decrements (up to grade 1 or 2 depending on organ) in organ function: depending on toxicology and expected route of elimination. Exclusions may also be based on human safety profiles of similar class agent
	Pregnancy	Exclude pregnant women and men or women of childbearing potential who will not use effective contraceptive measures
Special requirements	Tissue procurement	Protocols having mandatory collection of archival or fresh tissue must specify its availability and patient consent as part of entry criteria
	Blood sampling	Patients who cannot partake of PK studies for whatever reasons generally are excluded from first-in-man trials
	Oral administration	If the new agent is orally administered, entry is restricted to those that can take and absorb medications by this route

Consent	Only patients consenting are to be enrolled	Consent form to be used must be that approved by the ethical committee empowered to review for the treating institution Consent should contain all required elements (see Chapter 7)
Availability for follow-up	Patients must be available and willing to return to the cancer centre for trial related procedures	This may preclude entry of patients who live at great distance from the treating centre

where, in many cases, the tissue of toxicity (marrow) was also the tissue of malignancy. Finally, trials in special populations (as outlined in Chapter 5) will take place to define safe dosing in those at the extremes of age and with abnormal organ function.

For initial trials in solid tumours, further restriction of entry may take place: for example, phase I evaluation of an antibody to CA-125 likely would be restricted to patients with ovarian cancers that express that particular marker. For agents whose target is more widely distributed across histologies, such as epidermal growth factor receptor, entry may be restricted to those tumour types likely to express the target, such as was the case for the phase I study of gefitinib referred to earlier [3].

Disease extent In general, phase I trials are conducted in previously treated patients with recurrent local or metastatic disease for which no standard or curative therapy exists. Phase I trial entry also generally requires that disease in patients be clinically or radiologically documented, i.e. enrolment of patients whose *only* evidence of disease is an elevation of a serum marker is generally avoided, although may be allowed in some circumstances. Measurable disease according to standard response criteria is *not* required unless response assessment is an important secondary study endpoint.

Prior therapy Phase I trials of new cancer therapeutics generally enrol cancer patients who have received previous systemic therapy. It is debatable whether patients must have exhausted *all* possible forms of therapy: some would argue that as long as the only therapy(ies) otherwise available for patients is non-curative and without meaningful impact on the length of life, entry on to a phase I trial of a new agent is reasonable: after all such patients still have the other therapies available to them when/if their disease progresses on the phase I agent. Furthermore, phase I enrolment restricted to heavily pretreated patients may limit the generalizability of the final dose recommendation to untreated patients, particularly if the target organ of toxicity (such as bone marrow) has been impaired by the prior treatment. Thus, studies often specify that prior treatment may be quite extensive in the initial stages of the trial recruitment, but more limited as the recommended dose is nearing. This will be described in more detail in Chapter 7. Clear specification of the minimum and maximum number of prior systemic therapy regimens, as well as any restrictions on the amount of prior radiation or surgery should be included. Prior radiation may lead to increased susceptibility to the myelosuppressive effects of certain new therapies; in such instances restriction of entry to patients with prior radiation to a volume <25% of marrow containing skeleton is commonplace.

Depending on the expected toxic effects, limitations on the cumulative dose of certain specific agents may be required (e.g. limits on the total dose of prior taxane if new taxane being evaluated, or on the amount of prior anthracycline if a cardiotoxic agent is being assessed); such restrictions are also usually handled by mandating organ function within a fixed range of values.

3.2.1.2 Patient characteristics

Performance status Performance status is a crude general measure of the impact of illness on an individual's ability to be mobile and active. Several scales are available to categorize performance status, such as the World Health Organization [9], the Eastern Cooperative Oncology Group [10], or the Karnofsky [11]. Phase I trials should enrol patients with good to moderate performance status: those patients who are bedridden are *not* to be enrolled as their life expectancy is so short that adequate assessment of the effects of a new drug may not be possible. Furthermore, it will be difficult to distinguish between drug effects and disease effects if patients are in the final days of their illness.

Adequate organ function Until the toxic effects and pharmacological behaviour of any new agent are known, entry on to phase I trials is restricted to patients with adequate, predefined levels of organ function (measured by maximum allowable biochemistry values of liver and kidney function and by minimum levels of haematological parameters). Other drug-specific restrictions may also apply. For example, the patient must have no evidence of neurological or cardiac impairment beyond certain limits for agents that are predicted to have neurological or cardiac effects, respectively. Once the toxic effects and routes of elimination of a drug are better understood, separate trials in those with organ impairment are conducted to develop dosing guidelines (see Chapter 5).

Interestingly, in some trials it has become usual to allow modest degrees of hepatic enzyme elevation (e.g. 2× upper normal limit for aspartate amino-transferase or alanine aminotransferase) for general patient entry, but to permit higher levels for those whose abnormal values are due to liver metas-tases (e.g. up to 5× upper normal limit). This is not a particularly logical differentiation, however; if liver damage is evident, whether from metastatic disease or other causes, the same restrictions to entry should apply, particu-larly for first-in-man studies as hepatic dysfunction, regardless of mechanism, may impair clearance or metabolism of a drug. Docetaxel and anthracyclines are cases in point: both drugs have increased toxic effects when hepatic dysfunction due to metastatic involvement of the liver is documented.

Pregnancy As anticancer drugs affect cell proliferation, survival and differentiation, thus are either known or suspected to be genotoxic or teratotoxic, first-in-man studies must exclude pregnant and breast-feeding women and include a requirement for the use of effective contraception methods in all enrolled subjects.

3.2.1.3 Eligibility for special drug administration or procedures for the trial

Some trials include special measures of a drug or its effects in tumour or normal tissue samples. When this is required, entry criteria must be written appropriately to accommodate these tests. For example, if assessment of effects on target in tumour is required, fresh tumour biopsies will be necessary, and thus the patient must have tumour lesions accessible for biopsy *and* must consent to the biopsy procedures. In those trials where only archival tumour samples are needed, the entry criteria should specify that tumour blocks from previous surgery must be available for research.

When phase I trials of oral drugs are undertaken, entry criteria must reflect this and require that patients be able to take (and absorb) oral therapy. For agents requiring prolonged intravenous administration, patients must have an accessible intravenous site or indwelling line to be eligible.

3.2.1.4 Consent and availability

Although it may be self-evident, the entry criteria should specify that only patients consenting to all the trial-related procedures are eligible for enrol-ment. Further, as many phase I trials require repeated visits or prolonged outpatient treatment, only patients able to undertake these visits should be recruited. Thus for some trials, it may be necessary for patients to reside within a reasonable geographic distance of the hospital or clinic where the trial is taking place, even if only for the duration of the study.

3.3 Endpoints: pharmacodynamic effects of the drug

The *primary* endpoint in phase I trials is that which drives decisions about dose escalation and dose recommendation. In general, endpoints that assess a dose-related effect of the drug are 'PD' measures: ones that relate to the effect of the drug on the body. As noted earlier, PD effects include many measures: molecular changes, antitumour effects, and toxicity. Dosing for cancer drugs has traditionally been based on the highest dose that can be given with 'acceptable' and reversible toxic effects; thus toxicity has been the primary endpoint for these trials for decades [12–14]. The entry into the clinic of molecularly targeted agents with mechanisms of action that differ from those of cytotoxic chemotherapeutics has raised questions about the use of toxicity as the primary endpoint (see more below). Whatever is selected as the primary endpoint, other secondary measures are also incorporated into first-in-man studies. These include measures of PK behaviour, antitumour response (if the patient has measurable disease), and other PD studies as noted below and in Table 3.3.

3.3.1 Toxicity as the primary endpoint

Historically, most anticancer drugs have been cytotoxic chemotherapeutic agents. These target the process of DNA replication/cell division (either DNA itself, enzymes involved in DNA replication such as topoisomerase enzymes, or tubulin). As these targets are also present in all normal cells and are especially relevant in dividing cells, then it is logical that doses of cyto-toxics, which result in antitumour effects, are also likely to be doses that cause toxic effects on normal dividing tissues. Furthermore, antitumour effects were shown to be dose-related in early studies in the laboratory [15]. Thus, if toxic effects were dose-related as were antitumour effects (see Figure 3.1 for a

Table 3.3 Phase I trial endpoints* and measurement criteria

Endpoint	Measurement (examples)
Toxic effects	Standard toxicity criteria (e.g. CTCAE v 3.0; WHO)
PK	C_{max}, half-life, AUC, steady-state levels
Functional imaging effects	Change in tumour blood flow Change in glucose uptake
Molecular effects	Change in tumour target inhibition Change in downstream activation
Antitumour effects	Categorization of objective best response according to standard criteria (WHO, RECIST)

*All endpoints except PK may be considered as 'PD' effects, although this term is often used to refer only to molecular and functional imaging changes.

cartoon representation of this concept), then targeting the highest tolerable dose with the use of toxicity as the endpoint of phase I trials is a logical extension of these observations.

Besides the theoretical and laboratory evidence to support the use of this endpoint, a wealth of historical data now available also supports this strategy. The highest tolerable dose, based on toxic effects, is usually the optimally *effective* dose in clinical studies. Randomized trials in which lower doses of chemotherapy were given and compared with 'full' standard dose (and more toxic) treatment have shown superior outcomes in the full dose group (e.g. [16]).

Given the above, the standard primary endpoint for phase I trials of single agent cytotoxic therapeutics has been toxicity. To administer the drug in the highest tolerable dose in subsequent phase II and III studies also ensures that it is unlikely one would miss real antitumour activity should it exist, as it is implausible that higher doses would be less effective than lower doses.

3.3.1.1 Assessing toxic effects

Given the importance of toxicity measurement, not only in determining dose but also in describing the safety profile of cancer treatment in general, standardized assessment tools (Toxicity Criteria) have been developed to assure a common language of description of adverse effects from therapy. It should be noted that, although 'toxicity' is the term commonly used in medical literature, 'adverse event' is the more appropriate descriptor as the former implies a causative relationship from the drug and the latter remains neutral as to cause. Both terms will be used in this section, as the criteria developed have used the terms interchangeably.

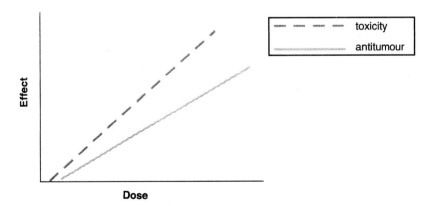

Figure 3.1 Dose–effect relationships for cytotoxic agents. Modified from: Eisenhauer EA (1998) Ann Oncol 9: 1047–52. Reproduced with permission.

The history of standardized tools for assessment of adverse events in cancer clinical trials began with the World Health Organization (WHO), which in 1981 published the first widely used toxicity criteria [9]. These and other criteria developed since that time categorize and quantify both symptomatic experiences of the patient as well as changes in organ function. The severity of events is described using a grading system whereby grade 0 means 'absent' or 'normal', grade 4 is life-threatening in severity, and grade 5 is fatal. The original WHO scale had a limited number of events from which to choose in describing patient outcomes. This shortcoming led to the development of the Common Toxicity Criteria (CTC) by the US National Cancer Institute in collaboration with other cancer clinical trials organizations in 1982. Subsequently, the CTC have been expanded and updated to reflect the effects of a wide spectrum of new anticancer agents. The most recent version (version 3) was released in 2003 and is known as the CTCAE (Common Terminology Criteria for Adverse Events), eliminating the word 'toxicity' from its title [17]. The CTCAE version 3.0 has over 200 adverse event *terms* divided into 28 *categories* of organ systems in contrast to the original WHO, which had only 28 *terms* in total. The CTCAE version 3.0 has been widely adopted by academic groups and pharmaceutical companies engaged in cancer clinical trials. Table 3.4 illustrates some of the differences between the original WHO criteria and the CTCAE version 3.0 using a few selected events as examples.

Each term in the CTCAE version 3.0 is mapped to a MedRA term: MedRA is the Medical Dictionary for Regulatory Activities Terminology, which has been developed under the auspices of the International Conference on Harmonization. The International Conference on Harmonization was initiated in an effort to harmonize regulatory requirements of governments around the world vis-à-vis pharmaceutical product development [18]. Preclinical and clinical topics are discussed and guidelines developed for review and adoption by member countries. A dictionary of international medical terminology (MedRA) was seen as an important aspect of this effort, especially for the collection and dissemination of adverse event (safety) information [19]. It is increasingly important that, whatever system is used to document adverse effects in clinical trials, it can be 'translated' into MedRA terminology as this facilitates submission of adverse event data to regulatory authorities around the world. CTCAE version 3.0 provides this capability hence its increasing use in oncology trials.

Toxic effects or adverse events are also commonly described by their *duration* as well as by the investigator's assessment of their *relationship* to treatment, although these descriptors are not usually integrated in the grading system *per se*; rather these parameters are assessed and documented as supplementary information to the adverse event if required.

3.3.1.2 Dose-limiting toxicity, maximum tolerated dose, and recommended phase II dose

In phase I cancer trials, doses of investigational treatment are escalated in cohorts of patients until predefined criteria are met. When toxic effects are the primary endpoint, those criteria are *dose-limiting toxic effects*.

Dose-limiting toxicity (DLT) is generally defined as severe, but reversible, organ toxicity. Phase I protocols must define those events with accompanying severity levels that will limit dose. Generally, precise laboratory levels or grades are defined as dose-limiting for haematological, renal, and hepatic events. Other events (other major organ effects) that may be dose-limiting are described in general terms only (e.g. 'any other grade 3 major organ toxicity'). Table 3.5 gives examples of common DLT definitions that are found in phase I protocols. For drugs that are given in a multidosing schedule (daily or weekly) within a cycle, DLT should also be considered to have occurred if patients miss more than a pre-specified number of doses due to toxicity, as inability to deliver full dose is, in itself, a marker of limiting effects.

When DLT is considered, not only is severity of the event taken into consideration, but also its *timing*. For an event to be considered dose-limiting it must occur within a pre-specified *period of time after dosing begins*. This time period is usually one cycle (for intravenous drugs given in an intermittent fashion) and may be 4–8 weeks for agents administered orally on a continuous basis. This is a typical condition that does *not* take into account cumulative toxicity. In the circumstance where cumulative toxicity from a phase I agent is likely, longer observation periods are required at each dose level.

Table 3.5 Examples of common dose-limiting toxicity definitions*

Type/event	Dose-limiting toxicity	Comments
General		During cycle 1 only
Absolute neutrophil count	Grade 4 ($<0.5 \times 10^9$/l) for > 5 days	Usually specify duration as well as grade. No standard agreement on the number of days: varies from 3 to 7
Platelets	Grade 4 ($<25 \times 10^9$/l)	
Complications of myelosuppression	Febrile neutropenia or grade 3 infection with grade 3 or 4 neutropenia Thrombocytopenic bleeding	Toxicity criteria have specific definitions for some of these terms
Hepatic	AST or ALT grade 3	
Other major organ toxicity	Grade 3	

*Grades used are based on CTCAE v 3.0.

The trial design defines how many patients out of those treated at a given dose level must experience DLT to halt further escalation: generally two patients out of a minimum of three or six must experience DLT for escalation to cease.

The dose level at which DLT is seen in the minimum number of patients required to halt further escalation is termed the *maximum tolerated dose (MTD)*. There is some confusion in the definition of this term, however: often in the USA and some other locales, the dose at which a prespecified number of

Table 3.6 Definitions of phase I terminology

Term	Abbreviation	Definition	Comment
Dose-limiting toxicity	DLT	Adverse event of severity or consequence that may limit dose escalation	
Maximum tolerated dose	MTD	Two common usages: 1. Dose at which pre-specified number of patients (usually 2 of 3 or 2 of 6 exhibit DLT). Dose escalation stops 2. Maximal safe dose: usually same as recommended phase II dose. Dose level at which critical number of DLT events is seen is higher, and has no standard term applied except it is 'above the MTD'	Definition commonly used in studies from Europe *Definition used in this book* Definition more commonly used in studies from the USA
Maximum administered dose	MAD	Term suggested to resolve confusion with MTD definitions: MAD is highest dose administered which has DLT in pre-specified number of patients (same meaning as MTD definition no. 1)	Not generally used as yet
Recommended phase II dose	RD	Dose recommended for further study in single agent trials.	Abbreviation is not standard but *will be used in this book* (May be synonymous with MTD when MTD definition no. 2 is used)

patients with DLT is seen is considered to be *above the MTD*. See Table 3.6 for definitions of common terms used in phase I design. To avoid this confusion it has been suggested that the dose at which escalation ceases because of the observation of a critical number of DLT events should be referred to as the *maximum administered dose (MAD)*, rather than the MTD. Despite this suggestion, 'MTD' continues to be widely used and has more than one definition.

The *recommended phase II dose* (RD) is, generally, a dose level below that at which escalation has stopped because of critical numbers of patients with DLT. Toxic effects at this dose level are expected and may be severe in some patients, but their frequency is lower than at the level above. In those places where the highest dose given is defined as being *above* the MTD, such as the USA, the recommended phase II dose may be referred to as the MTD. Given this semantic confusion, it is very important for protocols and phase I publications to define clearly the terms used in a particular study. In Table 3.6, these definitions and synonyms are described and the ones that will be utilized in this book are highlighted for clarity.

3.3.2 Non-toxicity measures as primary endpoints

Many novel agents targeting multiple intracellular and extracellular pathways (so called 'non-cytotoxic agents'; sometimes referred to as 'cytostatics', 'molecular targeted agents', or 'biologic agents') are being developed as anti-cancer therapeutics. A plethora of rational targets have been identified and agents affecting them are now in the clinic or about to enter clinical evaluation. See Table 3.7 for a sampling of representative targets and related inhibitory agents. As is clear, there are many such new drugs, and more are expected in the coming decade as new targets for cancer therapy are discovered and validated. These agents may differ in their preclinical dose–effect relationships from those of cytotoxics [20]. Once the putative target is 'saturated' by adequate doses of drug, it would be expected that the antitumour effects should plateau as well. Toxic effects, however, may not follow this same relationship if the level of target is higher in normal tissues or if *non*-target effects of the drug produce toxicity. Drugs such as anti-sense oligodeoxynucleotides, for example, can produce complement activation at high doses, an effect that is related to the structural class, not to the target of the drug [21]. These concepts are illustrated in the cartoon, Figure 3.2, which should be contrasted with the relationships for cytotoxic agents sketched in Figure 3.1.

Because achieving maximal toxicity may not be necessary for maximal efficacy (which will occur, logically, when the target is saturated by its inhibitor), a great deal has been written about which endpoints could substitute for toxicity to define the recommended doses of such agents [22–24].

Table 3.7 Examples of new targets and agents in recent clinical evaluation

Target	Agent
Farnesyl tranferase	BMS-214662
	R1155777 (tipifarnib)
	SCH 66336 (lonafarnib)
Raf kinase	BAY 43–9006 (sorafenib)
EGFR	ZD1839 (gefitinib)
	OSI-774 (erlotinib)
	C225 (cetuximab)
	EMD 72000 (matuzumab)
HER2	trastuzumab
ABL/c-kit	STI-571 (imatinib mesylate)
Angiogenesis: VEGF	bevacizumab
Angiogenesis: VEGFR	ZD6474
	PTK787 (vatalanib)
	SU11248 (sunitinib)
Angiogenesis: other	endostatin
BCL-2	G3139 (oblimersen)
DNA methyltransferase	MG98
Matrix metalloproteinase	BMS-275291
MEK	CI-1040
mTOR	CCI-779 (temsirolimus)
	RAD 001(everolimus)

The sections below describe some of the commonly suggested alternative endpoints for use in phase I studies of non-cytotoxic agents. Each is described

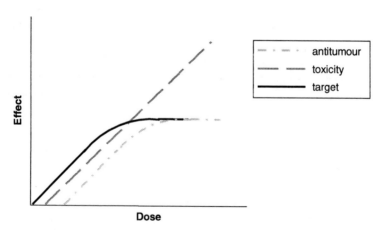

Figure 3.2 Dose–effect relationships for non-cytotoxic, targeted agents. Modified from: Eisenhauer EA (1998) *Ann Oncol* 9:1047–52. Reproduced with permission from ESMO.

with some examples given and this section ends with a summary of the experience to date.

3.3.2.1 Measures of target effect

This is the most rationally appealing endpoint to use for agents that have been developed to inhibit a specific target. Such measures are often referred to as PD effects (although strictly speaking any measure of what the drug does to the body is a PD effect). There are a number of challenges to be faced, however, if measures of target inhibition are to be used to define dosing in patients.

Which tissue? Logically, measurement of target inhibition should be undertaken in the tissue in which it is most important: tumour. To do this would entail serial tumour biopsies: at least two (before and at some point after treatment has begun), but more than two may be required to assess the variability in baseline measure and to define optimally the time course of inhibition and recovery. This presents obvious logistical challenges, as it would mean that all patients on the phase I trial would need to have accessible tumour and consent to repeat biopsies. This requirement would limit the numbers of patients available and consenting to such studies. Furthermore, if target-related changes in tissue are to be the primary endpoint, those patients whose tissue biopsy is inadequate or who, for reasons of disease progression or refusal, do not have follow-up biopsies, would have to be replaced on the dose level to which they were recruited.

For these reasons, some have suggested using normal tissues to measure changes in molecular effects. Depending on the target, peripheral blood mononuclear cells (the most appealing as repeat 'biopsy' entails nothing more than repeat blood sampling), buccal mucosa, or skin are some options. If normal tissue is sampled, ideally the validity of the tissue being evaluated and the assay being used will have been assessed in animal models prior to initiation of the study. That is, the tissue will have been shown in animals to express the target and to exhibit a dose-related (or PK-related) inhibition with treatment that parallels that seen in tumour in the same animals (see Chapter 2).

Examples from the clinical literature suggest that it is possible to repeatedly sample buccal mucosa and peripheral blood mononuclear cells [25,26]. Skin biopsies have also been undertaken repeatedly [3,27]. Repeated tumour biopsies are possible [28,29] but the sampling may not always be adequate (biopsy may be necrotic, have normal tissue included, or be an insufficient sample) to do the planned assays. To highlight some of these points, examples of assays undertaken in various tumour or normal tissues as part of phase I trials are shown in Table 3.8.

Which assay? Seldom is it the case that, at the time of the first-in-man study of a new agent, there is a validated commercial Good Laboratory Practice (see

Table 3.8 Examples of phase I trials incorporating serial molecular tissue measurements

Agent/ schedule	Target	Tissue sampled	Endpoints assessed	Outcomes	Dose recommendation	First author/ reference
BMS214662, 2 i.v. schedules: 1-h and 24-h i.v.	Farnesyl transferase (FT)	PBMCs	FT activity (radioenzyme)	1 h: 80% inhibition for <6 h at doses >118 mg/m^2 24 h: 40% inhibition for <24 h at doses >275 mg/m^2	Toxicity basis of dose recommendation: 1 h: 209 / mg/m^2 24 h: 275 mg/m^2	Tabernero [28]
		Tumour	FT activity	'Similar to PBMCs' (data not shown in article	PD data support dose recommendation	
			Apoptosis (TUNEL)	1 h: dose-related apoptosis 24 h: apoptosis in some patients, not dose related		
			MAPK and signalling pathway molecules (IHC)	No affect on MAPK pathway measures No affect on Ki67		
SCH66336, oral b.i.d. × 7 days	Farnesyl transferase (FT)	Buccal mucosa	Prelamin A farnesylation	75% inhibition at doses 350 mg, 100% at 400 mg (not tolerable)	Toxicity basis of dose recommendation: 350 mg p.o. b.i.d. × 7 days PD data support dose recommendation	Adjei [25]
MG98 2-h i.v. t.i.w., 3 of 4 weeks	DNA methyl-transferase 1 (DNMT1)	PBMCs	DNMT1 mRNA	No consistent changes from baseline. No dose-related trends.	Toxicity basis of dose recommendation: 360 mg/m^2	Stewart [26]
Gefitinib, oral daily	EGFR tyrosine kinase inhibitor	Skin	EGFR and pathway molecules (IHC)	Inhibition of EGFR activation in all patients, all doses	Toxicity basis of dose recommendation PD data show effect of drug, but no dose effect	Baselga [3]

PBMC, peripheral blood mononuclear cell; b.i.d., twice daily; t.i.w., three times a week.

Appendix I for references) quality assay of the desired molecular change available for general use. Thus, most such assays are carried out in research laboratories. It is critical when the trial endpoint will be based on laboratory test results that assay development and validation be done *before* the clinical trial begins. Critical questions include the actual measure that will constitute 'the' endpoint (e.g. level of expression of a protein or phosphorylation of protein?) and the method of measurement (mRNA or protein?). Test–test reproducibility should be assessed and variables of practical importance, such as how to process, fix and store tissue (Snap frozen? Fixed then frozen? Fixed then paraffin? Conditions for storage?) need clarification as well. Furthermore, it may not be clear when choosing to measure the impact of a molecularly targeted agent what is the most critical measure of effect. Should the assay focus, for example, on the phosphorylation of a kinase or on the downstream impact of kinase phosphorylation? Sometimes a multitude of assays may be undertaken. This gives the appearance of 'fishing' for one that will give the results expected/hoped for: a dose-related (or PK–parameter-related) change in measurement indicating a drug–dose effect. When multiple assays are done, however, it is plausible that they may not be concordant. Which to believe, if any, is problematic, unless one is designated as the 'primary' endpoint for decision making and that designation is based on solid preclinical data.

How much inhibition in what proportion of patients? It is equally important to have some estimate of the magnitude of target inhibition (or of the desired molecular effect) that is required to have an impact on tumour growth. Beyond this, what proportion of patients should have this effect with a given dose in order to conclude that dose should be recommended? There is not a great deal of literature addressing this issue and, once more, some extrapolation from preclinical experiments is required to guide the clinical evaluation, emphasizing again the importance of relevant preclinical studies.

What if the target ... is not the target? Despite great scientific rigour in the identification of both targets and agents with putative inhibitory effects, sometimes the agent has effects that are mediated by a mechanism other than that originally believed. Under these circumstances, assays of the putative target may mislead the investigator into believing either the dose is sufficient when it is not, i.e. if higher doses are required to affect the 'real' target, or insufficient when it in fact is, as the 'real' target is adequately inhibited. For example, when BAY 43–9006 (sorafenib) was first brought into clinical testing it was stated to be a 'specific' inhibitor of raf-1 kinase [30]. Subsequently, it was reported to have nanomolar inhibitory capability for several other kinases relevant to the malignant phenotype: vascular endothelial growth factor receptor 2 and 3, PDGFR-B, Flt3 to name a few [31]. It is speculated that its activity in some tumours (renal cell carcinoma, for example) is mediated by its effects on these other targets, not raf. Had measures of raf signalling inhibition been the primary endpoint of phase I evaluation for this agent (in fact toxic effects were the endpoint of phase I trials), it is possible the drug may not have proven to inhibit this pathway sufficiently, and this could have affected decisions about its development. As noted, because toxic effects were used as the phase I endpoint for dose recommendation, the discovery of 'new' targets after phase I trials were initiated was not of great relevance in making those decisions, though it has had an impact on the understanding of why BAY 43–9006 is showing activity in some tumour types such as renal cell carcinoma. This example serves to illustrate how the knowledge about the target of a new agent can evolve considerably early in its development. Thus, locking oneself into making decisions about dosing, or even about subsequent development, for a drug solely on the basis of measures of proof of target effect, may lead to erroneous decisions if the target ... is not the target after all.

Sample size   Although this will be discussed in greater detail below and in Chapter 6, it is worth noting that designs that focus on an endpoint of *avoidance of an adverse outcome in a small proportion of patients* (e.g. toxicity) may enrol fewer patients per dose level than those where the endpoint is the *occurrence of a favourable outcome in a majority of patients* (e.g. target inhibition). As described by Korn *et al.* [22], for a trial to show a dose response in target inhibition from 40% at one dose level to 90% inhibition at a higher dose, 17 patients would need to be treated at each level (and all would need to be evaluable for the measurement).

Examples of phase I studies where more than the usual one to three patients per dose level were enrolled when a 'biological' measure was the primary endpoint include early trials of aromatase inhibitors (see [32] for the example of anastrozole). In this particular example, measurement of oestradiol levels in peripheral blood was the endpoint and six to eight patients were enrolled per dose level. Another example is the phase I trial of O6-benzylguanine where the primary endpoint inhibition was of O6-alkylguanine in 90% of patients. The design required up to 13 patients per dose level [33].

Target effect as primary endpoint *versus* proof-of-principle studies   It is important to note that, while using measure(s) of target effect as a *means of defining dose* faces several challenges as noted above, one may still include such assays in phase I trials simply as a means of proof-of-principle, or proof of concept. The difference is that proof-of-principle studies seek primarily to investigate if the drug has its designed molecular effect, in normal (or tumour) tissue and these PD effects are incorporated into the trial as a secondary objective. Such trials are *not* designed to use measures of the magnitude of that effect to define dose, but to use these outcomes as supportive evidence of target modulation by the agent. Proof-of-principle studies may not require that all patients or all dose levels undergo evaluation. Not all patients will be required to consent to biopsies or have accessible tumour lesions, and decisions to escalate dose will not depend on a rapid turn around from the laboratory. This is a subtle difference, as a trial in which nothing more than proof-of-principle is planned may generate data that confirm or even establish a dose recommendation. Conversely, trials in which measures of target effect are the planned primary endpoint clearly also are proof-of-principle as they will study the impact of drug on molecular endpoints. Thus the difference between these concepts is more one of *planned intent and prospective design* (primary versus secondary endpoints) than in output.

3.3.2.2 Pharmacokinetic measures

Another measure that can be considered as an alternative to toxicity for the primary endpoint in phase I trials is the assessment of PK parameters. As measurement of the drug disposition during phase I trials is a standard aspect of their conduct, achievement of a target area under the curve, a minimum trough level, or a steady-state plasma level of drug above a predefined value may be utilized to define recommended dose. Generally, surpassing this minimum level is desirable, to assure adequate drug delivery at the level of the tissues.

Ideally, preclinical *in vivo* data of PK data from an efficacy tumour model are required to define the minimum plasma values or target levels for extrapolation to humans. Unfortunately, many preclinical PK studies are done only in the toxicology evaluation of the compound, not as part of the efficacy evaluation. The latter is most informative, and should also replicate the schedule and route of administration that will be studied in the trial. Knowledge of the IC_{50} (inhibitory concentration of 50%) from *in vitro* work is complementary but cannot substitute completely for the *in vivo* data, which more closely mirror the clinical setting, albeit with some imperfections. Furthermore, it is important in calculating the 'target' PK value that will determine if the recommended dose has been achieved or surpassed, to factor in the relative amounts of protein-bound/free drug, which may differ between species. Finally, it goes without saying that there must be a validated assay for measurement of the drug levels available for trials in which a PK measure is the primary endpoint. In fact, it can be argued that the requirement for a validated assay should apply to all phase I studies, regardless of the primary endpoint.

Several trials [34–37], notably those employing monoclonal antibodies or anti-sense oligodeoxynucleotides, have relied on PK measurements to define dose (see Table 3.9 for examples). It is not clear from reading the reports of these studies whether this measure was the planned primary endpoint at the outset when the protocol was written or if it became the endpoint when other measures, such as toxic effects, were not documented.

3.3.2.3 Functional imaging

Functional imaging has the potential to provide *in vivo* assessments of the impact of new agents on tumours and normal tissues, making this an interesting approach to defining recommended doses of drugs. Technology used in trials to date has included dynamic contrast enhanced magnetic resonance imaging (DCE-MRI), functional (or dynamic) computed tomographic (CT) scanning, positron emission tomography (PET), and ultrasound (US). The greatest area of interest has been in the use of one or more of these in the study of angiogenesis inhibitors and vascular targeting agents, where parameters such as tumour blood flow and perfusion in relation to drug dose have been assessed [38–43]. Although the field is still evolving, as seen in Table 3.10, several studies have been undertaken with results suggesting that both DCE-MRI and $[^{15}O]H_2O$ PET can show dose-related differences in measures of perfusion or flow with some of the investigational agents assessed. DCE-MRI has been adopted more widely in recent trials because of the practical challenges in PET associated with the delivery of ^{15}O given its very short half-life. Functional CT has the appeal of being an even simpler and more accessible technology than DCE-MRI, but it has not been as widely studied. There is no common standard 'language' yet developed for acquiring, analysing, and reporting functional imaging data, although that is in process with some specific recommendations in place for MRI assessment [44]. Until there is wide agreement on the precise prescription for how and when to repeat these dynamic evaluations in the course of a study and how to analyse and report study results, it is somewhat challenging to compare results across trials. Further, it is not clear yet if information from such trials is able to determine the optimal (recommended) *biologic dose* or simply demonstrate a *biologic effect* of the drug [45]. If DCE-MRI, or other functional imaging measures, is to substitute for the standard toxicity endpoint in dose-seeking trials, the technique requires validation (that is, the dose defined by the technology as optimum should be compared for efficacy with the dose defined by other means such as toxicity) and standardization so that it may be deployed in all centres using standard protocols.

In addition to assessing measures of vascularity and flow, functional imaging, most commonly ^{18}F-flourodeoxyglucose (FDG) PET, may also be

Table 3.9 Examples of phase I trials utilizing pharmacological measures to recommend dose

Agent/schedule	Target	Starting dose	Highest dose	Outcomes	Dose recommendation	Author/reference
BAY 12-9566, oral in a variety of schedules (once daily, b.i.d., t.i.d. and q.i.d)	Matrix metallo-proteins	100 mg o.d.	800 mg bid	Saturable absorption. PK for doses of 400 mg t.i.d., 400 mg q.i.d. and 800 mg b.i.d. similar At 800 mg p.o. b.i.d. Css BAY 12-9566 = $135\pm29\mu g/1$ (target range: $60-150\mu g/1$) MTD not reached	Based on safety, saturable behaviour, convenience, and achievement of 'target' Css, 800 mg p.o. b.i.d. recommended	Hirte [34]
Endostatin, daily i.v. bolus (20-min infusion)	Angiogenesis	15 mg/m^2	600 mg/m^2	AUC at 300 mg/m^2 = $677\pm172\mu g/ml/min$ Target AUC (active in Lewis lung): 600– μg/ml/min MTD not reached Drug supply precluded further escalation	Doses of 300–600 mg/m^2 doses were safe and achieved target AUC. Authors circumspect on whether this is 'recommended' dose and schedule	Herbst [35]

(Continued)

Table 3.9 *Continued*

Agent/schedule	Target	Starting dose	Highest dose	Outcomes	Dose recommendation	Author/reference
ISIS 5132, 21-day i.v. infusion	c-raf kinase	0.5 mg/kg/day	5.0 mg/kg/day	At 2 mg/kg/day, Css 5132 = 110 nM At 4 mg/kg/day, Css 5132 = 420 nM (*in vitro* IC_{50} was 100 nM) MTD not reached	Based on safety and plasma concentration data, dose of 4 mg/kg/day recommended	Cunningham [36]
C225 (cetuximab), i.v. single dose and weekly single agent	Epidermal growth factor receptor	5 mg/m²	400 mg/m²	Dose-dependent (saturable) PK Systemic clearance saturated at doses in range of 200–400 mg/mg² At 200 mg/m² C225 levels sustained above 200 nmol/l Preclinical data suggest levels >30 nmol/l active MTD not reached	Based on safety and PK data, 200 mg/m² was recommended dose	Baselga [37]

Table 3.10 Examples of phase I trials with imaging endpoints

Agent	Class	Imaging technique(s)	Endpoints assessed	Outcomes	Author/reference
Endostatin, daily i.v.	Angiogenesis inhibitor	$[^{15}O]H_2O$ PET	Tumour blood flow	Some suggestion of decrease flow at higher doses on day 28, but not day 56	Herbst [38]
		$[^{18}F]$ FDG PET	Tumour metabolism	As above for blood flow	
Endostatin, daily i.v.	Angiogenesis inhibitor	Dynamic CT	Microvessel density as assessed by CT attenuation	No dose effect, but 4/21 patients had some evidence of decrease	Thomas [39]
		DCE-MRI	Blood flow/vascularity	No changes seen	
		Ultrasound	Blood flow/vascularity	No changes seen	
		$[^{18}F]$ FDG PET	Tumour metabolism	No overall or dose-dependent trend	
PTK787, daily oral	VEGFR tyrosine kinase inhibitor (angiogenesis inhibitor)	DCE-MRI	Change from baseline in bidirectional transfer constant (Ki) to assess permeability and vascularity	Dose related and AUC-related decrease in Ki	Morgan [40]
Combretastatin, A4 phosphate, every 3 weeks i.v.	Vascular targeting agent	DCE-MRI	Tumour blood flow (gradient peak)	Significant decrease at recommended maximum dose (60 mg/m^2) in 6 of 7 patients	Dowlati [42]
Combretastatin, A4 phosphate, weekly x 3 i.v.		DCE-MRI	Tumour blood flow/vascular permeability as assessed by change in transfer constant, K^{trans}	Reduction in K^{trans} in 6/16 patients at doses ≥ 52 mg/m^2	Galbraith [42]
Combretastatin A4 phosphate		$[^{15}O]H_2O$ PET	Tumour perfusion	Dose dependent reduction in perfusion. Mean decrease 49% at doses ≥ 52 mg/m^2	Anderson [43]

PET, positron emission tomography; CT, computerized tomography; MRI, magnetic resonance imaging; DCE, dynamic contrast enhanced; FDG, fluorodeoxyglucose.

used to assess metabolic activity in tumour masses. Metabolically active tumours take up the sugar and the uptake decreases as tumours become metabolically inactive prior to regressing. Thus [18]FDG-PET has most often been considered as an option for showing antitumour activity, rather than one that can help identify dose relationships, though the two may be connected [46]. The observation of imatinib's profound and early effects on PET scans of gastrointestinal stromal tumours heralding classic objective antitumour responses [47] is but one of many examples that have established a fairly good relationship between early changes in [18]FDG PET and eventual objective response. The same relationships have not been established between PET changes and recommended dose. It may be the case that a dose–effect in metabolism identified by PET can be generally shown, but this has not been firmly established. Thus, to use [18]FDG PET changes to define recommended dose in a heterogeneous group of patients on a phase I trial is premature.

Of importance, however, is the fact that this technology may also be exploited to study other PD and PK parameters in tumours *in vivo*. Besides [18]FDG, other labelled compounds, such as thymidine, have been studied [48] as markers of tumour proliferation. PET clearly has the potential to be used for non-invasive molecular imaging such as measuring drug distribution to tumour *in vivo* as well as measuring the effect of drugs on their targets in tumour masses. Research programmes such as that in Manchester UK (Wolfson Molecular Imaging Centre, Director Dr P. Price) are studying methods to achieve these goals since if feasible and practical, determining drug dosing for new anticancer drugs could be profoundly altered as a result.

3.3.3 Experience with the use of alternative endpoints

Non-cytotoxic targeted agents are not, in fact, theoretical beasts: numerous such agents have been evaluated in first-in-man studies. As many more are likely to enter the clinic in the next one to two decades, it is useful to consider how the phase I evaluation was undertaken with those that have completed study and to consider what can be learned from this experience. A recent review of 31 targeted agents evaluated in 57 phase I trials in solid tumours was published [49]. Study abstracts or full publications available up to March 2003 were reviewed; the actual protocols for the trials were not available so it was not possible to determine what the intended primary phase I endpoints were. Nonetheless, in practice, toxicity was the most common reason for halting dose escalation and the most common basis for phase II dose recommendation (35 of 50 trials in which a phase II dose was recommended). Blood level measurements were the second most common basis for dose recommendation (nine of 50) (Table 3.11). Interestingly, only five of the trials in this review

Table 3.11 Survey of 57 phase I trials of targeted agents: basis of phase II dose recommendation

Recommended phase II dose?			No. of trials	No. of agents
Not stated			5	5
Not recommended			2	1
Recommended			52	27
	Primary basis	Toxicity	35	19
	of recommendation:	PK	9	7
		Other trial results (toxicity)	2	2
		Clinical activity	1	1
		PBMC findings	1	1
		Tumour (target or response)	1	1
		Convenient schedule	1	1
	Total trials		57	

*From the review of Parulekar and Eisenhauer [49] but data have been updated based on erratum published in *J Natl Cancer Inst* 2004; **96**(21): 1640. Reprinted with permission from Oxford University Press.

incorporated tumour biopsies to assess the molecular impact of treatment; 16 trials performed serial biopsies of normal tissue. In only two studies (one in tumour, one in peripheral blood mononuclear cells) was the finding in tissue the primary basis of dose recommendation. In many other cases, however, findings from tissue samples supported the dose recommended on the primary basis of either toxic effects or blood level determinations. Imaging studies were also infrequently incorporated and in no case formed the sole basis of dose selection. While this review was not comprehensive, it was extensive and suggests that, despite the discussion about alternative endpoints, particularly tissue effects of drug, for determining phase II dose recommendations, it is not yet the case that these are being utilized as primary endpoints in phase I trials. Rather, observation of toxic effects continue to be the major reason for halting dose escalation and the basis for phase II dose recommendation.

Is this a problem? It may not be if, in fact, toxic effects are due to a target effect in normal tissue. For example, epidermal growth factor receptor inhibitor skin toxicity is a dose-related effect, which has been correlated with inhibition of target and downstream molecular measures in tumour biopsy studies [3,27]. Furthermore, the increases in blood pressure seen with inhibitors of vascular endothelial growth factor and its receptor are in keeping with its mechanism of action [50–52]. Thus, it is a reasonable strategy to use toxicity as the endpoint for establishing the dose range of a drug, particularly when the toxicity is due to the drug's effect on target in normal tissues, as was the case for the examples cited. If further information on the effect of doses within that range on other PD outcomes (such as molecular or imaging measures or antitumour response) is important for drug development decisions, then conducting additional trial(s) of larger patient numbers of uniform histology with accessible tumour tissue may be a useful approach. In fact, there are several examples where this has been done: randomized phase II trials of the epidermal growth factor receptor inhibitor gefitinib (ZD1839) evaluated two doses at the low end and the middle of the dosing range in which antitumour effects (objective response) was the primary endpoint [53,54]; another epidermal growth factor receptor inhibitor, EMD72000 (matuzumab), was evaluated first in a dose-seeking trial, then in subsequent trials a few dose levels were selected for evaluation of both imaging and biopsy studies [27,55,56]. This approach could allow assessment of the 'alternative' endpoints designed to measure molecular or imaging effects in a more uniform population with a smaller range of doses. The resulting information could be used to reinforce, or change, the recommended dose from the initial phase I trial.

3.3.4 Summary of endpoints

Traditional phase I trials utilize measurement of toxicity as the primary endpoint for decisions about halting dose escalation and recommended single agent dosing. The use of toxicity as the endpoint for trials of cytotoxic agents was originally based on the philosophy that high doses of drugs would be required to have maximal impact in a fatal disease and also on lab observations of a dose–effect relationship for both toxicity and for efficacy, making toxicity a useful 'surrogate' measure to identify doses that were likely to be effective. In addition, its use has been strongly reinforced by the long history of cancer drug development, which has affirmed that dosing to the highest levels tolerable results in maximal efficacy in many human clinical trials.

The era of novel molecular targeted therapeutics ('non-cytotoxic' agents) has provided an opportunity for review and debate about utilizing toxic effects as the main 'driver' for dose recommendation at the end of phase I trials [49]. Assessment of target effects on normal and tumour tissue and measures of functional imaging, related to dose and PK effects, have been promoted as means of rational selection of optimal doses of targeted therapies. Notwithstanding the desire to move in this direction, evidence to date suggests that, as trials of such drugs have been undertaken, toxicity (and to a lesser degree assessment of blood levels of drug) continues to drive decision making in dose escalation and in dose recommendation. Attempts to assess other measures have clearly been made in many trials, and results from these tests frequently have supported the dose recommendation made on the basis of toxicity, but rarely have they supplanted it.

It is useful to consider why as a community, phase I investigators and trial sponsors have thus far remained largely bound to the use of toxicity as the primary endpoint in phase I trials. The following provides some factors that may account for this.

First, there are practical considerations in repeated sampling of tumours, normal tissue or in conducting expensive imaging evaluations, which are self-evident. Secondly, in the trials performed to date, the assays, their analysis and interpretation were in their infancy when the new agents first went into human trials. Thus there was undoubtedly considerable, and reasonable, uncertainty about how much weight to put on the results of these assays in the first generation of studies to use them. Finally, assessment of toxicity was not only familiar and standardized, but also was required in any case: whatever the primary endpoint selected on theoretical grounds, toxic effects must be documented as part of first-in-man studies.

Thus, when or if there is uncertainty about the validity of the alternative primary endpoints discussed above, the observation of toxic effects, particularly those that may be due to an effect of the drug under study on the target in normal tissue, can allow a reasonable means of making dose decisions. Dosing to toxicity makes it unlikely the doses selected will be too low, although they may be higher than necessary. Other measures, such as imaging changes, blood levels of drug, and molecular changes in sampled tissues were thus included largely as secondary endpoints, perhaps as proof-of-principle that the drug was doing what it was intended to (as discussed earlier).

It is plausible that, with time and experience, the heavy reliance on assessment of toxicity to drive dosing recommendations will be supplanted by some type of composite endpoint that includes observations of toxicity but also integrates one or more direct measures of molecular effect and ties these in with PK observations.

Until then, if knowledge about the molecular impact of a novel agent on its putative target is required or highly desirable for future drug development decisions, a rational approach would be to establish a dosing range of safety using toxicity (or measures of blood levels, if toxic effects do not occur) in a standard phase I design, and then carry out a subsequent trial(s) in which a more homogeneous group of patients are assigned to a small number of doses across the range (e.g. the toxicity-recommended dose and one to three levels below it). In this second study (which some have labelled 'phase Ib') molecular effects on normal or malignant tumour lesions could be measured or

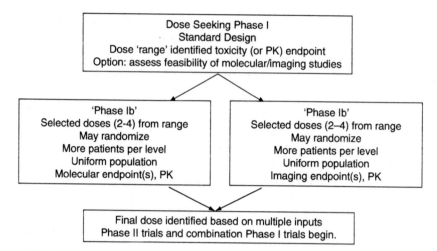

Figure 3.3 Proposed sequential integration of non-toxicity endpoints in drug development.

functional imaging undertaken and PK studies done to narrow down the dose to one that is based on assessment of the biological effects of the doses studied, as well as their relationship to PK measures. If the first dose ranging study incorporates molecular or other measures these could be seen as secondary endpoints to refine methodology and obtain preliminary proof-of-principle data. As noted earlier (see EMD 72000 examples) this strategy is already being deployed in the development of some new agents. This approach is illustrated in Figure 3.3.

3.4 Trial design

When a new agent is studied in patients for the first time, it is probable that more than one schedule of administration will be evaluated, unless preclinical studies make it clear that only a single schedule is worthwhile. Thus, many intravenous agents will be evaluated in a repeated dosing (or prolonged infusion) schedule as well as in a single dose schedule and for oral agents, continuous and intermittent dosing schedules are evaluated. Furthermore, there may often be more than one clinical trial evaluating each schedule.

There are a variety of designs used to conduct first-in-man phase I trials, but they have in common several features: selection of a 'safe' starting dose, sequential dose escalation in small cohorts of patients (and sometimes within cohorts), and determination of a recommended dose based on a pre-specified primary endpoint. Good phase I design should yield a relatively precise determination of the recommended dose and must address the competing issues of safety and efficiency: individual patients should not be exposed to doses of drug that are likely to be excessively toxic; at the same time, the recommended dose should be arrived at in a timely fashion with as few patients as possible treated at doses likely to be subtherapeutic. While efficiency is enhanced by higher starting doses, fewer patients per dose level, and large escalation steps, patient safety is enhanced by lower starting doses, more patients per dose level (to assure it is really a safe dose), and smaller dosing increments [14]. Good designs balance these competing variables.

3.4.1 Starting dose

The starting dose for phase I first-in-man trials is based on animal toxicology where the drug has been given in the same schedule as will be assessed in humans (see Chapter 2). Generally, the most sensitive of two species is identified and the dose is almost always administered on a milligram per metre squared (mg/m^2) basis in patients, requiring conversion from the usual animal dosing, which is given on a per body weight basis (see below). Although there is some controversy about the use of body surface area-based dosing in later drug development, it is agreed that, at least for estimation of the starting dose, using a body surface area-based calculation is standard [57]. Thereafter, whether one uses flat dosing increments (common for oral agents where tablets are of fixed dose amount), or one continues to employ body surface area to derive dose increments varies. For intravenous drugs, phase I trials generally utilize body surface area-based dose increments.

If mice are the most sensitive species, the starting dose usually considered 'safe' is one-tenth the mouse-equivalent LD10 (0.1 MELD10: one-tenth the dose that causes 10% lethality in mice; the murine LD10 may also be referred to as the murine MTD). If one-tenth the MELD10 is substantially more toxic in a second species, generally one-third or less of the lowest toxic dose (TDL) or of the no observed adverse effect level (NOAEL) equivalent dose in that species is selected as the human starting dose. The question of whether higher starting doses might be both safe and reduce trial time for phase I trials has been addressed by some [14,58,59], and the evidence suggests that for most agents that do *not* exhibit interspecies differences in toxicity, starting doses may safely be somewhat higher (e.g. 0.2 MELD10). However, more aggressive dose escalation schemes (see below) largely overcome the advantage of a higher starting dose, so most have not adopted this. A practical issue when determining the starting dose is how to convert doses to equivalent doses between species. Table 3.12 gives conversion factors for species most commonly used in toxicology testing. A worked example is also shown.

Table 3.12 Conversion factors for animal dosing to human dosing.* (Examples of conversions in italics below each)

Animal species	Animal dose units		To convert dose in mg/kg to mg/m² multiply by factor listed
Mouse	mg/kg		3
	20 mg/kg	*=*	*60 mg/m²*
Dog	mg/kg		20
	3 mg/kg	*=*	*60 mg/m²*
Rat	mg/kg		6
	10 mg/kg	*=*	*60 mg/m²*
Monkeys	mg/kg		12
	5 mg/kg	*=*	*60 mg/m²*
Guinea pig	mg/kg		8
	8 mg/kg	*=*	*64 mg/m²*
Rabbit	mg/kg		12
	5 mg/kg	*=*	*60 mg/m²*

*From *Guidance for Industry and Reviewers: Estimating the Safe Starting Dose in Clinical Trials for Therapeutics in Adults Healthy volunteers.* US Department of Health and Human Services, Food and Drug Administration, December 2002.

3.4.2 Escalation plan

Chapter 6 deals in dose escalation designs in great detail, so only general remarks will be made here. Phase I escalation designs have evolved from the historically common 'modified Fibonacci scheme', which enrolled new cohorts of patients at higher doses in ever diminishing increments using a mathematical pattern. Most new designs, enrol new cohorts at large dose intervals at the beginning of dose escalation [14] and at smaller dose intervals as the MTD approaches, but the switch in interval size is not arbitrary: toxicity, pharmacological, or other measures are used to guide escalation to the next step. Both empirical and statistical methods for dose escalation are used, as outlined in detail in Chapter 6. However the dose escalation plan is described in the protocol, there should be included the option for creation of 'intermediate' dose levels based on emerging observations so that this action can be undertaken without the need for formal protocol amendment.

Dose escalation proceeds until a prespecified endpoint is reached. If toxicity is the primary endpoint; escalation continues until a minimum number, usually two of three, or two to three of six patients, experience a dose-limiting event. When this happens, the next lower dose level is expanded to gain more information as it will likely be the recommended dose. If that dose, in turn, shows more DLT events than acceptable, further de-escalation is undertaken. Intermediate levels may be useful as the investigators narrow in on the final recommended dose, if it appears it will fall between dose levels. This is most likely to happen if the dose below the MTD shows little or no toxicity.

If the primary endpoint is a pharmacological measure, escalation will continue until a minimum level is achieved in the proportion of patients described in advance in the protocol, provided other events (e.g. toxicity) do not intervene. It is important to realize that use of pharmacological measures to make decisions regarding dose escalation means that the results of PK analysis must be available after each dose level in *real time*. Furthermore, if PK data suggest the behaviour of the compound is non-linear or if levels plateau (due to saturation in absorption of oral drug for example), this will necessitate some renewed thinking about how to adjust the design or schedule. Chapter 10 offers some practical advice about how to respond to such observations and how to write the protocol in such a way that investigators can be responsive to data as it is generated during the course of the study.

3.4.3 Patient entry

An important aspect of patient enrolment on to phase I trials is that it is staggered: not all patients are entered at once, but rather in steps, as information about safety or other endpoint measures emerge.

3.4.3.1 Cohort size

The number of patients entered per dose level has roots in empiricism: although historically three patients minimum per level have been recruited, as few as one patient per level may be enrolled (Chapter 6 also describes how some designs incorporate patient numbers into escalation steps). When toxicity is the primary endpoint, entry of one patient per dose level in the first few dose levels has become commonplace [14]. However, this may not be advisable if the *class* of the new drug being studied is one with previously documented wide interpatient variability in toxic effects; for example, antimetabolites represent a class where there is considerable interpatient variability [60]. In these circumstances, the usual minimum of three patients per dose level is more appropriate as decisions about the safety of a given dose may require more than one patient's experience following drug exposure.

As escalation proceeds beyond the first few dose levels, usually the number of patients per level increases to three, once toxicity of a minimum degree (e.g. grade 2) has been seen in at least one patient. Thereafter a minimum of three patients in each cohort are recruited, expanding to six in the event one of three has a DLT in the protocol prescribed observation period (usually one cycle or 4–8 weeks of chronic therapy). When toxicity is not the primary endpoint, or when the drug being studied is expected to have wide interpatient variability, at least three patients per dose level are recommended. Patients who fail to complete the observation period necessary to assure DLT is not seen, or who fail to complete at least 80–90% of the treatment prescribed for *non*-toxicity reasons (e.g. early drop-outs for disease progression) must be replaced on that dose level.

Finally, as noted earlier, it is advisable to expand the cohort (e.g. a total of six to 10 patients) receiving what is believed to be the recommended dose and to include patients who are representative of those likely to receive the drug in phase II trials. This expanded cohort allows increased confidence in the safety and appropriateness of the final recommended dose.

All the 'rules' mentioned above must be clearly defined in the protocol document: examples will be given in Chapter 7 later in this book.

3.4.3.2   Intrapatient dose escalation

It is clear that patients on the initial stages of phase I trials will be assigned to receive doses that are subtherapeutic. This has been cited as one of the ethical issues associated with phase I trials as most patients enter the studies with at least a hope that the treatment offered may benefit them [61,62]. Approaches to enhancing the proportion of patients *overall* in a phase I trial who are exposed to 'therapeutic' dose levels includes not only limiting enrolment on lower dose levels, but also allowing escalation within individual patients (intrapatient dose escalation). That is, the protocol may be written in such a way so that not only are new patients enrolled at ever increasing doses based on safety or other assessments of the preceding dose level, but those patients already on the trial may also be escalated to higher dose levels provided they have not exhibited any substantial toxicity themselves. Which level they escalate to may be the highest level already demonstrated to be safe in a newly recruited cohort *or* to the level that is open for new patient recruitment.

Although intrapatient escalation has not been routinely utilized in phase I trials, there is certainly increasing interest in it. In an article on phase I designs by Simon *et al.* [63], simulations of a number of different possible designs were conducted. The various designs included not only different dose escalation methods but also varying numbers of patients per dose level and whether or not, within a given design, intrapatient escalation was permitted. When intrapatient dose escalation was modelled into the design, escalation of an individual patient to the next dose level was 'allowed' if no toxicity >grade 1 was seen in the preceding cycle at their assigned dose level. The authors concluded that, on the basis of their simulation data, intrapatient escalation was safe, though it did not appreciably shorten the study duration. However, it did allow fewer patients to be 'undertreated' in comparison with standard interpatient escalation approaches.

Although the idea of intrapatient dose escalation is appealing, it does not seem to be widely applied. There are some theoretical and practical objections to it. Those patients undergoing intrapatient escalation who experience significant toxicity at their escalated dose may be difficult to sort out: is it the administered dose that cycle or the cumulative dose causing the problem? Although the Simon study carries some reassurance about the safety of this approach, the data used for the simulations were based on only nine agents (in a total of 20 phase I trial datasets). Secondly, the 'rules' about when escalation can occur are not consistent: some require information about the safety of the drug at the next dose level to be known in the new cohort of patients before allowing patients enrolled at lower dose levels to be escalated. Clearly this would mean that patients would have to be on treatment *at least* two cycles, to allow newly recruited patients a chance to be treated at the next higher dose, before intrapatient escalation could take place. Many phase I patients will have progressed by that point in time. Thus, practically speaking, very few patients could be escalated if safety of the next dose level would need to be assured before intrapatient escalation. Thirdly, how such patient data are to be counted in terms of the trial report is unclear: should the observations for patients who have doses escalated be reported together with the data on others at their initial dose, their escalated dose or some blend of the two? Finally, it is argued that as the actual chance of benefit (in terms of response rate) on a phase I trial is low (in the range of 5%) [64–67], the added benefit likely to accrue to an *individual* patient by escalation of one dose level is very small indeed. In other words, if the low overall rate of response in phase I trials is the problem, it seems implausible that intrapatient dose escalation will have a huge impact on the probability of benefit. The only article to examine this systematically [67], found that response rates in trials with no intrapatient escalation were slightly lower (3.2%) than those permitting intrapatient escalation (5.3%), suggesting there might be a small positive impact of this strategy on response rates.

Thus, despite the appeal of escalating patients to higher doses than they were assigned initially, should safety criteria be met, some issues remain with its routine application in phase I protocols. Many phase I protocols continue to be written prohibiting intrapatient escalation as it is believed to have minimal impact on trial efficiency while bringing with it concerns about practical issues and safety. Others are quite content to allow intrapatient escalation within their protocols. Whatever is allowed within a given protocol, it is important to continue to require a minimum number of *newly* recruited patients at each dose level, and to base further dose escalation decisions upon the behaviour of the drug in these individuals, rather than to confuse the determination of MTD by a mix of escalated and new patients.

3.5 Summary

The primary goal of phase I trials is to establish the recommended dose of a new agent or new combination regimen. Cancer patients comprise the population usually enrolled on such trials, although in some instances first-in-man trials of specific drugs may have a brief exposure in healthy volunteers before trials in patients begin. Subjects must be selected to have adequate organ function, performance status, and must provide informed consent for the study including all its extra investigations and follow-up. Although there is interest in exploring new endpoints to define recommended doses (such as tissue changes in molecular pathways relevant to the agent's mechanism of action) toxicity, the traditional endpoint for phase I trials, remains the most commonly utilized primary measure to define dose.

Phase I design involves dose escalation in small cohorts of patients beginning at a safe starting dose based on animal toxicology and proceeding until toxic effects or other findings limit further escalation. When toxicity is the primary endpoint, the recommended dose is slightly below that producing dose-limiting effects in an unacceptable proportion of patients; when other measures are to be the basis of dose recommendation, they should be described in advance in the protocol and based on justification from preclinical models. It is advisable that the recommended dose be studied in an expanded cohort of patients whose pretreatment characteristics are similar to those of patients that will be enrolled in phase II studies to have greater confidence in the safety of the dose recommendation. When drug development decisions depend on the data of ancillary molecular or functional imaging studies, it is proposed that trials directed to these specific questions be conducted once the dose-ranging phase I trial is complete, and should be based on adequate preclinical data of PK–PD relationships. These 'phase Ib' studies would enrol larger cohorts of patients of the same histology and treat them at a handful of dose levels in the dose range of interest in order to address the molecular or imaging questions with adequate controls and sufficient power.

Other important aspects of phase I trials include: (a) ethical considerations; (b) designs for trials in special populations (those patients at extremes of age or having abnormal organ function); and (c) options for their statistical design. These topics are covered in the following chapters.

References

1. Yates RA, Dowsett M, Fisher GV, Selen A, Wyld PJ (1996). Arimidex (ZD1033): a selective, potent inhibitor of aromatase in postmenopausal female volunteers. *Br J Cancer* 73(4): 543–8.

2. Swaisland H, Laight A, Stafford L, *et al.* (2001). Pharmacokinetics and tolerability of the orally active selective epidermal growth factor receptor tyrosine kinase inhibitor ZD1839 in healthy volunteers. *Clin Pharmacokinet* **40**(4): 297–302.

3. Baselga J, Rischin D, Ranson M, *et al.* (2002). Phase I safety, pharmacokinetic, and pharmacodynamic trial of ZD1839, a selective oral epidermal growth factor receptor tyrosine kinase inhibitor, in patients with five selected solid tumor types. *J Clin Oncol* **20**: 4292–302.

4. Millar AW, Brown PD, Moore J, *et al.* (1998). Results of single and repeat dose studies of the oral matrix metalloproteinase inhibitor marimastat in healthy male volunteers. *Br J Clin Pharmacol* **45**: 21–6.

5. Wojtowicz-Praga S, Torri J, Johnson M, *et al.* (1998). Phase I trial of marimastat, a novel matrix metalloproteinase inhibitor, administered orally to patients with advanced lung cancer. *J Clin Oncol* **16**(6): 2150–6.

6. Quirt I, Bodurtha A, Lohmann R, *et al.* (2002). Phase II study of marimastat (BB-2516) in malignant melanoma: a clinical and tumor biopsy study of the National Cancer Institute of Canada Clinical Trials Group. *Invest New Drugs* **20**(4): 431–7.

7. Evans JD, Stark A, Johnson CD, *et al.* (2001). A phase II trial of marimastat in advanced pancreatic cancer. *Br J Cancer* **85**(12): 1865–70.

8. Maloney DG, Grillo-Lopez AJ, Bodkin DJ, *et al.* (1997) IDEC-C2B8: results of a phase I multiple-dose trial in patients with relapsed non-Hodgkin's lymphoma. *J Clin Oncol* **15**(10): 3266–74.

9. Miller AB, Hoogstraten B, Staquet M, Winkler A (1981). Reporting results of cancer treatment. *Cancer* **47**: 207–14.

10. Oken MM, Creech RH, Tormey DC, *et al.* (1982). Toxicity and response criteria of the Eastern Cooperative Oncology Group. *Am J Clin Oncol* **5**: 649–55.

11. Karnofsky DA, Burchenal JH (1949). The clinical evaluation of chemotherapeutic agents in cancer. In: Macleod CM, ed. *Evaluation of Chemotherapeutic Agents*, pp. 199–205. Columbia University Press, New York.

12. Carter SK (1977). Clinical trials in cancer chemotherapy. *Cancer* **40**: 544–57.

13. Geller NL (1984). Design of phase I and II clinical trials in cancer: a statistician's view. *Cancer Invest* **2**: 483–91.

14. Eisenhauer EA, O'Dwyer PJ, Christian M, Humphrey JS (2000). Phase I clinical trial design in cancer drug development. *J Clin Oncol* **18**: 684–92.

15. Skipper HE, Schabel FM Jr, Wilcox WS (1964). Experimental evaluation of potential anticancer agents. XIII. On the criteria and kinetics associated with 'curability' of experimental leukaemia. *Cancer Chemother Rep* **35**: 1–111.

16. Tannock IF, Boyd NF, DeBoer G, *et al.* (1988). A randomized trial of two dose levels of cyclophosphamide, methotrexate, and fluorouracil chemotherapy for patients with metastatic breast cancer. *J Clin Oncol* **6**(9):1377–87.

17. Common Terminology Criteria for Adverse Events. Available at: http://ctep.cancer.gov/forms/CTCAEv3.pdf [last accessed August 2005]

18. International Conference on Harmonisation. Website of history and information is at: http://www.ich.org [last accessed August 2005]

19. MedRA (Medical Dictionary for Regulatory Activities Terminology) available at: http://www.medramsso.com [last accessed August 2005]

20. Eisenhauer EA (1998). Phase I and II trials of novel anti–cancer agents: endpoints, efficacy and existentialism. *Ann Oncol* 9: 1047–52.

21. Jason TL, Koropatnick J, Berg RW (2004) Toxicology of anti-sense therapeutics. *Toxicol Appl Pharmacol* 15: 66–83.

22. Korn EL, Arbuck SG, Pluda JM, Simon R, Kaplan RS, Christian MC (2001). Clinical trial design for cytostatic agents: are new approaches needed? *J Clin Oncol* 19: 265–72.

23. Gelmon KA, Eisenhauer EA, Harris AL, Ratain MJ, Workman P (1999). Anticancer agents targeting signaling molecules and cancer cell environment: challenges for drug development? *J Natl Cancer Inst* 91: 1281–7.

24. Parulekar WR, Eisenhauer EA (2002). Novel endpoints and design of early clinical trials. *Ann Oncol* 13 (Suppl. 4): 139–43.

25. Adjei AA, Erlichman C, Davis JN, *et al.* (2000). A phase I trial of the farnesyl transferase inhibitor SCH66336: evidence for biological and clinical activity. *Cancer Res* 60: 1871–7.

26. Stewart DJ, Donehower RC, Eisenhauer EA, *et al.* (2003). A phase I pharmacokinetic and pharmacodynamic study of the DNA methyltransferase 1 inhibitor MG98 administered twice weekly. *Ann Oncol* 14: 766–74.

27. Vanhoefer U, Tewes M, Rojo F, *et al.* (2004). Phase I study of the humanized epidermal growth factor receptor monoclonal antibody EMD72000 in patients with advanced solid tumors that express the epidermal growth factor receptor. *J Clin Oncol* 22: 175–84.

28. Tabernero J, Rojo F, Marimon I, *et al.* (2005) Phase I pharmacokinetic and pharmacodynamic study of weekly 1-hour and 24-hour infusion BMS-214662, a farnesyltransferase inhibitor, in patients with advanced solid tumors. *J Clin Oncol* 23: 2521–33.

29. Goss G, Hirte H, Miller WH Jr, *et al.* (2005). A phase I study of oral ZD 1839 given daily in patients with solid tumors: IND.122, a study of the Investigational New Drug Program of the National Cancer Institute of Canada Clinical Trials Group. *Invest New Drugs* 23(2): 147–55.

30. Lyons JF, Wilhelm S, Hibner B, Bollag G (2001). Discovery of a novel Raf kinase inhibitor. *Endocr Relat Cancer* 8: 219–25.

31. Wilhelm S, Carter C, Tang LY, *et al.* (2003). BAY 43–9006 exhibits broad spectrum anti–tumour activity and targets Raf/MEK/ERK pathway and receptor tyrosine kinases involved in tumour progression and angiogenesis. *Clin Cancer Res* 9 (Suppl.): A78.

32. Plourde PV, Dyroff M, Dwosett M, Demers L, Yates R, Webster A (1995). ARIMIDEX®: a new oral, once-a-day aromatase inhibitor. *J Steroid Biochem Mol Biol* 53: 175–9.

33. Friedman HS, Kokkinakis DM, Pluda J, *et al.* (1998). Phase I trial of O6-methylguanine for patients undergoing surgery for malignant glioma. *J Clin Oncol* 16: 3570–5.

34. Hirte H, Goel R, Major P, *et al.* (2000). A phase I dose escalation study of the matrix metalloproteinase inhibitor BAY 12–9566 administered orally in patients with advanced solid tumours. *Ann Oncol* 11: 1579–84.

35. Herbst RS, Hess KR, Tran HT, *et al.* (2002). Phase I study of recombinant human endostatin in patients with advanced solid tumors. *J Clin Oncol* 20: 3792–803.

36. Cunningham CC, Holmlund JT, Schiller JH, *et al.* (2000). A phase I trial of c-*raf* kinase anti-sense oligonucleotide ISIS 5132 administered as a continuous intravenous infusion in patients with advanced cancer. *Clin Cancer Res* 6: 1626–31.

37. Baselga J, Pfister D, Cooper MR, *et al.* (2000). Phase I studies of anti-epidermal growth factor receptor chimeric antibody C225 alone and in combination with cisplatin. *J Clin Oncol* **18**: 904–14.

38. Herbst RS, Mullani NA, Davis DW, *et al.* (2002). Development of biologic markers of response and assessment of antiangiogenic activity in a clinical trial of recombinant human endostatin. *J Clin Oncol* **20**: 3804–14.

39. Thomas JP, Arzoomaniam RZ, Alberti D, *et al.* (2003). Phase I pharmacokinetic and pharmacodynamic study of recombinant human endostatin in patients with advanced solid tumors. *J Clin Oncol* **21**: 223–31.

40. Morgan B, Thomas AL, Drevs J, *et al.* (2003). Dynamic contrast-enhanced magnetic resonance imaging as a biomarker for the pharmacological response of PTK787/ZK222584, an inhibitor of the vascular endothelial growth factor receptor tyrosine kinases, in patients with advanced colorectal cancer and liver metastases: results from two phase I studies. *J Clin Oncol* **21**: 3955–64.

41. Dowlati A, Robertson K, Cooney M, *et al.* (2002). A phase I pharmacokinetic and translational study of the novel vascular targeting agent Combretastatin A-4 phosphate on the single-dose intravenous schedule in patients with advanced cancer. *Cancer Res* **62**: 3408–16.

42. Galbraith SM, Maxwell RJ, Lodge MA, *et al.* (2003). Combretastatin A4 phosphate has tumor antivascular activity in rat and man as demonstrated by dynamic magnetic resonance imaging. *J Clin Oncol* **21**: 2831–42.

43. Anderson HL, Yap JT, Miller MP, Robbins A, Jones T, Price P (2003). Assessment of pharmacodynamic vascular response in a phase I trial of Combretastatin A4 phosphate. *J Clin Oncol* **21**: 2823–30.

44. Leach MO, Brindle KM, Evelhoch JL, *et al.* (2003). Assessment of antiangiogenic and antivascular therapeutics with MRI: recommendations for appropriate methodology for clinical trials. *Br J Radiol* **76** (Special Issue No. 1): S87–91.

45. Rehman S, Jayson GC (2005). Molecular imaging of antiangiogenic agents. *Oncologist* **10**: 92–103.

46. Laking GR, Price PM, Sculpher MJ (2002). Assessment of the technology for functional imaging in cancer. *Eur J Cancer* **38**: 2194–9.

47. Stroobants S, Goeminne J, Seegers M, *et al.* (2003).[18]FDG-Positron emission tomography for the early prediction of response in advanced soft tissue sarcoma treated with imatinib mesylate (Glivec®). *Eur J Cancer* **39**: 2012–20.

48. Wells P, West C, Jones T, Harris A, Price P (2004). Measuring tumor pharmacodynamic response using PET proliferation probes: the case for 2-[(11)C]-thymidine. *Biochim Biophys Acta* **1705**: 91–102.

49. Parulekar WR, Eisenhauer EA (2004). Phase I trials designs for solid tumor studies of targeted, non-cytotoxic agents: theory and practice. *J Natl Cancer Inst* **96**: 990–7.

50. Thomas AL, Morgan B, Drevs J, *et al.* (2003). Vascular endothelial growth factor receptor tyrosine kinase inhibitors PTK787/ZK222584. *Semin Oncol* **30** (3, Suppl. 6): 32–8.

51. Miller KD, Chap LI, Holmes FA, *et al.* (2005). Randomized phase III trial of capecitabine compared with bevacizumab plus capecitabine in patients with previously treated metastatic breast cancer. *J Clin Oncol* **23**: 792–9.

52. Hurwitz H, Fehrenbacher L, Novotny W, *et al.* (2004). Bevacizumab plus irinotecan, fluorouracil, and leucovorin for metastatic colorectal cancer. *N Engl J Med* **350**: 2335–42.

53. Fukuoka M, Yano S, Giaccone G, et al. (2003). Multi-institutional randomized phase II trial of gefitinib for previously treated patients with non-small cell lung cancer. *J Clin Oncol* 21: 2237–46.

54. Kris MG, Natale RB, Herbst RS, et al. (2003). Efficacy of gefitinib, an inhibitor of the epidermal growth factor receptor tyrosine kinase, in symptomatic patients with non-small cell lung cancer: a randomized trial. *JAMA* 290: 2149–58.

55. Salazar R, Tabernero J, Rojo F, et al. (2004). Dose-dependent inhibition of the EGFR and signalling pathways with the anti-EGFR monoclonal antibody (Mab) EMD 72000 administered every three weeks (q3w). A phase I pharmacokinetic/pharmacodynamic (PK/PD) study to define the optimal biologic dose (OBD). *J Clin Oncol*, 2004 ASCO Annual Meeting Proceedings (Post-Meeting Edition). 22: No.14S (Suppl.): 2002.

56. Trarbach T, Beyer T, Schleucher N, et al. (2004). Final results of a randomized phase I pharmacokinetic and pharmacodynamic study of weekly EMD 72000 (matuzumab), a humanized anti-epidermal growth factor receptor (EGFR) monoclonal antibody, in subjects with advanced gastrointestinal cancers. *Ann Oncol* 15(Suppl. 3): iii101 (Abstr. 378).

57. Ratain MJ (1998). Body-surface area as a basis for dosing of anticancer agents: science, myth or habit? *J Clin Oncol* 16: 2297–8.

58. Penta JS, Rozencweig M, Guarino AM, Muggia FM (1979). Mouse and large-animal toxicology studies of twelve antitumour agents: relevance to starting dose for phase I clinical trials. *Cancer Chemother Pharmacol* 3: 97–101.

59. Penta JS, Rosner GL, Trump DL (1992). Choice of starting dose and escalation for phase I studies of antitumour agents. *Cancer Chemother Pharmacol* 31: 247–50.

60. Seymour L, Eisenhauer E (2001). A review of dose-limiting events in phase I trials: antimetabolites show unpredictable relationships between dose and toxicity. *Cancer Chemother Pharmacol* 47: 2–10.

61. Ratain MJ, Mick R, Schilsky RL, Siegler M (1993). Statistical and ethical issues in the design and conduct of phase I and II clinical trials of new anticancer agents. *J Natl Cancer Inst* 85: 1637–43.

62. Kodish E, Stocking C, Ratain MJ, Kohrman A, Siegler M (1992). Ethical issues in phase I oncology research: a comparison of investigators and institutional review board chairpersons. *J Clin Oncol* 10: 1810–16.

63. Simon R, Friedlin B, Rubinstein L, Arbuck SG, Collins J, Christian MC (1997). Accelerated titration designs for phase I clinical trials in oncology. *J Natl Cancer Inst* 89: 1138–47.

64. Decoster G, Stein G, Holdener EE (1990). Responses and toxic deaths in phase I clinical trials. *Ann Oncol* 1: 175–81.

65. Von Hoff DD, Turner J (1991). Response rates, duration of response and dose response effects in phase I studies of antineoplastics. *Invest New Drugs* 9: 115–22.

66. Sekine I, Yamamoto H, Kunitoh H, et al. (2002). Relationship between objective responses in phase I trials and potential efficacy of non-specific cytotoxic investigational new drugs. *Ann Oncol* 13: 1300–6.

67. Roberts TG, Goulart BH, Stallings SC, et al. (2004). Trends in the risks and benefits to patients with cancer participating in phase I clinical trials. *JAMA* 292: 2130–40.

Chapter 4

Ethical issues in phase I cancer trials

Elizabeth A. Eisenhauer

4.1 Introduction

There are international and national standards addressing the ethical conduct of clinical trials and the protection of human subjects in research. The *Nuremberg Code* (1947) [1] and the *Declaration of Helsinki* (initially published in 1964 and revised numerous times since) [2] defined principles to govern biomedical research and protect the rights, safety, and well-being of trial subjects. The Belmont report in the USA [3] defined three ethical principles that underpin human subjects research, drawing on these earlier documents. These are: *Respect for Persons* (individuals are to be treated as autonomous beings, capable of making informed choices; and those with diminished autonomy must be offered protection), *Beneficence* (maximize the possible benefits and minimize harms) and *Justice* (treat research participants fairly and distribute the benefits and burdens of research equitably).

The *Guideline for Good Clinical Practice* of the International Conference on Harmonization [4], adopted by most jurisdictions including the European Union, Japan, United States, and Canada reaffirms the principles of the Nuremberg Code and the Declaration of Helsinki. Further, it details the process of ethical committee review of research, the content of informed consent forms, the obligations of the investigator and the sponsor in clinical trials, the required elements of clinical research protocols and the documents that must be in place prior to beginning a clinical trial. All of these elements and processes apply to phase I cancer trials. The following sections do not provide a comprehensive review of clinical trial ethical issues; rather they will highlight those aspects of particular importance in first-in-man and other phase I oncology trials.

4.2 General ethical issues in phase I oncology trials

Beyond the general aspects of research conduct referred to above, phase I first-in-man trials in oncology have been the focus of special ethical scrutiny for a number of reasons, well-summarized in a recent overview by Agrawal and Emanuel [5]: (a) there is concern that the *risk–benefit ratio* for many cancer drugs does not justify phase I studies; (b) secondly, that *disclosure of information*, i.e. the informed consent process, is inadequate; and (c) finally, because subjects are cancer patients whose disease is no longer curable and for whom other therapeutic options are very limited, the population has been seen as '*vulnerable*' and in need of special protection. Each of these concerns will be discussed in the sections that follow. In all cases, the discussion focuses only on first-in-man phase I trials.

4.2.1 Risk/benefit

There are no universal standards to apply to the question of risk/benefit in phase I oncology trials (or for that matter in oncology trials in general). Although the benefit, in terms of antitumour effect, for a *specific* agent undergoing its first-in-man phase I study is *unknown*, the benefit that can be *expected*, based on hundreds of phase I trials, can be estimated. Several major reviews have shown that benefit, as measured by objective response, is in the range of 5% overall [6–9], with up to 60% of all phase I trials having at least one objective response observed (and about 10% of trials having overall response rates in excess of 10%). Although it can be argued that objective response may not equate with 'benefit' in the most abstract sense, it is certainly an objective measure of change that is acceptable to the US Food and Drug Administration and the broader community for accelerated approval of new cancer drugs [10]. Furthermore, the response rate documented in these reviews of about 5% is in keeping with that expected from certain 'standard' single agent oncology therapeutics, such as gemcitabine in pancreatic cancer [11] or erlotinib in non-small cell lung cancer [12]. Thus the 'benefit' as assessed by this objective means is small but certainly could be considered quite acceptable by some external standards. Moreover, other benefits may accrue to patients enrolled on phase I studies besides objective tumour shrinkage, though these are more challenging to document. In a review of patients enrolled on cancer phase I trials, Daugherty *et al.* documented that 70% of patients expected to receive psychological benefit by participating (though no follow-up data are presented to show it transpired) [13]. As reviewed by Agrawal and Emanuel [5], some investigators have observed improvement in the quality of life of patients over the period of time they were on phase I cancer trials, but given the design of such studies it is not clear if this is related to the agent itself, related to the frequent medical interactions (and thus opportunities for symptom control for example) that phase I trials entail, or related to benefits from the hopeful beliefs held by patients enrolled on such studies (see more on this below). However, as argued by Agrawal and Emanuel, regardless of whether observed quality of life improvements are truly a result of the intervention of the phase I drug or not, 'participating in phase I trials and focusing on quality of life are not necessarily—and should not be—inherently incompatible goals'. [5]

The other aspect of the risk/benefit ratio is, of course, the risk of serious adverse effects to patients receiving a new agent for the first time. Once again, this risk cannot be accurately quantified for a specific agent as it enters phase I trials, as no human data are available, but adequate preclinical data and good trial design (safe starting dose, careful dose escalation, ongoing safety monitoring) mitigate this risk. In terms of 'real data', a recent review found that overall, the risk of toxic death in phase I trials is about 0.5%; and the risk of this outcome is even lower (0.06%) in trials conducted in the recent past (1999–2002) [9], suggesting the true risk of toxic death is extremely low in today's phase I trials. Thus, the expected risk/benefit ratio, based on objective data, of a properly designed and conducted phase I trial is acceptable using the aforementioned endpoints. Clearly data from historic series are informative but not absolutely predictive of what the risk is to an individual patient on an individual phase I trial. However, the historical summary data are reasonable sources of information upon which an informed discussion can be held.

4.2.2 Disclosure of information: informed consent

Another subject of ethical debate surrounding phase I cancer trials is that of informed consent. Several authors have documented high expectations of benefit in patients consenting to phase I trials, which, given the data cited above, could be interpreted to indicate that the informed consent process was inadequate. Daugherty *et al.* found that 85% of patients enrolled on a phase I trial chose to do so because of possible therapeutic benefit [13]. Cohen *et al.* have found that a similar proportion (87%) of subjects on phase I trials believed the treatment might cure them [14]. It is argued therefore that, if

80% or more of patients on phase I trials believe they might experience therapeutic benefit, and the true response rate expected is only about 5%, then the patients must have been misinformed. However, discordance between actual prognosis and belief in benefit may not necessarily represent misinformation. A review of consent forms from 272 oncology phase I trials (63% having industry funding of some sort) from the US National Cancer Institute-designated cancer centres was recently published [15]. Trials were included if they were conducted in the 1999 calendar year. This review found that only *one* of the 272 consent forms stated that subjects were *expected* to benefit. The remainder indicated either that there would be no benefit to participating (4%), that benefit was uncertain (94%) or were silent on the subject (2%). Ninety-two per cent of consent forms indicated that the trial's main purpose was dose-escalation, safety, or toxicity. Thus in this review, the consent forms almost never promised direct benefit. This information seems at odds with the reported motivation by patients for enrolling on such studies. Clearly, the consent forms reviewed came from only US trials so perhaps there are limits to the generalizability of these conclusions. However, the adoption of International Conference of Harmonization Good Clinical Practice guidelines (which contain explicit instructions on consent form content) around the world implies that the content of consent forms should be similar in multiple jurisdictions. Furthermore, the consent form document is not equivalent to the entire process of informed consent: the discussion between the investigator or other health care professionals and the patient may have different content. However, when this has been examined more directly, through either recording of conversations, surveys on informed consent discussion content, or structured patient information interviews, the data support the notion that the majority of conversations regarding phase I trials correctly identify the investigational nature of the therapy, and the unknowns in risk and benefit that might accrue to the patient [16,17]. Further, even if the motivation to join the study may be possibility of benefit for many patients, some research suggests that this *hope* for benefit is not the same as actually believing it *will* happen: in Daugherty's series 85% of patients were motivated to join a phase I trial because of possible therapeutic benefit but only 22% *believed* they would receive any therapeutic benefit by participating (70% said they believed they would, however, receive psychological benefit). This divide between patient's expectation or hope of benefit and the real probability of benefit has been termed a 'therapeutic misconception' and is often taken as a sign of failure of the informed consent process. However as argued by Weinfurt *et al.*, this may not be the case: it may in fact reflect linguistic issues [18]. When patients have a frequency-type piece of information given them, they may respond using belief-type statements. That is, the belief and hope that may be recalled in citing reasons for joining a phase I trial (most information in such publications is obtained after a decision was taken to accept a trial, not at the time) may not reflect the information given (or even understood) but rather the hoped-for outcome of the decision. Agrawal and Emanuel characterize this as a 'motivation to maintain hope in a difficult situation rather than a misunderstanding of the information' [5]. A relationship has been observed between the presence of hope, overestimation of prognosis and good measures of coping in cancer patients participating in phase I trials [19]. It is plausible that the motivations described by patients for their enrolment in phase I trials reflect the fact that maintaining hope is important to them and the trial provides a vehicle for hope's expression: even if the factual information they received and understood made it clear therapeutic benefit was an improbable outcome.

4.2.3 Vulnerable population?

The observation that hope may motivate consent to phase I enrolment is one of the reasons some argue that cancer patients who are phase I candidates are, as a group, 'vulnerable' and worthy of special protection by ethics committees or other bodies. The basis of this argument is not clear: seriously ill patients of all types are faced daily with important decisions regarding treatment options, which, if they are adequately informed and competent, it is presumed and *expected* they will make for themselves. It isn't clear what is different about advanced stage cancer patients *per se* in this regard. Thus those that argue vulnerability must be doing so, not from the perspective of the patient group as a whole (who, after all, could choose to accept alternative treatments or supportive care if no phase I trial were available without being argued 'vulnerable'), but rather the *nature of the choice put before them* (phase I trial yes or no). This argument is not credible, as it seems to stem from the opinion that if patients agree to such trials, and think they might benefit, they are either ill-informed (which the data cited earlier suggest is not the case) or unable to take decisions for themselves. There is no evidence to support the latter argument, nor is it plausible to suppose a special condition of cancer patients renders them incapable of weighing risks and benefits wisely. To deny competent patients the right to make *informed* decisions about their care or about participation in legitimate clinical research is counter to the principles of Nuremberg and Helsinki referred to earlier. That a healthy person cannot *understand* the decision of a patient to enrol in a phase I trial doesn't mean the patient is vulnerable or incompetent; rather that the frames of reference for those healthy and those ill are inherently different.

4.3 Ethical considerations in exclusion criteria

As is described in Chapter 3, inclusion and exclusion criteria must be carefully considered as one designs a phase I first-in-man trial. The fact that access to phase I agents is restricted to only a subset of patients can be argued to be unethical if it is even remotely possible the new drug may help. This argument is discussed in the UNESCO report on Ethical Considerations Regarding Access to Experimental Treatment and Experimentation on Human Subjects [20]. This line of reasoning is based on the principle of justice, where the burden of research (and thus access to research options) ought to be fairly distributed. However, this argument can be countered on several fronts.

First, eligibility criteria serve the dual purpose of ensuring patient safety (for example individuals with impairment of the very organs thought to be important in drug metabolism might suffer serious toxic effects) and also allowing recruitment of a population most likely to *address the primary study question*: defining the recommended dose. This is accomplished by recruiting patients who are likely to survive long enough for the required follow-up. Patients with very poor performance status, those with significant co-morbidity or organ impairment may die soon after treatment is given so they cannot contribute meaningfully to the study question and it will not be clear if their death might be treatment related. While early death can occur on phase I studies even when appropriate inclusion criteria are in place, it is less frequent than would be the case if criteria were much more broadly written.

Secondly, and more importantly, it cannot be argued that restrictive enrolment is discriminatory if the 'treatment' has not yet demonstrated any evidence of efficacy. While it may be wrong to withhold *effective* treatment from those who could benefit, phase I agents are of *unknown* toxicity and efficacy. In fact, the opposite position can be argued: that it is unethical to expose *large* numbers of patients to a drug unless it is known to be both safe and effective.

Finally, practically speaking, at the time first-in-man phase I trials are initiated, the availability of drug is extremely limited: usually supplies for the first few studies is available, but no more, so widespread prescription would not be feasible without extra resource.

Thus exclusion criteria, provided they are based on reasonable medical and physiological parameters (and not social, economic, or other parameters) are not inherently unethical.

4.4 Consent for tissue procurement and invasive procedures

Increasingly, early clinical trials of all types include analyses of tissue or imaging studies to evaluate potential signs of a new agent's biological effects on molecular and other endpoints. It has always been understood that a phase I trial would include extra investigations such as more frequent blood samples or standard radiological studies, but the growing use of more invasive procedures merits special consideration.

Two questions are at the centre of the discussion. First are the ethical and consent issues around undertaking invasive procedures that are non-therapeutic, in particular repeated biopsies of tumour or normal tissue. Secondly, are the ethical and consent issues surrounding research studies on tissue and its possible banking for future, unknown, research.

With respect to the former, as in all research procedures, there is a requirement to balance the incremental *risk* such procedures pose (such as bleeding), against the potential *benefit* for discovery of useful information that helps inform decisions about how best to use the drug. Studies including fresh tumour sampling must have clearly written eligibility criteria to ensure that patients are appropriately selected to minimize risk (for example, patients should have easily accessible lesions, not in an organ or tissue site where bleeding is anticipated to be a sizable risk). Although risk can be quantified, there is essentially no possibility of direct benefit to the patient through having research studies undertaken on their tumour or normal tissue sample, so it is extremely important that the research questions proposed must be both truly meaningful and also require the use of patient material to answer. With respect to informed consent, the same principles apply as for all human subjects research: patients must be informed about the procedural risks, the lack of therapeutic benefit expected from the procedure, the scientific reason for requesting it, and consent must be given freely. This raises the question about whether trials incorporating fresh biopsy studies should always be written so as to make the biopsy aspect optional with a consent process separate from that of the main study consent. There is no clear direction given about this: each study must be evaluated individually. As not all cancer patients will be eligible for enrolment on phase I trials in any case, further restriction of entry criteria to include only those who have lesions to biopsy and consent to undergo this procedure may be reasonable in some circumstances. However, if this is planned, there needs to be strict attention paid to the consent form and planned consent process: patients should not be coerced into undergoing invasive procedures in order to get what they may hope to be a useful therapy.

As described, the justification for conducting these additional studies is based on the importance of the knowledge to be gained through them. Therefore, both the protocol and consent form must detail how the tissue will be investigated, or how the specialized imaging studies will be used, to gain meaningful information vis-à-vis the study goals.

This brings us to the second question: How any tissue procured in these studies will be handled, stored, and what research investigations will be undertaken. Concern is several fold: about the nature of the investigations to be conducted on the tissue; the storage and use of the tissue in future, unspecified, research projects; assurance of privacy and confidentiality; and the patient's rights regarding commercialization of discoveries.

It is clear that patients must be informed about what laboratory investigation is planned for their tissue (whether freshly biopsied or archived from earlier diagnostic or treatment procedures). However, there is variability among experts and government authorities with respect to the *detail required* in providing this information: some require consent forms to have a detailed listing of all planned laboratory tests, and would not permit additional studies without re-consent. Others accept more general language, provided the *intent* of the testing is clear, for example for phase I trials when mechanistic questions about the new agent are being addressed: 'laboratory studies will be undertaken to help determine if the drug has effects on my cancer cells as predicted' or 'laboratory studies will be undertaken to understand better how the drug works in killing cancer cells and whether this is related to the dose of the drug'. In these examples, even though the language is vague, the use is directed toward a specific set of research questions.

If the text above were *all* the information supplied in the consent form, it would not be possible to use the tissue to study other general questions of cancer biology or other non-malignant disease without the patient's re-consent. Therefore, if it is anticipated there will be tissue remaining after the planned phase I study questions are addressed, the options for storage and future study of that tissue must be provided to the patient for consideration and consent. Will leftover tissue be stored in a tissue bank, returned to the hospital from which it came (if applicable), or destroyed? Even though the tissue is no longer part of the patient, research on it, particularly if linked to (even anonymized) individual characteristics, is considered 'human subjects' research [21], and thus requires informed consent. To enable future research (in cancer or other diseases) on stored tissue, it is common practice to request consent for this possibility *at the time the original consent for study-related research is given*. The use of this approach is variable and not all hospitals or ethical committees are agreed on it: some argue that new consent is required each time a new laboratory research study is proposed and are uncomfortable with prospective consent being given to 'any future study' (see, for example, [22] and the footnote on p. 85 of reference [23]). However, two recent reviews suggest the majority of patients who donate their tissue for a specific research project are also agreeable to having it used for future, unspecified, research (including research on different diseases) [24,25]. If future research includes the possibility of testing for germ-line genetic changes, this normally requires *explicit* description and consent because identification of a heritable mutation could have far reaching impact on the patient and/or the family if they could be identified. In order to encompass all the possible options for stored tissue, it has been recommended that the consent form contain a checklist of options so the patient can indicate their preferences [23]. This approach has the advantage of simplicity and efficiency, but is only useful if patients are reminded to complete it in full.

Phase I investigators should familiarize themselves with the local views on this complex subject and develop consent forms accordingly in order to avoid delays in the ethical review process for their study.

The study protocol and consent form must address not only what research will/might take place on tissue but also where tissues will be stored and how anonymity will be assured. Plans for patient confidentiality and privacy protection should be carefully scrutinized by the ethical committee in order to ensure compliance with applicable laws or regulations.

Finally, the consent form must also address two other issues: whether there is a possibility the patient's tissue will be *sold*, and whether the patient can expect any *payment* in the case a discovery is made based on the results of the research on their tissue that leads to successful commercialization. Many jurisdictions prohibit the sale of human tissues or body parts.

Regulation of the use of banked human tissue is in evolution, so the foregoing serves only to highlight some of the issues in a general fashion. Although tissue freshly removed from patients (or accessed from pathology archives) for investigation as part of phase I trials is unlikely to result in large numbers of stored specimens, investigators must still be knowledgeable about and comply with the various local or national regulations that apply to the storage and future use of biological samples. Contracts for clinical trials that include biological sample procurement must provide clarity and compliance for these issues as well.

Useful documents to read include the guidances on the subject from the US Office for Human Research Protection [26], the US National Bioethics Advisory Commission Report [23], the Australian National Statement on Ethical Conduct in research Involving Humans Part 15: Use of Human Tissue samples [27], The Opinion of the European Group on Ethics and New Technologies to the European Commission on Ethical Aspects of Human Tissue Banking [28], the recently enacted United Kingdom Human Tissue Act [29], the Canadian Tri-Council Policy (specifically section 15) [30], and an article comparing the laws in the United States and Europe vis-à-vis the use of human biological samples in research [31].

4.5   Ethical review and informed consent as processes

As noted earlier there are several international codes of conduct that speak to the proper process for ethics committee review of protocols as well as the consent form content (see Table 7.10 for a checklist of essential elements based on one of these documents). Besides the international codes, many countries (and even institutions) have their own regulations that stipulate in greater detail the constitution and function of ethical review committees and the content of consent forms. These apply equally to all phases of clinical investigation.

It is important to note that both ethical review and consent are ongoing processes, not one-time events in the story of a study or a patient. In first-in-man oncology trials in particular, it is important to keep the ethics committee informed of emerging safety information from the study. When, even before an annual report is due, study data shows that the drug is producing important toxic effects, normally the consent form would be modified to reflect these so the ethics committee and new patients will be aware of the risks of treatment.

In terms of patient interactions, initial consent to the study may be best accomplished in two or more meetings with the investigator and study team. Having the consent process performed in stages allows time for the patients and family to 'digest' the information, develop additional questions and seek outside (e.g. family physician) advice about participating. Indeed, a review of studies exploring what activities or tools enhance research participants' understanding in informed consent, found that one of the most effective ways of improving the understanding of research subjects was to have a study team member or neutral educator spend more one-on-one time with study participants [32].

Ongoing contact with the patient is, of course, standard during the treatment phase of first-in-man studies, but in addition to seeking information from the patient on how he or she is tolerating the drug, such encounters also offer the opportunity to provide the patient with updated information on drug safety if it is available. Indeed, the investigator is *obliged* to make the patient aware of significant new findings that might affect his/her willingness to continue the study drug, and to document such discussions in the medical record. For phase I trials, this generally means new information about serious toxicity (which may, depending on the nature of the effect and the ethical committee advice, require formal re-consent). However, in addition to providing information about serious toxicity, the patient should also be informed about other toxic effects, for example, nausea, fatigue, skin rash, that the cumulative study data suggest are treatment related. This continuous provision of new information fosters strong relationships between patients and the investigator, and offers the opportunity for the patient to become truly a part of the study team.

4.6 Summary

As for other types of human subjects research, phase I oncology trials must be underpinned by three fundamental ethical principles articulated in the Introduction: *Respect for Persons, Beneficence,* and *Justice.* Although some have argued that cancer patients eligible for these trials may be a vulnerable group and in need of special protection, there is no evidence to support this contention. Cancer patients are capable of making informed choices about their care, including decisions about enrolment on clinical trials. First-in-man trials do have some special aspects, however: they involve administration of agent(s) with unknown effects having the potential for toxicity, the primary goal of the study is not efficacy, and the trial may include non-therapeutic invasive procedures.

The arguments and evidence supplied in this chapter provide background to the reader regarding the special issues faced by ethical committees and investigators in assuring ethical conduct of phase I trials. Educators, investigators, ethical committee members, and institutions must have in place procedures not only to assure appropriate consent form content and protocol review, but also appropriate training for and oversight of the informed consent process for those engaged in patient recruitment. Trials themselves must be founded on good science, appropriate and adequate preclinical data, display acceptable risk/benefit, and have embedded in them ongoing monitoring of patient safety to minimize risks to subjects as new information emerges in the course of the trial. The review of research by an independent ethical review committee helps to assure the balance in risk/benefit and adherence to the principles and regulations that govern human subjects research. When there is doubt about a course of action, acting in the best interests of the individual patient should take precedence over the concerns for the study. Respect for and protection of patients remains the cornerstone of ethical conduct in clinical research.

References

1. The Nuremburg Code: http://www.hhs.gov/ohrp/references/nurcode.htm [last accessed August 2005]
2. World Medical Association Declaration of Helsinki: ethical principles for medical research involving human subjects (2000). *JAMA* **284**: 3043–5. and also: http://www.wma.net/e/policy/pdf/17c.pdf [last accessed August 2005]

3. The Belmont Report. Ethical Principles and Guidelines for the Protection of Human Subjects of Research. The National Commission for the Protection of Human Subjects of Biomedical and Behavioral Research Available at: http://www.hhs.gov/ohrp/human-subjects/guidance/belmont.htm [last accessed August 2005]

4. International Conference on Harmonization, Guidelines for Good Clinical Practice: http://www.ich.org/MediaServer.jser?@_ID =482&@_MODE=GLB [last accessed August 2005]

5. Agrawal M, Emanuel EJ (2003). Ethics of phase I oncology studies: reexamining the arguments and data. *JAMA* **290**: 1075–82.

6. Decoster G, Stein G, Holdener EE (1990). Responses and toxic deaths in phase I clinical trials. *Ann Oncol* **1**: 175–81.

7. Von Hoff DD, Turner J (1991). Response rates, duration of response and dose response effects in phase I studies of antineoplastics. *Invest New Drugs* **9**: 115–22.

8. Sekine I, Yamamoto H, Kunitoh H, *et al.* (2002). Relationship between objective responses in phase I trials and potential efficacy of non-specific cytotoxic investigational new drugs. *Ann Oncol* **13**: 1300–6.

9. Roberts TG, Goulart BH, Stallings SC, *et al.* (2004). Trends in the risks and benefits to patients with cancer participating in phase I clinical trials. *JAMA* **292**: 2130–40.

10. Dagher R, Johnson J, Williams G, Keegan P, Pazdur R (2004). Accelerated approval of oncology products: a decade of experience. *J Natl Cancer Inst* **96**: 1500–9.

11. Burris HA 3rd, Moore MJ, Andersen J, *et al.* (1997). Improvements in survival and clinical benefit with gemcitabine as first-line therapy for patients with advanced pancreas cancer: a randomized trial. *J Clin Oncol* **15**: 2403–13.

12. Shepherd FA, Rodrigues Pereira J, Ciuleanu T, *et al.* (2005). Erlotinib in previously treated non-small-cell lung cancer. *N Engl J Med* **353**: 123–32.

13. Daugherty C, Ratain MJ, Growchowski E, *et al.* (1995). Perceptions of cancer patients and their physicians involved in phase I trials. *J Clin Oncol* **13**: 1062–72.

14. Cohen L, de Moor C, Amato RJ (2001). The association between treatment-specific optimism and depressive symptomatology in patients enrolled in a phase I cancer clinical trial. *Cancer* **91**: 1949–55.

15. Horng S, Emanuel EJ, Wilfond B, Rackoff J, Martz K, Grady C (2002). Descriptions of benefits and risks in consent forms for phase I oncology trials. *N Engl J Med* **347**: 2134–40.

16. Rodenhuis S, van den Heuvel WJA, Annyas AA, Koops HS, Sleijfer DT, Mulder NH (1984). Patient motivation and informed consent in a phase I study of an anticancer agent. *Eur J Cancer Clin Oncol* **20**: 457–62.

17. Tomamichel M, Sessa C, Herzig S, *et al.* (1995) Informed consent for phase I studies: evaluation of quantity and quality of information provided to patients. *Ann Oncol* **6**: 363–9.

18. Weinfurt KP, Sulmasy DP. Schulman KA, Meropol NJ (2003). Patient expectations of benefit from phase I clinical trials: linguistic considerations in diagnosing therapeutic misconception. *Theor Med Bioeth* **24**: 329–44.

19. Helft PR, Hlubocky F, Wen M, Daugherty CK (2003). Associations among awareness of prognosis, hopefulness, and coping in patients with advanced cancer participating in phase I clinical trials. *Support Care Cancer* **11**: 644–51.

20. UNESCO International Bioethics Committee (1996): Ethical Considerations regarding access to experimental treatment and experimentation on human subjects. Available at: http://portal.unesco.org/shs/en/file_download.php/9eaaa3ba669f5235ec154da-f86e9f2e7experimentationCIB4_en.pdf [last accessed August 2005]

21. Clayton EW (2005). Informed consent and biobanks. *J Law Med Ethics* **33**: 15–21.

22. Sade RM (2002).Research on stored biological samples is still research. *Arch Intern Med* **162**: 1439–40.

23. National Bioethics Advisory Commission. Research involving human biological materials: ethical issues and policy guidance. Available at http://bioethics.georgetown.edu/nbac [last accessed August 2005]. Direct pdf file: http://www.georgetown.edu/research/nrcbl/nbac/hbm.pdf [last accessed August 2005]

24. Chen DT, Rosenstein DL, Muthappan P, *et al.* (2005). Research with stored biological samples: what do research participants want? *Arch Intern Med* **165**: 652–5.

25. Malone T, Catalano PJ, O'Dwyer PJ, Giantonio B (2002). High rate of consent to bank biologic samples for future research: the Eastern Cooperative Oncology Group experience. *J Natl Cancer Inst* **94**: 769–71.

26. Office for Human Research Protection (OHRP) and Department of Health and Human Services (HHS), Guidance on research involving coded private information or biological specimens. Available at: http://www.hhs.gov/ohrp/humansubjects/guidance/cdebiol.pdf [last accessed August 2005]

27. Australian National Statement on Ethical Conduct in research Involving Humans Part 15: Use of Human Tissue samples http://www7.health.gov.au/nhmrc/publications/humans/part15.htm [last accessed August 2005]

28. The Opinion of the European Group on Ethics and New Technologies to the European Commission on Ethical Aspects of Human Tissue Banking http://europa.eu.int/comm/european_group_ethics/docs/avis11_en.pdf [last accessed August 2005]

29. The United Kingston Human Tissue Act (2004). http://www.opsi.gov.uk/acts/acts2004/20040030.htm [last accessed August 2005]

30. The Canadian Tri-Council Policy Statement: Ethical Conduct for Research Involving Humans http://www.pre.ethics.gc.ca/english/policystatement/policystatement.cfm [last accessed August 2005]

31. Baeyens AJ, Hakimian R, Aamodt R, Spatz A (2001/2002). The use of human biological samples in research: a comparison of the laws in the United States and Europe. *Bio-Sci Law Rev* **5**: 155–60.

32. Flory J, Emanuel E (2004). Interventions to improve research participants' understanding in informed consent for research: a systematic review. *JAMA* **292**: 1593–1601.

Chapter 5

Special populations and interaction studies

Chris Twelves

Special populations: introduction

Given the differences between patients with cancer, as well as the range of novel agents being evaluated both as single agents and in combination, it is inevitable that a 'one size suits all' approach cannot be applied to phase I cancer trials. For ethical reasons, in general, patients should not be excluded on the grounds of gender, ethnicity, or age. There may, however, be a need for separate studies in particular patient groups. This is especially true in relation to patients with liver or renal impairment.

Patients are selected carefully for phase I trials to reduce the risks to which they are exposed. These patients usually have relatively normal liver and renal biochemistry, are over the age of 18, with fewer concurrent problems and associated concomitant medications than those seen in routine clinical practice. Although it is not considered appropriate to exclude older patients or those from ethnic minorities, in practice such patients are usually under-represented in clinical trials. The safety profile, pharmacokinetic characteristics, and dose recommendations from a standard phase I trial may not, therefore, be universally applicable.

Many factors including altered organ function, age, gender, ethnicity, body size, enzyme polymorphisms, drug interactions, and food (in the case of oral drugs) may influence the maximum tolerated dose (MTD) or recommended dose (RD) in a phase I trial. Most often, this is due to altered pharmacokinetics affecting systemic drug exposure. In other cases there may be altered pharmacodynamics, such that end organ sensitivity is affected. In most special populations, such as patients with liver dysfunction, the question is whether a dose lower than that identified in the standard phase I trial is needed. In others, such as paediatric patients, an increased drug dose may be required to achieve equivalent systemic exposure. It would be time-consuming and inordinately costly to carry out a phase I trial of all new agents in every special population alongside the standard phase I trial. Equally, it would be inefficient to address these issues only when a drug has completed its clinical development, as this may delay approval or limit the patient population for whom it is indicated. Therefore, the relevant 'special populations' should be identified early during the development of a new drug in order that specific studies can be conducted soon after the drug has been characterized and a dose recommended in a standard population, but before large-scale phase III studies are undertaken.

The aim of a phase I trial in a special population is to enable the new drug to be used safely and at a potentially effective dose in the relevant population. First it needs to be established whether or not dosing is an issue in that population. Where that is the case, a safe but potentially effective and clinically relevant dosing scheme should be established. These are complex studies because of the nature of the patient population and the need for extensive pharmacokinetic sampling.

5.1 Organ impairment studies

Patients eligible for first-in-man phase I trials usually have relatively normal liver and renal biochemistry, whereas in routine clinical practice renal impairment and abnormal liver biochemistry tests are common in patients with cancer.

Some of these issues are illustrated by the anthracyclines, where optimal dosing of anthracyclines in patients with liver metastases remains unclear, with many clinicians not following current recommendations [1]. These recommendations followed the observation by Benjamin *et al.* [2] of increased toxicity with doxorubicin in eight patients with liver metastases and abnormal liver biochemistry tests; dose reductions in six subsequent patients abrogated this excess toxicity. Although these dose reductions, based primarily on serum bilirubin, were recommended, they were never validated. Subsequent studies largely failed to confirm a relationship between abnormal liver biochemistry and either toxicity or pharmacokinetics [3] and there is concern that some patients may be exposed to an increased risk of toxicity while others receive suboptimal therapy. Accordingly, different anthracycline dosing strategies have been adopted [4–6].

5.1.1 Renal and hepatic impairment

There is increasing awareness that renal or hepatic impairment can significantly affect the pharmacokinetics and safety of anticancer drugs. Thus regulatory authorities and clinicians are paying increasing attention to this issue in drug development. Guidelines for industry have been developed by government authorities and the NCI Organ Dysfunction Group has made specific recommendations for oncology trials.

Many drugs are eliminated by the kidneys, so the potential for renal impairment to influence both the pharmacokinetics and tolerability of anti-cancer drugs is clear. Renal function may be directly affected in patients with cancer, for example where there is ureteric obstruction. More often, renal function deteriorates as the result of ageing. In other cases renal impairment is caused by nephrotoxic chemotherapy, e.g. cisplatinum, or concomitant medication, e.g. non-steroidal anti-inflammatories. Renal impairment, especially when severe, can also affect safety and efficacy indirectly through changes in absorption, metabolism, and protein binding.

The liver also has important effects on drug disposition so patients with hepatic impairment constitute another important special population. In contrast to renal dysfunction, the most common cause of hepatic dysfunction is metastatic disease in the liver. Not only are liver metastases common in several of the common adult cancers, but these patients also have a relatively poor prognosis. The presence of liver metastases is the single most important prognostic factor for patients with breast cancer [7], and prognosis worsens progressively with increasingly abnormal liver biochemistry tests [8]. Other causes of hepatic dysfunction include excessive alcohol consumption, hepatitis B or C infection and other less common primary liver diseases. Liver function may be preserved even in the presence of extensive disease due to its considerable metabolic reserve and, in the case of established cirrhosis, the regeneration of hepatocytes. Mechanisms that may contribute to altered pharmacokinetics and pharmacodynamics in patients with hepatic dysfunction include impaired hepatocellular function, reduced biliary elimination, and decreased protein binding.

Specific studies may be needed in patients with renal or hepatic impairment because they are excluded from most early trials. The definition of 'acceptable' renal and hepatic tests varies. Standard phase I trial eligibility criteria for renal function typically specify a serum creatinine $<1.5\times$ upper limit of normal (ULN) or creatinine clearance >60 ml/min. Acceptable liver tests are typically serum bilirubin normal or $\leq1.5\times$ ULN, aspartate aminotransferase/alanine aminotransferase $\leq5\times$ ULN in the presence of liver metastases or $\leq2.5\times$ ULN in their absence. The basis for greater flexibility in patients who do not have liver metastases is unclear, but may be rationalized by the poor prognosis and limited capacity for hepatocyte in patients with metastatic disease.

Guidance has been published by the US Food and Drug Administration (FDA) for the conduct of studies in patients with renal [9] or hepatic [10] impairment. Corresponding guidelines are available from the European Medicines Agency (EMEA) for renal [11] and hepatic impairment [12]. In each case these recommendations are generic, and not specific to cancer therapy. They also approach such studies as being primarily pharmacokinetic in nature rather than tolerability studies. These guidances recognize that the greater uncertainties surrounding the assessment of hepatic function relative to renal function make it more difficult to offer definitive dose recommendations for patients with hepatic impairment.

The NCI Organ Dysfunction Group provides specific instructions for oncology trials and a valuable template protocol for renal impairment studies [13].

When are organ impairment studies needed? The first decision to be made is whether an organ impairment study is necessary. FDA guidelines on the circumstances under which a renal or hepatic impairment study may be needed are summarized in Table 5.1(a) and Table 5.1(b), respectively. Such studies are not obligatory in all circumstances, provided a justification is provided to the regulatory authorities. Specifically, they are unlikely to be important where the organ concerned plays little or no part in drug elimination, especially where the therapeutic index is wide, and if the drug will not be used in patients with renal or hepatic impairment.

If an organ impairment study is required, at what stage in development should it be carried out? The EMEA emphasizes the desirability of addressing

Table 5.1 (a) When renal impairment studies may be important, and (b) When hepatic impairment studies may be important

---

(a)

The drug is likely to be used in patients with renal impairment

Renal impairment is likely to significantly alter the pharmacokinetics of a drug and/or its active/toxic metabolites

A dose adjustment is likely to be necessary for safe and effective use in such patients

The drug and/or its metabolites have a narrow therapeutic index

Excretion and/or metabolism are primarily renal

A drug has both high hepatic clearance and significant protein binding

(b)

The drug is likely to be used in patients with hepatic impairment

Hepatic metabolism and/or excretion accounts substantially (>20%) to the metabolism and/or elimination of a drug and/or its active/toxic metabolites

Hepatic elimination and/or its active/toxic metabolites accounts for <20%, but there is a narrow therapeutic index

If the route of metabolism is unknown and it cannot be shown that hepatic elimination is minor

---

organ impairment prior to opening phase III studies to avoid unnecessary restrictions to eligibility criteria in those studies. By contrast, the FDA recommendations imply that renal impairment studies will be carried out after standard phase III trials have demonstrated the safety and efficacy of a drug in patients with relatively normal renal function. Indeed, in some cases the realization that organ impairment is an issue comes through a standard phase III trial. Nevertheless, where renal impairment is identified as a probable issue earlier in the development of a drug, there is a strong case for doing the study sooner so that dose recommendations can be made for these patients as part of the initial approval process.

Design of organ impairment studies General study designs have been proposed by the FDA and EMEA (Table 5.2); the NCI Organ Dysfunction Group propose modifications specifically for oncology trials.

Aims The primary aim of a renal dysfunction study, stated by both the EMEA and FDA, is to determine whether the pharmacokinetics of a drug, and/ or its active metabolites, are altered to such an extent as to require a different dose to that established in a standard trial population. The definition of a 'clinically significant' alteration in kinetics will depend, among other factors, on the therapeutic index of a compound and the between subject variability in pharmacokinetics in a standard population.

Table 5.2 Food and Drug Administration (USA)/European Medicines Agency definitions of organ impairment studies

Type of study	
Full	Definitive study
	Full range of organ impairment
	Equal numbers in each impairment group
	May include a normal 'control' group
Reduced/staged	If anticipated that organ impairment is not clinically relevant
	Two groups studied initially (normal and impaired)
	If initial study shows *no* effect of impairment, close study
	If initial study *does* show an effect of impairment, evaluate intermediate impairment groups
Population pharmacokinetics	Based on previously conducted phase II/III trials
	Should include patients with relevant degrees of organ impairment
	Need to adjust for imbalances between patients with and without organ impairment
Dialysis	Relevant only for renal function; unlikely to be important for most anticancer drugs

The aims of a study in patients with hepatic impairment are similar, but the complexities of how liver dysfunction affects drug metabolism and the difficulty of measuring hepatic function in a meaningful way may limit the robustness of recommendations. Indeed, while encouraging such studies, the EMEA acknowledges they may serve primarily to identify patients at risk and to stimulate further research.

The NCI Organ Dysfunction Group interpret these general aims in the context of conventional phase I trial design. Their primary aims are (a) to establish the MTD and DLTs, and (b) to characterize the pharmacokinetics and pharmacodynamics, of the study agent in patients with varying degrees of organ dysfunction.

Classification of renal dysfunction Renal dysfunction is classified according to glomerular filtration rate (GFR). This can be measured directly by widely available tests, e.g. ^{51}Cr-EDTA, or ^{99}mTc- DTPA, but inulin clearance and ^{125}I-iothalamate clearance, which are arguably the best measures of renal function, are also available. A simple alternative is to estimate creatinine clearance using a formula such as those of Cockcroft and Gault [14], Jelliffe [15], or Wright et al. [16].

These formulae are less accurate than direct measurement of GFR, probably underestimating GFR by 20–30%. Specifically, the Cockcroft–Gault formula has not been validated in those with very severe renal impairment, children, or patients older than 85 years [17]. The NCI Organ Dysfunction Group emphasizes the need for accurate estimation of creatinine clearance and that it be stable, recommending creatinine clearance be calculated from at least two separate 24-hour urine collections.

Definitions of renal dysfunction are shown in Table 5.3. The NCI Group recommends body surface area (BSA)-adjustment of creatinine clearance to

Table 5.3 Measures of renal impairment

Group	Description	Estimated creatinine clearance—FDA/EMEA (ml/min/1.73m^2)	Estimated creatinine clearance—NCI (ml/min/1.73m^2/BSA)
1	Normal renal function	>80 ml/min	≥60 ml/min
2	Mild renal impairment	50–80 ml/min	40–59 ml/min
3	Moderate renal impairment	30–50 ml/min	20–39 ml/min
4	Severe renal impairment	<30 ml/min	<20 ml/min
5	Requiring dialysis	End-stage renal disease	Any

FDA/EMEA, Food and Drug Administration (USA)/European Medicines Agency; NCI, national Cancer Institute; BSA, body surface area.

increase the accuracy of estimation and because many anticancer drugs are dose according to BSA:

BSA-indexed Cr Cl = creatinine clearance (ml/min) × (1.73/actual BSA)

Classification of hepatic dysfunction This is more difficult. Several systems are used to classify liver dysfunction, but none has been adequately validated as a marker of clinically relevant changes in drug metabolism.

The Child–Pugh classification (Tables 5.4 and 5.5) is the most widely used measure of hepatic function, although it was developed as a prognostic marker in patients undergoing transection of hepatic varices rather than predicting drug elimination [18]. It is based on clinical (encephalopathy and ascites), and biochemical (bilirubin, albumin, and prothrombin time) signs of liver failure. The Child–Pugh classification has several practical limitations in patients with cancer. A subject with no clinical or biochemical signs of liver disease scores 5 and is in the 'mild' liver impairment category; conversely the score may be affected by extrahepatic disease, e.g. peritoneal or cerebral metastases. There will also be few circumstances in which a patient with cancer who has severe liver dysfunction by the Child–Pugh classification should be treated either in standard practice or a liver impairment trial as this would usually reflect the patient being very near to the end of their life. Finally, the Child–Pugh classification does not link to conventional eligibility criteria for cancer trials based on liver biochemistry tests. As a result, the group of patients who have no signs of hepatic failure but have liver biochemistry tests outside the usual

Table 5.4 Scoring system for the Child–Pugh classification

Assessment	Degree of abnormality	Score
Encephalopathy	None	1
	Moderate	2
	Severe	3
Ascites	Absent	1
	Slight	2
	Severe	3
Bilirubin (mg/dl)	<2	1
	2.1–3.5	2
	>3.5	3
Albumin (g/dl)	>3.5	1
	2.8–3.5	2
	>3.5	3
Prothrombin time (seconds > control)	0–3.9	1
	4–6	2
	>6	3

Table 5.5 Child–Pugh categories of liver dysfunction

Group	Description	Child–Pugh score
A	Mild liver dysfunction	5–6
B	Moderate liver dysfunction	7–9
C	Severe liver dysfunction	10–15

limits, which constitutes the group most relevant for hepatic impairment studies, are not identified by the Child–Pugh scheme.

Other, more sophisticated and direct measures of liver function do exist. Where the metabolism of a drug is understood in detail it may be possible to co-administer a specific probe, for example, if the drug is a CYP 3A4 substrate. Other exogenous markers of liver function have also been proposed but all have limitations [19]. Indocyanine green clearance is only weakly correlated with doxorubicin clearance [20] and the metabolism of lignocaine to monoethylglyci-nexylidide by the cytochrome (CYP) P450 system did not correlate with epirubi-cin clearance [21]. Antipyrine, and galactose clearance have also been used, but bromosulphthalein clearance has been largely abandoned due to toxicity.

Approaches based on standard liver biochemistry tests as suggested by the NCI Organ Dysfunction Working Group have been evaluated in hepatic impairment cancer trials (Table 5.6). They have the advantage of being simpler, more clinically relevant and also linking directly to other trials where they are standard eligibility criteria [22–24]. Compared with the Child–Pugh classification, this classification of four groups based on serum bilirubin and aspartate aminotransferase levels gave a more even distribution of patients across the dysfunction categories [24]. Specifically, fewer than half the patients in the Child–Pugh Group A were classified as having normal hepatic function and more than half had mild or moderated impairment using the biochemical classification.

Table 5.6 Biochemical classification of liver dysfunction

Group	Description	Liver biochemistry tests (NCI Organ Dysfunction Group)
1	Normal liver function	Bilirubin ≤ ULN AST ≤ ULN
2	Mild liver dysfunction	Bilirubin 1–1.5 × ULN or AST > ULN
3	Moderate liver dysfunction	Bilirubin 1.5–3 × ULN Any AST
4	Severe liver dysfunction	Bilirubin 3–10 × ULN Any AST

Despite recognizing the limitations of the Child–Pugh classification, the regulatory authorities propose its use, albeit in conjunction with other more appropriate markers of liver dysfunction. In practice, this may entail using a biochemical classification to categorize patients with cancer while recording their Child–Pugh score.

Types of study The various types of organ dysfunction study are shown in Table 5.2. A 'full' study as defined by the FDA and EMEA, and the design proposed by the NCI Organ Dysfunction Group, all specify treatment of patients with a full range of organ impairment. Although the regulatory authorities permit use of a well defined historical 'control' group with normal organ function, a control group within the trial is preferred. As far as possible, the control subjects should match the patients with organ impairment rather than be healthy volunteers. In practice, recruitment of cancer patients into the control group is likely to be considerably easier than into the impaired function groups. At the other extreme, in a renal impairment study patients on dialysis would often be excluded as the study population should be one in which the drug is likely to be used.

For renal impairment studies, the reduced/staged design is suggested where there is good reason to believe that organ impairment does not affect pharmacokinetics sufficiently to warrant dose modifications. Because of the difficulties in assessing liver function, the FDA suggests that a study comparing 'control' patients with those in the moderate Child–Pugh category would generally be appropriate. This is, however, unsuited to cytotoxics where treating only 'control' patients and those with poor renal or hepatic function runs the risk of severe toxicity. It may, however, be appropriate for targeted, biological therapies.

Population pharmacokinetic studies from phase II and III trials can be used to evaluate the impact of organ function. Such an analysis is, however, only helpful in so far as the study population included sufficient patients with a wide range of renal or hepatic impairment, and the accepted measures of organ function have been recorded. Because patients with significant organ impairment are usually excluded from such trials, population pharmacokinetics or analysis of standard trial may highlight the need to carry out a specific renal or liver impairment study but will not be a substitute for such a study.

Study design Most renal and hepatic impairment studies in oncology will be adapted from the 'full' design. The NCI Organ Dysfunction Group provides a specific protocol template, but other trial designs are possible within the regulatory guidelines.

In practice, these studies are a challenge in oncology because of the difficulties identifying patients with renal or hepatic impairment, who are sufficiently fit to enter the study but for whom more other appropriate treatment is not available. One consequence of this is that organ impairment trials will usually need to be carried out in several centres or by a co-operative group with expertise in early clinical trials.

Treatment plan Patients will be stratified according to their degree of renal or hepatic impairment as described above. Other eligibility criteria are similar to those of other early clinical trials in oncology.

The mode of drug administration will depend on the agent being evaluated, and usually mirror the planned use of the drug. Cytotoxic or targeted agents normally given orally over a prolonged period of time may also be studied after a single dose, provided kinetics are known to be linear and time-independent; this will generate pharmacokinetic but not tolerability data. In most cases a multiple-dose study is preferred where this is the schedule under clinical development.

There are differing approaches to the starting dose and dose escalation. The NCI Organ Dysfunction Group envisage a comprehensive approach, with parallel dose escalation schemes across a range of cohorts each with differing renal function. This implies up to four or five parallel phase I liver and renal impairment trials, respectively, each with several dose levels. This may prove very time-consuming and expensive as accrual to these trials can be difficult.

In practice, the RD in patients with normal renal or hepatic function (RD_{normal}) will usually be known from standard phase I and II trials when an organ impairment study is designed. Another approach is, therefore, to escalate the degree of renal impairment in patients being treated in a sequential manner. This can be done by treating an initial group with normal renal or hepatic function at the RD_{normal}, then treating a cohort with mild impairment at the same dose. If RD_{normal} is tolerated by patients with mild organ impairment, a cohort with moderate impairment is then treated at the same dose. On the other hand, if RD_{normal} is not tolerated, the dose would be de-escalated to predetermined dose levels in a separate cohort of patients with mild renal dysfunction until a tolerable dose was identified. Having established a reduced but tolerable dose (RD_{-x}), a cohort of patients with moderate renal dysfunction would be evaluated and the process repeated, starting at the reduced dose found tolerable in those with mild dysfunction.

Irrespective of the study dose escalation scheme, dose-limiting toxicity (DLT) will be defined in the usual way and evaluated specifically over the first cycle of treatment. Although baseline elevation in renal biochemistry tests do not constitute DLTs, changes in renal function with a temporal relation to administration of the study drug would be considered as DLTs. The usual phase I cohort size of '3 + 3' can be applied to organ impairment studies.

The NCI group propose a more flexible, sophisticated model in which once initial estimates of tolerability and pharmacokinetics have been made in a cohort of three to six patients, an expanded cohort of 12–15 patients should be treated to confirm these findings in each renal impairment group. MTD and RD within each renal impairment group are defined according to standard phase I practice.

Pharmacokinetics and pharmacodynamics Detailed pharmacokinetic evaluations of the parent drug and/or its active metabolites, are fundamental to these studies. Hence, organ impairment studies can only be carried out at centres with the staff and resources to take, process, and store blood (and in some cases urine) samples reliably.

Mathematical models may be constructed relating renal function, usually creatinine clearance, to the relevant pharmacokinetic or clinical parameters. The pharmacokinetic parameters of interest are usually clearance of the drug and/or active metabolites, dose-normalized area under the concentration–time curve (AUC) or dose-normalized peak concentration; renal clearance can be calculated from urinary excretion data. Where appropriate, for example where protein binding is high, free drug concentrations may be measured. The model aims to predict pharmacokinetics from renal function as a quantitative basis for rational dose recommendations.

In the regulatory context, if a sponsor is to claim that dose adjustment for renal impairment is not required on the basis that pharmacokinetics are not altered this requires a statistical rationale. The FDA describes one approach by which 'no effect' boundaries for the ratio of key pharmacokinetic measurements from patients with impaired and normal renal function, respectively. The 'no effect' boundaries should be defined prior to the study, based on information from previous studies on within- and between-patient pharmacokinetic variability and pharmacokinetic/pharmacodynamic relationships. If, for example, the 90% confidence interval for the ratio of defined pharmacokinetic measurements fell within these boundaries it could be claimed that there was 'no effect' of renal impairment on pharmacokinetics and no pharmacokinetic basis for dose modification. An alternative approach also described would be to assume a priori 'no effect' boundaries of 70–143% for C_{max} or 80–125% for AUC without further justification, accepting that this may reflect the limitations of small sample size in renal impairment studies and wide between-patient variability may preclude meeting these boundaries.

Relating pharmacokinetics to impaired hepatic function has generally proved more difficult, but such relationships should be investigated. Where there is an obvious, twofold or greater increase in drug exposure, the FDA recommends dose reductions. Similar considerations apply in concluding there is 'no effect' for hepatic dysfunction as for renal impairment.

Pharmacodynamic parameters in a phase I trial may be direct measures drug–target interactions or, more often, standard toxicity assessments. These pharmacodynamic effects may be more important than altered pharmacokinetics, especially in patients with liver impairment. In an organ dysfunction trial DLTs will be assessed as usual, defining a dose level as tolerable or otherwise in each cohort for each renal or hepatic impairment category. The importance of clinical toxicities in this context is emphasized by the NCI Organ Dysfunction guideline where establishing the MTD and DLTs in patients with varying degrees of organ dysfunction is the key aim.

Examples of organ impairment studies in oncology To date there have been relatively few organ impairment studies in oncology and many of those that have been performed do not follow the current guidelines. In part, this is because many important cytotoxics, such as carboplatin and the anthracyclines, were developed and in clinical use before these guidelines were defined. Secondly, the difficulty of such studies in oncology may make the strict implementation of the guidelines impractical. Finally, clinical drug development continues long after regulatory approval, and dosing strategies may be pursued by clinicians not directed towards regulatory submission.

The best example of dosing according to renal function is carboplatin, but this emerged only after it had entered routine use in the clinic. Drug exposure, as reflected by the AUC, predicts carboplatin toxicity more accurately than dose in mg/m^2. The kidneys are the major route of elimination for carboplatin, and its renal clearance is very similar to the GFR. A formula was proposed, validated and subsequently adopted basing carboplatin dose on a target AUC and GFR that replaced BSA dosing in everyday practice [25]. Some examples are shown in Table 5.7 [26–32].

Much effort has been directed towards anthracycline dosing in patients with liver dysfunction. Results of initial studies were conflicting, but following more systematic evaluation dose modifications for epirubicin have been proposed based on serum aspartate aminotransferase [6] or weekly administration [4]. The need for docetaxel dose modification in patients with liver dysfunction became apparent from a population pharmacokinetic analysis, leading to dose recommendations based on liver biochemistry tests [33]. Other examples are shown in Table 5.8 [30,34–36].

Conclusions There are particular challenges doing organ dysfunction trials, but they are important in bridging the gap between the standard clinical trial population and the patients treated routinely in the clinic. FDA and

Table 5.7 Selected renal dysfunction studies

Drug	Study design	Outcome	Reference
Raltitrexed	Cr Cl 'normal' or <65 ml/min All received standard dosing	Strong correlation between drug clearance and Cr Cl Increased toxicity in patients with renal impairment 50% dose reduction recommended	Judson et al. (1998) [26]
Oxaliplatin	Multiple categories of renal impairment and range of doses	Renal impairment increased platinum exposure	Takimoto et al. (2003) [27]
	Normal or Cr Cl <60 ml/min	No relationship between renal impairment and acute treatment toxicities	Massari et al (2000) [28]
Topotecan	Patients grouped by degree of renal impairment	Topotecan clearance reduced Increased clinical toxicities Reduced starting dose for patients with 'moderate' impairment	O'Reilly (1996) [29]
Gemcitabine	Creatinine 1.6–5.0 mg/dl Multiple dose levels studied	Increased toxicity even at reduced doses No specific dose recommendations	Venook et al. (2000) [30]
Gemcitabine	Doses 500–1000 mg/m^2 Four renal impairment levels based on EDTA-Cr Cl	No reduction in drug clearance No increase in toxicity	Delaloge et al. (2004) [31]
Capecitabine	Normal, mild (50–80 ml/min), moderate (30–50 ml/min) or severe (<30 ml/min) renal impairment 1 cycle at standard dose	Increased exposure to specific metabolites Increased toxicity in moderate/severe renal impairment Dose recommendations approved	Poole et al. (2002) [32]

Cr Cl, creatinine clearance.

EMEA guidelines suggest when and how such studies should be done. Systematic organ impairment studies, combining pharmacokinetic and clinical evaluation, will usually be carried out between several trial sites. Once dose recommendations have been made for patients with renal or hepatic impairment they should be prospectively validated.

Table 5.8 Selected liver dysfunction studies

Drug	Study design	Outcome	Reference
Paclitaxel	3 categories, defined by increased AST +/or bilirubin 3- and 24-h infusions used	Small patient numbers Confounded by different infusion schedules General recommendation that doses be reduced	Venook et al. (1998) [34]
Gemcitabine	Classified ◆ AST ≤2 × normal and bilirubin <1.6 mg/dl ◆ bilirubin 1.6–7.0 mg/dl	Tolerated by patients with raised AST Increased risk of toxicity and increase in AST in patients with raised bilirubin	Venook et al. (2000) [30]
Oxaliplatin	Dose escalated in 5 groups defined by degree of liver impairment Different starting doses for the 5 groups	Full oxaliplatin dose of 130 mg/m² tolerated by all categories of liver impairment	Doroshow et al. (2003) [35]
Capecitabine	Classification by increases in liver biochemistry tests Standard dose administered to all groups	No clinically significant changes in kinetics in patients with mild/moderate impairment	Twelves et al. (1999) [36]

5.2 Age and early clinical trials

The average age of patients entering phase I studies is usually about 60 years. In part this reflects the fact that cancer is largely a disease of older adults, and a similar age distribution is seen in phase II and III trials. Patients under the age of 18 are usually excluded from cancer trials, this is perhaps due more to potential legal issues in gaining consent for complex trials from minors than because of speculation that dosing requirements may differ in young adults. The issues are different in younger children, especially those less than 1 year old. There is a particular need for early clinical trials in children if advances in treating childhood cancers are to be furthered [37]. Concern about the under-representation of older patients is again not restricted to phase I trials. It is, however, of particular concern in oncology because the median age of patients treated in clinical practice is substantially higher than that of those in whom dosing, tolerability, and efficacy have been established. There will, therefore, often be a need for separate dose-finding studies in both the paediatric and geriatric populations.

5.2.1 Paediatric patients

Background Cancer in children differs in many ways from the disease in adults. The incidence of paediatric cancer is relatively low, with just 1 in 600 children diagnosed with cancer before their 15th birthday. Over the last 40 years improvements in survival have been more marked in children than adults. Nevertheless, cancer remains a major cause of death in children, with a disproportionately large number of years of life lost through children dying from cancer. On the other hand, with the majority of children with cancer now being cured, long-term treatment-related morbidity poses particular problems.

In contrast to adult cancer, and in particular the geriatric population, entry to clinical trials through co-operative groups is standard practice in paediatric oncology. Cancer drug development does, however, present specific practical and ethical challenges in children. In addition, paediatric tumours are quite distinct histologically and in terms of their molecular biology. Although traditional screening programmes have identified drugs with activity against cancers in children, the NCI 60-cell panel does not include paediatric cancers. Xenograft models and transgenic models of paediatric malignancies are now being developed [38].

New anticancer drugs are invariably developed first in adults, but children are not simply small adults. They differ in terms of their physiology, and the sensitivity of target organs. Moreover, children differ from each other depending on their stage of development; the physiology of a neonate is quite different from that of an adolescent. For example, the ratio of BSA to weight is substantially higher in young children than in adults. Use of BSA adjustment may have contributed to infants treated with vincristine, asparaginase, and prednisone experiencing a high frequency of neurotoxicity [39]. Drug metabolism may be impaired in neonates; for example, clearance of doxorubicin is reduced in children under the age of 2 years [40]. Likewise, renal function is markedly reduced in neonates. In later childhood drug metabolism may be more rapid than in adults, necessitating higher doses per unit of BSA or weight to achieve the same pharmacokinetic exposure or pharmacodynamic effects. Other physiological differences include total body water being higher and drug binding by plasma proteins lower, in neonates; gastric pH and motility also change with age and may alter drug exposure following oral administration.

The importance of conducting specific paediatric phase I trials is illustrated by comparing the MTD of anticancer drugs in children and adults. Traditionally, children appeared to tolerate higher doses of cytotoxics, with MTDs exceeding those in adults by 10–200% [41]. More recently, phase I trials in children have identified MTDs equivalent to or lower than in adults. This may reflect, at least in part, children now being more heavily pretreated before entering phase I trials. While DLTs are generally the same in children and adults, there are exceptions; myelosuppression was dose-limiting for dexrazoxane in adults, whereas hepatotoxicity was the DLT in children.

Guidance has been published for the conduct of studies in children by the FDA [42] and the EMEA [43]; these recommendations are generic and not specific to cancer therapy. The FDA has also issued specific guidance for industry in relation to paediatric oncology studies [44].

Ethics of phase I trials in children Definitions of childhood vary, and paediatric studies may include patients up to the age of 21, although more often the upper age limit is 18 years. Early clinical trials in children raise specific ethical issues, but it is in the younger patients that these concerns are greatest. Children are unable themselves to give informed consent, but the Declaration of Helsinki and its revisions enable research in children by permitting their participation if parents or legal guardians give formal consent in line with national legislation. The FDA and EMEA both stipulate that written informed consent should, however, be obtained from the child. It is important that, wherever possible, language is used that the child can understand, and that are aware of their right to decline participation in the trial and their right to withdraw.

For parents, giving informed consent on behalf of a vulnerable child with advanced cancer, for whom there is usually no further effective treatment, to enter a dose-finding study of a compound with potentially serious or fatal toxicities raises many issues [45,46]. Paediatricians perceive potential clinical benefit, altruism, and maintenance of hope as key factors influencing parents' decision that their child enter a phase I trial [47]. Ethical difficulties, relating to consent and risks of toxicity in particular, were perceived by a higher proportion of UK- than US-based paediatricians (83% and 48%, respectively).

Although response rates in paediatric phase I trials are low, such studies are generally safe. A review of paediatric phase I studies described 56 single agent trials in 1606 children, published between 1978 and 1996 [48]. The overall response rate was 7.9%, but varied between tumour types being highest in neuroblastoma or acute myelogenous leukaemia and lowest in osteosarcoma and rhabdomyosarcoma. Although 7% of patients died on study, only 0.7%

died from drug toxicity compared with 5.6% from progressive disease. On-study mortality rates were constant over the period studied, but response rates appeared higher in the period 1990–96 than 1978–1989 (10.3% and 5.8%, respectively).

The EMEA states explicitly that, to minimize the risk of distress to the child, trials should be designed and performed only by those experienced in the treatment of children.

When in the development of a new drug should paediatric studies be done? A general principle is established by the EMEA that, in order to minimize risk to children, safety studies should be carried out first in animals as part of routine preclinical development, then adults and only then in children. However, if a compound is being developed initially for the treatment of a childhood-specific illness, paediatric development may start ahead of any exposure in adults (Table 5.9).

Design of paediatric phase I studies The term 'children' covers a wide range of ages, with differing maturity and physiology. Not all children of a given age have the same degree of maturity, but a definition of age groups has been proposed by the EMEA (Table 5.10).

There are many similarities with adult phase I trials. The key aims of a paediatric phase I study are to: (a) define the recommended phase II dose; (b)

Table 5.9 Timing and aims of paediatric studies

Indication	Timing of paediatric studies	Aims
Disease exclusively affecting children	Trials in children can start before any adult human exposure	To demonstrate efficacy and show the safety profile
Disease affects children mainly, with particular severity or a different natural history	Trials in children needed early, following demonstration of safety and reasonable (phase I/II) efficacy in adults	To demonstrate efficacy and show the safety profile
Disease occurs in adults and children for which currently no treatment	Trials in children needed early, following demonstration of safety and reasonable (phase I/II) efficacy in adults	To demonstrate a safe and effective dosage schedule; to detect unforeseen or unique effects in childhood
Disease occurs in adults and children for which there currently is treatment	Trials in children usually follow completion of adult phase III trials	To demonstrate comparable safety, efficacy, or convenience in children relative to existing treatment; to determine a safe, effective dosage schedule; to detect unforeseen or unique effects in childhood

Table 5.10 Food and Drug Administration (USA)/European Medicines Agency classification of age groups

Age	Special features
Preterm (<36 weeks gestation) and term newborn (0–27 days)	Not generally applicable to paediatric oncology
Infants and toddlers (age 28 days to 23 months)	Rapid CNS maturation and development of immune system Drug metabolism cannot be extrapolated directly from body weight Rapid growth and wide variations in development within the group Evaluation of toxicity and efficacy difficult
Children (age 2–11 years)	Important milestones of psychomotor development Significant pharmacokinetic differences; metabolism per unit weight differs from adults Less rapid growth, but wide between-patient variations in development Flexible approach to evaluation of toxicity and efficacy
Adolescents (age 12–17 years)	Period of sexual development and rapid growth; variations in physique, psychosocial and sexual development Differences between the sexes Non-compliance a potential problem Assessment of toxicity and efficacy as in adult trials

define toxicities and specifically DLTs; (c) study pharmacokinetics and pharmacodynamic correlates; and (d) observe any preliminary evidence of antitumour activity.

At their broadest, eligible patients will be aged less than 18 or 21 years, but specific younger age groups are often defined. As for adult patients, children will have histologically/cytologically proven malignancy that is refractory to standard therapies or for which there is no curative treatment. They should have recovered from prior therapies, have adequate organ function and performance status with a life expectancy of at least 6–8 weeks. Informed consent, where necessary from the parent or guardian, is a prerequisite. Patients are usually treated in cohorts of three to six children, and toxicity recorded in the usual way, with DLTs, MTD, and RD defined as in adult studies.

Specific features of paediatric studies There are, however, significant differences between adult and paediatric phase I trials. For children aged 10 years or younger the Lansky scale evaluates activities appropriate for their age, such as the amount of time spent at play [49]. The Karnofsky or ECOG (Eastern Cooperative Oncology Group) performance status scales can be used for children older than 10 years. A formula has been derived to calculate GFR from serum creatinine specifically in children [50].

In most cases a drug will have been evaluated in adults and knowledge gained from those studies informs later paediatric studies. Rather than starting at one-tenth of the murine LD_{10}, the paediatric starting dose is often set at 80% of the adult MTD or RD. The use of BSA to adjust dose may be inappropriate, especially in those children less than 1 year of age or weighing less than 10 kg for whom dosing according to body weight should be considered. Rather than using a 'Fibonacci' scheme, dose escalation in paediatric phase I studies is typically by 20–30% increments. Pharmacologically guided dose escalation has been used to a limited degree [51], but within-patient dose escalation is not usually permitted. Studies usually require no more than five dose levels [52] and these modifications should increase the proportion of children treated at higher, and potentially therapeutic, dose levels.

Pharmacokinetic studies are important because of the potential differences in drug distribution and exposure at different stages of development. The volume of blood that can safely be sampled is limited in small children, but with high sensitivity of modern assay methodologies using samples as small as 20–100 µl, this should not preclude detailed characterization of pharmacokinetics. Interestingly, the FDA included cytotoxics among the 'hit and run' agents where they stated serum assays to be of 'little or no value'. They concluded that requirements for assay methodology may be relaxed or waived in favour of measuring biological effect. Given the difficulties of measuring biological activity in a meaningful way, most clinicians would consider pharmacokinetic studies an integral part of paediatric phase I trials. The EMEA recognizes that where a broad paediatric study has been completed there may not be sufficient patients in each age group to define differences in tolerability or efficacy. Under those circumstances pharmacokinetic data may be important in identifying differences between the age groups.

5.2.2 Elderly patients

Background Several studies have shown that older patients are underrepresented in clinical trials. A large analysis of Southwest Oncology Group trials over a 10-year period showed that, although about 65% of patients with cancer are aged over 65, that age group constituted only 25% of trial entry overall [53]. Expressed another way, trial participants aged 30–64 years of age represented 3.0% of the incident patients in that group, compared with 1.3% for those aged 65–75 years, and 0.5% for patients of 75 and over [54]. This underrepresentation is likely to be more, rather less, marked in early phase trials.

There are several possible reasons why older patients are less likely to enter trials [55]. In some countries, lack of reimbursement for experimental treatments can be an issue; the practicalities of additional hospital visits may also deter older, less independent patients from study entry. More generally, strict trial eligibility criteria will exclude a substantial proportion of older patients, not directly because of their age but because of organ function or co-morbidity. Concerns that older patients may tolerate chemotherapy less well may deter clinicians from approaching them about trials. Paradoxically, failure to include such patients in dose-finding studies will make the safe and effective treatment of older patients more difficult. The question of whether age does predict for increased risk of toxicity has been questioned [56]. Although toxicity may be no greater in older patients treated in phase II trials [57], by definition these patients would have to have met study entry criteria. Other studies claim that there is indeed an increased risk of toxicities in older patients (reviewed in [58]).

A plausible explanation for these apparently contradictory conclusions is that it is the variable consequences of ageing, rather than age itself, that increases the risk of toxicity. Older patients may be predisposed to toxicity through having a worse performance status [56] and coexisting medical conditions. This leads to an increased number of concomitant medications and risk of drug–drug interactions [59]. Organ function often deteriorates with increasing age. For example, GFR falls by about 1 ml/min for each year a patient is over 40 [60]. The implications of renal impairment in relation to early trials were discussed above; the standard Cockcroft–Gault formula is, however, not validated for patients over the age of 85. In these patients the Wright formula [16] appears more accurate especially in patients with renal impairment [17]. Other age-related physiological changes include: altered gastric pH, emptying and motility; changes in liver mass, perfusion and metabolic activity; lower cardiac output and reserve; reduced plasma proteins, total body water, and fat-free mass.

Increased age may also confer increased pharmacodynamic sensitivity to a drug, the kinetics of which are not altered. Docetaxel pharmacokinetics are unaltered in patients aged 65 or over, but these patients were much more likely to experience grade 4 or febrile neutropenia than younger patients [61]. Likewise, patients aged over 65 years are twice as likely to experience severe diarrhoea, although pharmacokinetics of irinotecan and SN-38 are similar to those in younger patients [62].

The frequent presence of other underlying diseases, concomitant medication, and resulting increased risk of drug interaction may all contribute towards this being a special population.

General guidelines The EMEA and FDA have published guidelines in support of studies in the geriatric population, with emphasis on phase III studies [63,64]. The general principle is that drugs should be studied in those age groups in which they will be used. In the context of oncology, this means a greater emphasis on the older population. The current guidelines define the geriatric population as patients over the age of 65. In the context of Western population demographics this is rather conservative and recruitment of patients aged 75 and above is encouraged. Phase III trials should include sufficient numbers of older patients that clinically important differences can be identified, with a minimum of 100 proposed for drugs to be used in the elderly. Inclusion of older patients within the main phase III trial, rather than separate studies in geriatric patients, is preferred as this facilitates comparison of tolerability with that in younger patients.

Many important age-related differences are due to altered drug exposure, for example those secondary to deteriorating renal function. Emphasis is, therefore, placed on comparing pharmacokinetics between the older and younger patients. A 'pharmacokinetic screening approach' is seen as a limited study measuring, for example, steady-state drug levels in geriatric and younger patients in a phase II or III trial. This approach has the advantage of assessing a broader range of age-related factors rather than age alone. 'Formal pharmacokinetic studies' may be carried out in a smaller, specific pharmacokinetic study, either as an alternative to the screening approach or to investigate more fully potential differences identified in a screening study. Organ impairment and drug–drug interactions are more likely, but not exclusive to, the elderly population. Specific pharmacokinetic studies described elsewhere are likely to be especially relevant to older patients.

Oncology dose-finding studies in the elderly Because most cytotoxic anticancer drugs have a narrow therapeutic index, but are widely used in older patients who represent the majority of patients, dosing in this population is highly relevant. The elderly are, however, a highly diverse population of patients by virtue of the differing extent to which they are be affected by age-related physiological changes, co-morbidity, and concomitant medications. The elderly are often frail, and it may be appropriate to carry out studies defined by performance status rather than chronological age [65,66].

Rather than focus specifically on trials restricted to the elderly, the emphasis should be on entering representative patient populations onto standard clinical trials in the first place. A reasonable approach is:

♦ To identify and enter increased numbers of older patients, who nevertheless satisfy the usual entry criteria, into phase I, II, and III trials.

- As the clinical and pharmacokinetic data bases, expand investigate the extent to which variability in tolerance may be explained directly by age-related physiological changes, co-morbidity, concomitant medications or age alone.
- Where risk factors such as organ dysfunction or performance status, which is often age-related, are identified within the 'standard' trial population, specific clinical/pharmacokinetic studies should be conducted as described elsewhere. These studies may include a higher proportion than usual of the elderly. Because patients entering organ impairment studies would generally be excluded from standard trials, this increases the likelihood that doses suitable for older patients will be defined.
- If reduced tolerance is observed in the elderly that cannot be explained, options include:
  - deriving empirical dose recommendations based on the clinical data base where that is possible;
  - conducting specific dose-finding studies in the elderly.

In practice, the main limitation is that standard eligibility criteria exclude many elderly, less fit patients from trials leading to regulatory submissions. Organ impairment and similar studies may abrogate this bias, but in practice much 'fine tuning' of treatment regimens will continue to be undertaken by academic groups. This is illustrated by experience with capecitabine in breast cancer. Bejetta *et al.* [67] carried out a study of capecitabine given initially at the standard dose of 2500 mg/m^2 orally days 1–14 of a 21-day cycle in women with breast cancer aged over 65 (median age 73). An unacceptably high incidence of toxicity led to a reduction in starting dose to 2000 mg/m^2. An unrelated renal impairment trial demonstrated the need for dose reductions in patients with creatinine clearance 30–49 ml/min [32]. When renal function was reviewed in the elderly study, all had renal impairment and half would now be recommended to receive the lower dose.

5.2.3 Summary and conclusions

It is important to evaluate the pharmacokinetics and tolerability of anticancer drugs in both paediatric and geriatric populations, especially where they have a narrow therapeutic index. Specific trials are needed in children, who cannot be considered small adults, and in whom there are particular ethical concerns. By contrast, the emphasis in older patients should be their inclusion into standard trials.

5.3 Interaction studies, including combination trials

Anticancer drugs are rarely taken in isolation, so it is important to demonstrate their tolerability and dosing in clinically relevant contexts. Most cytotoxics are taken in combination with other chemotherapy and in the past these combinations could be developed empirically. The increasing need for regulatory approval as a prerequisite for reimbursement makes formal dose-finding studies more important. Although biological or targeted therapies may have activity alone, the majority are also given in combination with established cytotoxics. Combinations of novel biological agents, and of new drugs with radiotherapy, are also becoming increasingly relevant. The ethical and practical issues surrounding the addition of a novel agent to an established drug are quite distinct from those of first-in-man, single agent phase I trials.

Food interaction and bioequivalence studies were not part of anticancer drug development in the era of intravenous cytotoxics, but are becoming routine as more oral cytotoxic and targeted drugs emerge. There is also greater awareness of the potential for interactions, not only between anticancer drugs, but also involving other medication that may alter drug metabolism. Again, this may necessitate specific trials early in the development of a new anticancer drug.

As with most early trials of new anticancer drugs, studies in healthy volunteers are often inappropriate. There will, however, be classes of drug such as non-genotoxic signal transduction inhibitors, where healthy volunteer studies are possible.

5.3.1 Food effect

Although it is possible to predict from the chemical characteristics of a new compound whether it is likely or not to be orally bioavailable, preclinical models do not accurately predict the degree of absorption. Likewise, despite a large literature on the effect of food on drug absorption, there is no way to predict its impact for a specific chemical entity. Such interactions may be clinically important as most anticancer drugs either have a low therapeutic index, in the case of cytotoxics, or are administered over a prolonged period, especially with biological agents.

The FDA issued Guidance for Industry in 2002, but these are not specific to oncology [68].

5.3.1.1 Background

There are several mechanisms by which food may affect drug absorption [69]. Food increases gastric pH, which may affect drug stability, and delays gastric emptying. Bile flow and splanchnic blood flow are also increased after food. There may also be a direct physical or chemical interaction between food and the drug.

Food is likely to have its greatest effect when a drug is taken soon after eating. The nature of the meal, in terms of its calorific and nutrient content, composition, and volume can also affect the nature and extent of any interaction. The FDA recommends high-calorie, high-fat meals, which are likely to have the greatest impact, for these studies. Similarly, the physical–chemical characteristics of a drug and its dosage form will influence the effect of food. Drugs that dissolve rapidly, are highly soluble and highly permeable, may be less prone to food effects. By contrast, there is more potential for food effects with intermediate-release or modified-release products because of the greater complexity of drug dissolution and absorption.

5.3.1.2 Types of study

There are three distinct types of food-effect study:

+ Food-effect bioavailability studies are usually carried out with novel compounds, to compare the rate and extent of absorption under fed and fasting conditions. This can guide recommendations for administration in subsequent trials but also in general clinical use. Although it may be convenient to administer a once daily oral compound after an overnight fast, if that compound subsequently needs to be given more frequently repeated fasting may not be feasible.
+ A conventional bioavailability study may facilitate the development of an oral formulation of an anticancer drug previously administered intravenously by the pharmacokinetics after intravenous and oral administration. This can establish whether there is clinically significant absorption of the oral dose form ahead of a decision to pursue a full oral development programme. It allows more rational selection of a starting dose, based on oral bioavailability and comparison with the pharmacokinetics and tolerability of the intravenous dose form, expediting the oral phase I study.
+ Finally, fed bioequivalence studies are performed to demonstrate that a new oral formulation has bioequivalence with the standard oral formulation.

For novel immediate-release and modified-release compounds, the FDA recommends that a food-effect bioavailability study be carried out early in development to inform selection of formulations for further development. Both fed and fasting bioequivalence studies are recommended for new formulations of immediate-release and modified-release compounds. An exception is made for immediate-release compounds under specific circumstances, such as the label specifying administration only on an empty stomach, where a fasted only study may suffice.

5.3.1.3 Study design

The optimal design of a food-effect study is a randomized, balanced, single-dose, two-treatment, two-period, two-sequence cross-over design. In each case there must be an appropriate interval, determined from knowledge of pharmacokinetics, for drug washout, between the two treatments:

- For a food-effect bioavailability study subjects take a single dose of drug under fed and fasted conditions, the sequence being determined randomly.
- In a conventional bioavailability study subjects receive a single dose of the drug administered both intravenously and orally, ideally with the sequence of administration randomized.
- For a fed bioequivalence study the test and reference oral dose forms are administered in randomized sequence following a test meal.

In each case samples, usually plasma, are collected for characterization of phamacokinetics, the comparison of which between the two treatment periods forms the basis for analysis.

It may be possible to incorporate bioavailability studies within a phase I trial. For example, a patient may receive a single dose of study drug with and without food on 2 successive weeks before starting regular oral dosing on the phase I trial another week later. A conventional bioavailability study can be carried if a single oral dose is administered one week, a single intravenous dose a week later and then the phase I intravenous study commenced. The disadvantages of such an approach include the possibility that toxicity may be seen during the bioavailability part of the study, complicating dose escalation; the additional complexity may impair or delay study recruitment; the additional blood sampling may raise concerns from ethics committees. Nevertheless, this approach has been used successfully to save time and expense. One compromise may be to study bioavailability only at a limited number of dose levels. Regulatory authorities will, however, expect to see food-effect bioavailability data at the doses intended to be marketed.

Subjects Eligibility criteria should specify that the patient be able to take oral medication, is not vomiting, and has not undergone surgical resection or have any other medical condition, such as malabsorption that would complicate interpretation of the study. It should, however, be remembered that where patients with upper gastrointestinal cancer may be candidates for inclusion later in development it may be important to know whether absorption of the drug is affected by gastrectomy or pancreatectomy.

The size of the study will depend on the anticipated magnitude of any interaction, but is generally anticipated to be a minimum of 12 subjects.

Test meal The FDA recommends that food-effect studies be conducted with meals that maximize the anticipated effects on gastrointestinal physiology, and hence on drug exposure, rather than reflect the average breakfast. The recommended meal is high in fat (which contributes approximately 50% of total calorie content), and calories (800–1000 calories). This corresponds to two eggs fried butter, two strips of bacon, two slices of toast with butter, four ounces (120 g) of hash brown potatoes, and 8 ounces of whole milk (almost 250 ml). Other meal compositions can be used, but a scientific rationale for any major deviation would be expected.

This meal specification has significant practical implications. First, it will usually require that the patient have breakfast at the hospital, and perhaps be admitted the night before. Secondly, close liaison with the hospital kitchen is needed to ensure that the specifications are met. Thirdly, the recommended breakfast is unlikely to represent the normal diet of a patient with advanced cancer, who may not be able to eat such a meal. One compromise is to specify a 'standard' breakfast in the protocol; this will more closely reflect reality but may not match the stated FDA preference.

For both the 'fasted' and 'fed' studies, it is recommended that the overnight fast be of at least 10 hours, with no food for at least 4 hours pre-dose or post-dose. Water is allowed, but not in the hour before or after drug administration. For the 'fed' study, subjects should start their meal 30 minutes before drug administration, complete it in 30 minutes or less, and take the study drug 30 minutes after the start of the meal. These restrictions may be inappropriate for patients with cancer; any other drugs or fluids they need to take over the study period should be recorded and the reason stated.

Pharmacokinetics Timed samples, usually plasma, are collected for characterization of phamacokinetics for the two treatment periods, i.e. with or without food (food-effect bioavailability), intravenous and oral (conventional bioavailability), or two different oral dose forms (fed bioequivalence).

Definitions for the interpretation of pharmacokinetic data are provided by the FDA, based on the ratio of the mean pharmacokinetic parameters on the two treatment periods. For example, food can be said *not* to have had an effect if the 90% confidence intervals for this ratio, under fed and fasted conditions, falls within the equivalence limits of 80–125% for AUC and C_{max}.

5.3.1.4 Examples of food-effect studies

The increasing number of oral anticancer drugs, both conventional cytotoxics and targeted biological therapies, is making food-effect studies more important. Where food does appear to impact on pharmacokinetics this may not translate into a clinically significant effect. For example, endocrine agents have a wide therapeutic index so the effect of food on exemestane kinetics is not clinically important [70]. In the case of 6-thioguanine, food reduced peak concentration and overall exposure, but did not affect red cell 6-thioguanine nucleotide levels after 4 weeks of treatment [71] so appeared not clinically important. A selection of food effect studies are shown in Table 5.11 [72–77].

5.3.2 Drug–drug interactions

Despite their narrow therapeutic index and the many concomitant medications taken by patients with cancer, surprisingly little attention has been paid

Table 5.11 Selected food-effect studies

Drug	Study design	Outcome	Reference
Vinorelbine	13 patients received standard single doses of oral vinorelbine with randomized two-way cross-over design, 2 weeks apart	Relative bioavailability increased by 22–28% after food	Rowinsky et al. (1996) [72]
Capecitabine	11 patients received capecitabine using single dose randomised two-way cross-over design, 1 week apart Kinetics of capecitabine and metabolites studied	C_{max} and AUC 1.04–2.47-fold lower when capecitabine taken after food Recommendation to take with food as in initial clinical trials	Reigner et al. (1998)[73]
UFT/leucovorin	25 patients evaluated using single dose randomized two-way cross-over design, 3 days apart	Administration with food resulted in C_{max} and AUC lower for 5-FU and uracil, but higher for leucovorin and 5-methyltetrahydrofolate Recommended that food should not be consumed 1 h before or after UFT/leucovorin	Damle et al. (2001) [74]
Topotecan	Randomized two-period, cross-over design	Food delayed time to C_{max}, but not C_{max} itself Food does not affect extent of absorption of topotecan gelatin capsules	Herben et al. (1999) [75]
Gefitinib	Healthy volunteers received single 50 mg dose, with or without food	C_{max} reduced by 34% and AUC by 14% when ingested with food No specific recommendation	Swaisland et al. (2001) [76]
Erlotinib	8 healthy volunteers randomized to receive 7 days fed or fasted then the alternate food state on day 8	Exposure (AUC and C_{max}) approximately 33% higher after high calorie, high fat meal	Rakhit et al. (2003) [77]

to drug interactions. In many cases drug interactions are not identified during the initial development of a drug but become apparent when it enters general clinical use. Recently, more attention has been paid to differences in drug metabolism, and in particular the role of the CYP P450 family of enzymes, as a source of interpatient variability in exposure. In most cases the question will be whether the metabolism of a novel anticancer drug is influenced by concomitant medications that induce or inhibit its metabolism. On occasions, however, the new agent itself may be a potential enzyme inducer or inhibitor and a study may evaluate whether it influences the metabolism of other drugs.

Drug interactions in oncology were reviewed in detail by Beijnen and Schellens [78].

5.3.2.1 Background

The CYP P450 family is involved in the metabolism of many established anticancer drugs. These enzymes are located primarily in the liver, where they are responsible for much hepatic drug clearance, but also within the gut mucosa, where they can influence drug absorption.

CYP3A4 appears to be the most important isoform and has been the most widely studied. Its activity varies by as much as 20-fold, due not only to genetic polymorphisms but also because it can be inhibited or inducted by concomitant medications. The activity of CYP P450 can be measured indirectly using the clearance of a 'probe' that is known to be metabolized by the specific isoform [79]. For example, after administering a trace dose of ^{14}C radio-labelled erythromycin the exhaled isotope reflects hepatic metabolism of erythromycin by CYP3A4. Docetaxel is metabolized by CYP P4503A, and its activity, determined by the erythromycin breath test, correlates with docetaxel clearance [80]. Another CYP3A4 probe, levels of a hydrocortisone metabolite in urine, has been used prospectively to individualize docetaxel doses and reduce pharmacokinetic variability [81].

Where drug interactions are a concern, patients taking potential inducers/ inhibitors may be specifically excluded from the phase I programme. This is understandable, but has significant drawbacks. First, the list of potential inducers and inhibitors is long and their clinical relevance unclear. Trial recruitment may, therefore be slowed unnecessarily if patents taking a long list of other medications are excluded. Secondly, this can lead to a RD being identified that has not been tested in patients taking specific concomitant medication, who would then be excluded from subsequent studies. It is important, therefore that potential interactions are explored. Arguably, this may best be done by including all patients, irrespective of concomitant medication, which could be included as a variable when evaluating toxicity, efficacy, and pharmacokinetics throughout the development process. Given the current level of concern regarding drug interactions, this inclusive approach may be unattractive, so it is important that specific drug interaction studies are carried out early in the development process to establish whether or not interactions are clinically important.

In drug development the main concern is over drug–drug interactions. In particular, many drugs can inhibit or induce CYP3A4 (see Table 5.12 for a list of commonly used agents), with the potential significantly increase or decrease exposure to an anticancer drug metabolized by CYP3A4. When studying potential interactions, an inducer and/or inhibitor of CYP3A4 may be given on separate occasions along with the study drug and the pharmacokinetics of the study drug evaluated.

5.3.2.2 Types of study

The FDA issued Guidance for Industry in 1999 [82]. This emphasizes the role of *in vitro* studies in identifying the clinical studies that should be undertaken. At a later stage in development, once a drug is in clinical use, detailed population pharmacokinetic analyses may help to characterize known

Table 5.12 Inducers and inhibitors of CYP450 isoenzyme

Inhibitors	
Amiodarone	Metronidazole
Cannabinoids	Mibefradil
Clarithromycin	Miconazole
Erythromycin	Nefazodone
Fluconazole	Nelfinavir
Fluoxitene	Norfloxacin
Fluvoxamine	Quinine
Grapefruit juice	Ritonavir
Cranberry juice	Saquinavir
Indnavir	Sertraline
Itraconazole	Trleandomycin
Ketoconazole	Zafirlukast
Omeprazole (weak)	
Inducers	
Barbituates	Phenobarbitol
Carbamazepine	Phenytoin
Cotrimoxazole	Primidone
Dexamethase	Rifabutin
Ethosuxamide	Rifampicin
Methadone	Troglitazone
Metyrapone	
Mexilitene	

interactions or to identify previously unknown interactions or genotypic variations.

Clinical studies of inhibitors/inducers of a particular CYP P450 enzyme system are not needed if that enzyme does not metabolize *in vitro* the novel anticancer drug under consideration. By contrast, where studies *in vitro* do show the anticancer drug to be metabolized by CYP P450, clinical studies with inhibitors/inducers of that particular enzyme system are required to quantify the potential importance of interactions.

Similarly, clinical studies to assess the impact of a novel anticancer on the metabolism of other drugs would be indicated only if an effect had been demonstrated *in vitro* on drug metabolizing enzymes.

Drug interaction studies can have several different designs, but all are based on studying the pharmacokinetics of the study drug in the presence and absence of an enzyme inhibitor/inducer.

- The study drug may be given to the same patient on two occasions, with and without the induce/inhibitor, the sequence either being randomized or not (randomized and one sequence cross-over designs, respectively).
- Two separate populations, one receiving study drug alone and the other the study drug and inducer/inhibitor (a parallel design) may be studied.

Such studies have similarities to the food-effect studies described above, but are likely to be more complex. First, the enzyme inducer/inhibitor must be given for a sufficiently long time, and at an adequate dose, to achieve its desired effect before assessing its effect on the pharmacokinetics of the study drug; enzyme inducers tend to take longer to exert their effect than inhibitors. Where appropriate, there needs to be an adequate washout period between two study treatments to allow clearance of the study drug and also for the effects of the inducer/inhibitor to resolve. Single doses of the study drug will often be the clinically relevant mode of administration and has practical advantages; where the therapeutic index is narrow there is a risk of toxicity unless the study drug dose is modified. Prolonged administration of an oral study drug, to achieve steady state before administration of the inhibitor/ inducer, may reflect its clinical use but is likely to result in a long and cumbersome study.

Subjects Because of their complexity, the need for extensive blood sampling and the expectation that the inhibitor/inducer will significantly alter drug exposure, drug interactions are evaluated in specific studies rather than within other early trials. The size of the study will depend on the anticipated magnitude of any interaction, but is generally anticipated to be a minimum of 12 subjects.

CYP450 inhibitors and inducers   A wide range of drugs can act as inducers or inhibitors (Table 5.11). Not all are, however, equally potent. Initial studies would usually be carried out with inducers/inhibitors that are both specific and potent. For example, with CYP3A4, ketoconazole is accepted as an appropriate enzyme inhibitor and rifampicin as an inducer. If they fail to modify metabolism of the study drug it is reasonable to conclude there is no significant interaction via CYP3A4. Should an interaction with a potent induce/inhibitor be demonstrated, it does not follow that less potent or specific inducers/inhibitors would have the same effect. Hence, specific studies with concomitant medications of particular interest (e.g. phenytoin where the study drug may be used in patients with brain tumours) may be appropriate.

Where the question being asked is whether the novel agent itself acts an enzyme inducer/inhibitor, the probe will be determined by the enzyme system in question. For example, midazolam and erythromycin are metabolized by CYP3A4 in the liver and liver/gastrointestinal. tract, respectively. Other potential probes include theophylline (for CYP1A2), S-warfarin (CYP2C9), and desipramine (CYP2D6).

Pharmacokinetics   Pharmacokinetics are characterized for the two treatment periods i.e. with and without the inducer/inhibitor. These can be expressed as the ratio of the mean pharmacokinetic parameters with 90% confidence intervals. The interpretation of any apparent differences will be influenced not only by the magnitude of that effect, but also by the pattern of toxicity, therapeutic index, and pharmacodynamic relationships of the study drug.

5.3.2.3   Examples of drug interaction studies

Most of the important CYP isoenzymes can be induced by corticosteroids and anticonvulsants. Interactions have also been reported between warfarin and several cytotoxics. Warfarin is metabolized by the CYP450 system but is also highly protein bound. Competition either for CYP metabolism on protein binding sites may explain these interactions. Other examples of drug interaction studies are shown in Table 5.13 [83–87].

5.3.3   Combination phase I trials

Most anticancer drugs are given in combination, and historically these combinations were derived effectively but empirically. However, regulatory rlequirements are increasing and there is often now a need for a drug to be approved for a specific indication in a particular combination for reimbursement. In addition, there is the hope that new, targeted, rationally designed anticancer drugs will be used with existing agents in a

Table 5.13 Selected drug interaction studies

Drugs	Study design	Outcome	Reference
Epirubicin/ cimetidine	8 patients received epirubicin $\pm$ cimetidine	Cimetidine increased AUC of doxorubicin ($P =$ NS) and doxorubicinol ($P < 0.05$) Mechanism unclear	Murray *et al.* (1998) [83]
Imatinib/ ketoconazole	14 healthy volunteers Single doses of imatinib $\pm$ single dose of ketoconazole in random sequence	Ketoconazole (CYP450 3A4 inhibitor) AUC of imatinib increased significantly	Dutreix *et al.* (2004) [84]
Trabectedin/ dexamethasone	Clinical study Supported by studies in rats	Hepatotoxicity of trabectedin reduced Effect seen only if dexamethasone given first Lower hepatic, but not plasma, trabectedin levels; mechanism unclear	Van Kesteren *et al.* (2003) [85]
Paclitaxel/ cisplatin	Paclitaxel 100 mg/m^2 and cisplatin 50–100 mg/m^2	Myelosuppression more severe with sequence cisplatin $\rightarrow$ paclitaxel Paclitaxel clearance 25% lower when given after cisplatin	Rowinsky *et al.* (1991) [86]
Doxorubicin/ paclitaxel	36 patients studied Effect of sequence, interval between administration and dose investigated	Dose dependent increase in doxorubicin concentration May be mediated by Cremophor EL vehicle	Gianni *et al.* (1997) [87]

more logical manner. These pressures and expectation have led to an increasing emphasis on specific phase I trials of two or three drug combinations, and in combination with radiotherapy. They can be categorized as (a) novel cytotoxic and established cytotoxic (or radiotherapy); (b) novel 'biological' and established cytotoxic (or radiotherapy); and (c) 'biological' and 'biological'.

There are important differences between first-in-man phase I trials and combination phase I trials and it is important to highlight these differences to all involved in the trials. The implications, in terms of stage of disease, subsequent treatment options, and prognosis may be quite different for patients entering the two types of phase I trial. Indeed, it may be unhelpful to use the term phase I trial in the context of a combination study because of its implications; the term 'dose-finding' may be more appropriate.

Combination trials are described here because an important aim of these studies is to identify potential interactions between the novel and established agents.

5.3.3.1 Background

Combination phase I studies have similarities to, but also significant differences from, the first-in-man studies described in Chapter 3; this section will concentrate on these differences. The crucial difference is that almost always the novel agent will have undergone a classical phase I trial prior to the combination studies. Hence, there is already at least some knowledge of dose, toxicity, pharmacokinetics, and antitumour activity for the new agent; the established drugs with which it is being combined will usually have completed their development and be well characterized.

The ideal combination is one that is based on the mechanisms of action of the two drugs, with preclinical evidence of synergy, activity of both drugs as single agents and an absence of overlapping toxicities. In practice, agents are often combined empirically based on clinical experience, preclinical studies and pragmatism. Study design (e.g. starting doses, schedule) is also largely based on existing clinical experience, although sequence of administration may be influenced by preclinical data.

Combinations of cytotoxics are often derived by adding a novel agent with activity against a particular tumour type to an established agent also active against that cancer. An absence of overlapping toxicities increases the attraction of a combination, but is often impractical as most cytotoxics cause myelosuppression. Ideally the choice of a combination should be supported by additive or synergistic activity in xenograft models. There is no single rationale for the combination of a targeted, biological therapy with a cytotoxic. Again, these combinations are chosen on primarily clinical grounds, with both drugs being active against the tumour type intended for further clinical development. Preclinical evidence of additive or synergistic activity is usually sought, but can be misleading. Whereas synergy with chemotherapy in xenografts was predictive of clinical activity in the treatment of breast cancer with trastuzumab, it was misleading with gefitinib and erlotinib in non-small cell lung cancer. The importance of combining targeted, biological agents is emphasized by the increasing awareness that inhibiting individual signalling pathways is unlikely to be optimal against most cancers. One approach is to target the same pathway at two different levels. Alternatively a combination may inhibit the target pathway and one with which there is cross-talk. Or the aim may be to target two separate pathways, both of which are known to drive a particular malignancy. These distinct approaches emphasize the need for clinically relevant models.

A final factor that may influence the choice of combinations by pharmaceutical companies is the desire to combine two or more of their own compounds. Often this is simply because it makes good financial sense. In other cases detailed knowledge of two novel agents may influence a development strategy, especially in the challenging situation where two unlicensed drugs are to be combined.

5.3.3.2 Aims

In common with classical phase I trials, the primary aim is to define a RD, here for a new drug in combination with established treatment. Toxicities will be monitored, in particular any unexpected adverse effects. Pharmacokinetics, which are invariably central to first-in-man studies, are not always included in combination trials. Antitumour activity is usually assessed in these studies, often in the hope of identifying a 'signal' for the efficacy of the combination.

The desire to characterize antitumour activity is, however, often misguided and can be misleading. The established element of the combination will, almost by definition, have proven antitumour activity so any responses that are seen cannot be attributed specifically to the combination. More worrying is the possibility that a perceived low level of activity may have a negative impact on the further development of a combination. A phase I trial will certainly not have sufficient patients for that conclusion to be reached. Moreover, patients will have been treated at different dose levels and may not represent a true 'phase II population'.

5.3.3.3 Patient population

Because the toxicity of each component of a combination phase I trial will have been characterized in some detail it is not a requirement that patients be those for whom there is no standard therapy. Likewise, because RDs are usually known for each element of the combination when given as single agents, the doses administered in combination are likely to have at least some antitumour activity.

In many cases the key eligibility criterion would be that the standard element of the combination 'be reasonable or appropriate' for the patient. Whereas first-in-man studies are usually open to patients with all tumour types, a combination study may recruit patients with specific tumour types, either as an explicit eligibility requirement, or implicitly through the regimen being 'reasonable or appropriate'. Where one or more component of the combination is directed at a specific target, it is reasonable to limit recruitment to patients expressing that target with the caveat that this may be misleading if the target has not been correctly identified. Likewise, as there is therapeutic potential from at least one element of the combination, it is possible to restrict the number of prior therapies that the patient has received. Indeed, if there is concern that heavily pretreated patients may be more liable to toxicity, it may be desirable that they are excluded as the starting doses for the combination may be potentially toxic as well as active. Requirements in terms of performance status, organ function will often be similar to those for first-in-man studies, unless prior clinical experience with the drug's evaluation indicates otherwise. Finally, consent remains paramount, as does the need for patients to be willing and able to meet the schedule of treatment and evaluations.

The patient populations for combination phase I are such that the referral pattern for these trials will be different from those for first-in-man studies. If only patients with advanced disease for whom there is no standard treatment is available are referred, many will not be eligible for a combination study. In practice, this means educating colleagues about the nature and eligibility criteria for combination phase I trials. Where patients with a particular tumour type form the majority of those entering a trial it is also important to work closely with the team routinely responsible for their care.

5.3.3.4 Endpoints

Toxicity is recorded in the same way as for first-in-man studies and in many cases, especially where cytotoxics are combined, remains the key endpoint. In such trials the components of a combination are escalated until the incidence of dose-limiting toxicities exceeds a defined threshold as described in Chapter 3; a lower dose is then defined as the RD for the combination.

Non-toxicity measures may also be endpoints, especially when novel, targeted agents form one or more part of the combination. The appropriate biological endpoint should have derived from preclinical studies and have been confirmed in single agent phase I trials ahead of combination studies. The appropriate endpoint, tissue, time-point for measurement, sample handling, and analytical method should be known, as should the relationship between dose (or blood levels) and the pharmacodynamic endpoint. It is then possible to pose the question 'can a novel biological agent be administered at doses that achieve the desired biological effect in combination with an established regimen?' within the phase I trial.

Pharmacokinetics are sometimes, but not always, important in phase I trials. The question will usually be whether there is an interaction between the agents being combined. It can be argued that pharmacokinetics should always be studied as this is probably the best, and may be the last, opportunity to define the kinetics of a combination before it is either developed further or abandoned; pharmacokinetic data can also be helpful if problems such as unexpectedly severe toxicity arise. It is, however, often expensive and time-consuming to evaluate fully the kinetics of all elements of a combination. Specific reasons for incorporating pharmacokinetic studies include: (a) the drugs being combined sharing, and therefore potentially competing for, the same metabolic pathway; (b) one or more drugs being a known CYP450 inducer/inhibitor; (c) where sequence of administration may alter drug exposure; or (d) a need to demonstrate that specific exposure has been achieved to confirm a pharmacodynamic endpoint.

These drug interaction pharmacokinetic studies are similar in design to those described in Section 5.2.2.2. This context pharmacokinetics can be studied at different levels:

◆ *A full study of both the novel and established agents.* This is important if a specific interaction is anticipated. It requires multiple cycles of blood sampling and that the kinetics of each drug be studied administered alone, then in combination. This places significant additional demands on patients and staff, as well as prolonging the time to complete accrual and evaluation of each cohort.

◆ *A limited study of the novel and/or established agents.* If the pharmacokinetics of one or more of the drugs under evaluation have previously been fully characterized and pharmacokinetics when given in combination are compared with historical data. This avoids the need for separate administration and sampling of the single agents and the combination, and is less demanding for all concerned.

◆ *A specific study to assess the effect of schedule.* Here patients will usually be treated and sampled on two separate occasions, representing the two sequences of administration, and comparisons made of pharmacokinetics using the two schedules.

◆ *For pharmacodynamic correlations.* The pharmacokinetics of the drug of interest will be studied in the clinically relevant context, i.e. as administered in the study.

5.3.3.5 Design

There is no single formula to determine starting doses in combination studies. Unlike first-in-man studies, starting doses for combinations are usually based on clinical experience regarding the nature of toxicity, the RD and therapeutic index and mechanism of action of the individual single agents as well as any potential drug interaction. The starting doses of each component of a regimen, expressed as a percentage of the single agent RD, may also not be the same.

Starting doses are, therefore, determined on a case-by-case basis. For example, if a novel and established cytotoxic have overlapping toxicities, the starting doses (e.g. 50% and 50% of the RD) will be more conservative than if this is not the case (e.g. 70% and 70% of the RD). If a biological agent, with a defined dose threshold for activity and wide therapeutic index is combined with a cytotoxic and there are no overlapping toxicities, the starting doses may be 100% and 70% of the RD, respectively.

Because the starting doses are usually closer to the subsequent combination RD than is the case with first-in-man studies, there are generally fewer escalation steps and dose escalations are generally modest (25–30%) in combination phase I trials. Likewise, initial single patient cohorts would not be appropriate; cohorts typically follow the pattern of three patients with an additional three if DLT is seen and expansion to 12 patients or more at the RD. Typically, only a single drug is escalated in each cohort. The dose of one drug may be held over several dose levels while the other is escalated; more often, each drug is escalated at alternate dose levels. Another consequence of combining two or more compounds is that more than one MTD and RD may be identified. For example, the starting doses for a novel and an established cytotoxic may be 50% and 50% of their single agents RDs, respectively; possible MTDs for the combination may be 100% and 70%, 60% and 100%, or 75% and 75%, respectively. Again, decisions will depend on the starting doses, pattern of toxicities and perceived importance of maximizing the dose of each element of the combination. If preclinical data indicate the possibility of an interaction between two drugs, or if the pattern of toxicities is unexpected, the alternative sequence of administration may be investigated, or an interval introduced between the administration of the two drugs.

5.3.3.6 Ethics

The ethical issues surrounding combination phase I trials follow the principles laid out in Chapter 4, but are quite different and less difficult than for first-in-man trials.

The key difference between combination and first-in-man phase I trials is that for the former there is already knowledge of the dose, toxicity, pharmacokinetics, and antitumour activity of each component. The concern in first-in-man studies that patients in early cohorts are exposed to very low doses with almost no chance of benefit but the risk of unexpected toxicity is much less of an issue for combination phase I trials. Indeed, because of their design, response rates are higher and the risk of toxicity greater, in combination phase

I trials. Because patients offered entry to combination studies will often have less advanced disease, they may be less 'vulnerable' than those in conventional phase I trials. It is, however, important that the patient information sheet for a combination phase I trial is explicit that the study treatment is not 'standard' and that the dose of the established component may not be optimal.

5.3.3.7 Summary

Combination dose-finding on phase I studies have much in common with first-in-man trials, but also many differences. These studies are becoming more important as more targeted biological agents are developed, intended for use in combination with established agents. Also, the need to seek regulatory approval for new combination cytotoxic therapies has brought such regimens into a more formal drug development structure. Examples of combination studies have not been listed as they are too numerous and too varied. A key point is to make best use of the clinical and preclinical data already available when designing these studies. Flexibility in terms of identifying the most appropriate patient population and clinical setting is also important.

References

1. Dobbs NA, Twelves CJ (1998). Anthracycline doses in patients with liver dysfunction: do UK oncologists follow current recommendations? *Br J Cancer* 77: 1145–8.
2. Benjamin RS, Wiernik PJ, Bachur NR (1973). Doxorubicin chemotherapy—efficacy, safety and pharmacologic basis of an intermittent single high-dosage schedule. *Cancer* 33: 19–27.
3. Brenner DE, Wiernik PH, Wesley M, Bachur NR (1984). Acute doxorubicin toxicity. Relationship to pre-treatment liver function, response and pharmacokinetics in patients with acute nonlymphocytic leukaemia. *Cancer* 53: 1042–8.
4. Twelves CJ, O'Reilly SM, Coleman RE, Richards MA, Rubens RD (1989). Weekly epirubicin for breast cancer with liver metastases and abnormal liver biochemistry. *Br J Cancer* 60: 938–41.
5. Twelves CJ, Richards MA, Smith P, Rubens RD (1991). Epirubicin in breast cancer patients with liver metastases and abnormal liver biochemistry: initial weekly treatment followed by rescheduling and intensification. *Ann Oncol* 2: 663–6.
6. Dobbs NA, Twelves CJ, Gregory W, Cruickshank C, Richards MA, Rubens RD (2003). Epirubicin in patients with liver dysfunction: development and evaluation of a novel dose modification scheme. *Eur J Cancer* 39: 580–6.
7. Gregory WM, Smith P, Richards MA, Twelves CJ, Knight RK, Rubens RD (1993). Chemotherapy of advanced breast cancer: outcome and prognostic factors. *Br J Cancer* 68: 988–95.

8. O'Reilly SM, Richards MA, Rubens RD (1990). Liver metastases from breast cancer: the relationship between clinical, biochemical and pathological features and survival. *Eur J Cancer* **26**: 574–7.

9. FDA Guidance for the conduct of renal impairment studies: http://www.fda.gov/cder/guidance/1449fnl.pdf [last accessed August 2005]

10. FDA Guidance for the conduct of hepatic impairment studies: http://www.fda.gov/cder/guidance/3625fnl.pdf [last accessed August 2005]

11. EMEA guidance for the conduct of renal impairment studieshttp://www.emea.eu.int/pdfs/human/ewp/14701304en.pdf [last accessed August 2005]

12. EMEA Guidance for the conduct of hepatic impairment studies: http://www.emea.eu.int/pdfs/human/ewp/063302en.pdf [last accessed August 2005]

13. NCI Organ Dysfunction Group template for renal dysfunction studies: http://www.ctep.cancer.gov/forms/Renal_dysfunction_temp2.doc [last accessed August 2005]

14. Cockcoft D, Gault M (1976). Prediction of creatinine clearance from serum creatinine. *Nephron* **16**: 31–41.

15. Jelliffe R (1973). Creatinine clearance: bedside estimate. *Ann Intern Med* **79**: 604.

16. Wright JG, Boddy AV, Highley M, Fenwick J, McGill A, Calvert AH (2001). Estimation of glomerular filtration rate in cancer patients. *Br J Cancer* **84**: 452–459.

17. Marx GM, Blake GM, Galani E, *et al.* (2004). Evaluation of the Cockroft-Gault, Jelliffe and Wright formulae in estimating renal function in elderly cancer patients. *Ann Oncol* **15**: 291–5.

18. Pugh RNH, Murray-Lyon IM, Dawson JL, Pietroni MC, Williams R (1973). Transection of the oesophagus for bleeding oesophageal varices. *Br J Cancer* **60**: 646–9.

19. Figg WD, Dukes GE, Lesesne HR, *et al.* (1995). Comparison of quantitative methods to assess hepatic function: Pugh's classification, indocyanine green, antipyrine and dextromorphan. *Pharmacother* **15**: 693–700.

20. Gillies HC, Rogers HJ, Ohashi K, Liang R, Harper PG, Rubens RD (1986). Correlation between elimination of indocyanine and doxorubicin or idarubicin. *Proc Am Soc Clin Oncol* **5**: 56.

21. Dobbs NA, Twelves CJ, Rizzi P, *et al.* (1994). Epirubicin in hepatocellular, carcinoma: pharmacokinetics and clinical activity. *Cancer Chemother Pharmacol* **34**: 405–10.

22. Twelves C, Glynne-Jones R, Cassidy J, *et al.* (1999). Effect of hepatic dysfunction due to liver metastases on the pharmacokinetics of capecitabine and its metabolites. *Clin Cancer Res* **5**: 1696–702.

23. Takimoto CH, Saif MW, Lorusso PM, *et al.* (2004). A pharmacokinetic (PK) dose escalation study of DX-8951f (DX) in adult cancer patients with hepatic dysfunction: A comparison of the NCI hepatic classification criteria and the Child-Pugh classification. *J Clin Oncol* **22**: 14S 2017.

24. Patel H, Egorin MJ, Remick SC, *et al.* (2004). Comparison of Child-Pugh (CP) criteria and NCI organ dysfunction working group (NCI-ODWG) criteria for hepatic dysfunction (HD): Implications for chemotherapy dosing. *J Clin Oncol* **7**: 1748–56.

25. Calvert AH, Newell DR, Gumbrell LA, *et al.* (1989) Carboplatin dosage: prospective evaluation of a simple formula based on renal function. *J Clin Oncol* **7**: 1748–56.

26. Judson I, Maughan T, Beale P, *et al.* (1998). Effects of impaired renal function on the pharmacokinetics of raltitrexed (Tomudex ZD1694). *Br J Cancer* **78**: 1188–93.

27. Takimoto CH, Remick SC, Sharma S, *et al.* (2003). Dose-escalating and pharmacological study of oxaliplatin in adult cancer patients with impaired renal function: a National Cancer Institute Organ Dysfunction Working Group Study. *J Clin Oncol* **21**: 2664–2672.

28. Massari C, Brienza S, Rotarski M, *et al.* (2000). Pharmacokinetics of oxaliplatin in patients with normal versus impaired renal function. *Cancer Chemother Pharmacol* **45**: 157–64.

29. O'Reilly S, Rowinsky EK, Slichenmyer W, *et al.* (1996). Phase I and pharmacologic study of topotecan in patients with impaired renal function. *J Clin Oncol* **14**: 3062–73.

30. Venook AP, Egorin MJ, Rosner GL, *et al.* (2000). Phase 1 and pharmacokinetic trial of gemcitabine in patients with hepatic or renal dysfunction: Cancer and Leukemia Group B 9565. *J Clin Oncol* **18**: 2780–7.

31. Delaloge S, Liombart A, Di Palma M, *et al.* (2004). Gemcitabine in patients with solid tumors and renal impairment: a pharmacokinetic phase I study. *Am J Clin Oncol* **27**: 289–93.

32. Poole C, Gardiner J, Twelves C, *et al.* (2002). Effect of renal impairment on the pharmacokinetics and tolerability of capecitabine (Xeloda) in cancer patients. *Cancer Chemother Pharmacol* **49**: 225–34.

33. Bruno R, Hille D, Riva A, *et al.* (1998). Population pharmacokinetics/pharmacodynamics of docetaxel in phase II studies in patients with cancer. *J Clin Oncol* **16**: 187–196.

34. Venook AP, Egorin MJ, Rosner GL, *et al.* (1998). Phase I and pharmacokinetic trial of paclitaxel in patients with hepatic dysfunction: Cancer and Leukemia Group B 9264. *J Clin Oncol* **16**: 1811–19.

35. Doroshow JH, Synold TW, Gandaran D, *et al.* (2003). Pharmacology of oxaliplatin in solid tumor patients with hepatic dysfunction: a preliminary report of the National Cancer Institute Organ Dysfunction Working Group. *Semin Oncol* **30**: 14–19.

36. Twelves C, Glynne-Jones R, Cassidy J, *et al.*(1999) Effect of hepatic dysfunction due to liver metastases on the pharmacokinetics of capecitabine and its metabolites. *Clin Cancer Res* **5**: 1696–702.

37. Weitman S, Carlson L, Pratt CB (1996). New drug development for pediatric oncology. *Invest New Drugs* **14**: 1–10.

38. Houghton P, Adamson PC, Blaney S, *et al.* (2002). Testing of new agents in childhood cancer preclinical models: meeting summary. *Clin Cancer Res* **8**: 3646–57.

39. Woods WG, O'Leary M, Nesbit ME (1981). Life-threatening neuropathy and hepatotoxicity in infants during induction therapy for acute lymphoblastic leukaemia. *J Pediatr* **98**:642–5.

40. McLeod HL, Relling MV, Crom WR, *et al.* (1992). Disposition of antineoplastic agents in the very young child. *Br J Cancer* **66**: S23–9.

41. Marsoni S, Ungerleider RS, Hurson SB, Simon RM, Hammershaimb LD (1985). Tolerance to antineoplastic agents in children and adults. *Cancer Treat Rep* **69**: 1263–9.

42. FDA Guidance for pediatric studies: http://www.fda.gov/cder/guidance/1449fnl.pdf [last accessed August 2005]

43. EMEA Guidance for pediatric studies: http://www.emea.eu.int/pdfs/human/ewp/046295en.pdf [last accessed August 2005]

44. FDA Guidance for pediatric oncology studies: http://www.fda.gov/cder/guidance/3765dft.htm [last accessed August 2005]

45. Deatrick JA, Angst DB, Moore C (2002). Parents' views of their children's participation in phase I oncology clinical trials. *J Pediatr Oncol Nurs* 19: 114–21.

46. Aleksa K, Koren G (2002). Ethical issues in including pediatric cancer patients in drug development trials. *Paediatr Drugs* 4: 257–65.

47. Estlin EJ, Cotterill S, Pratt CB, Pearson ADJ, Bernstein M (2000). Phase I trials in pediatric oncology: perceptions of pediatricians from the United Kingdom Children's Cancer Study Group and the Pediatric Oncology Group. *J Clin Oncol* 18: 1900–5.

48. Shah S, Weitman S, Langevin AM, Bernstein M, Furman W, Pratt C (1998). Phase I therapy trials in children with cancer. *J Pediatr Hematol Oncol* 20: 431–8.

49. Lansky S, List MA, Lansky LL, *et al.* (1987). The measurement of performance in childhood cancer patients. *Cancer,* 60: 1651–6.

50. Newell DR, Pearson ADJ, Balmanno K, *et al.* (1993). Carboplatin pharmacokinetics in children: the development of a pediatric dosing formula. *J Clin Oncol* 11: 2314–23.

51. Marina NM, Rodman J, Shema SJ, *et al.* (1993). Phase I study of escalating targeted doses of carboplatin combined with ifosfamide and etoposide in children with relapsed solid tumours. *J Clin Oncol* 11: 554–60.

52. Vassal G, Pein F, Goyette A, *et al.* (1994). Development of new anticancer agents in children: methodology, difficulties, and strategies. *Ann Pediatr* 41: 477–84.

53. Hutchins LF, Unger JM, Crowley JJ, Coltman CA, Albain KS (1999). Underrepresentation of patients 65 years of age or older in cancer-treatment trials. *N Engl J Med* 341: 2061–7.

54. Murthy VH, Krumholz HM, Gross CP (2004). Participation in cancer clinical trials. Race-, sex-, and age-based disparities. *JAMA* 291: 2720–6.

55. Aapro MS, Kohne CH, Cohen HJ, Extermann M (2005). Never too old? Age should not be a barrier to enrollment in cancer clinical trials. *Oncologist* 10: 198–204.

56. Gronlund B, Hogdall C, Hansen HH, Engelholm SA (2002). Performance status rather than age is the key prognositic factor in second-line treatment of elderly patients with epithelial ovarian carcinoma. *Cancer* 94: 1961–7.

57. Giovanazzi-Bannon S, Rademaker A, Lai G, Benson AB 3rd (1994). Treatment tolerance of elderly cancer patients entered onto phase II clinical trials: an Illinois Cancer Centre study. *J Clin Oncol* 12: 2447–52.

58. Repetto L (2003). Greater risks of chemotherapy toxicity in elderly patients with cancer. *J Support Oncol* 1 (Suppl. 2): 18–24.

59. Terret C, Albrand G, Droz J, *et al.* (2004). Multidimensional geriatric assessment reveals unknown medical problems in elderly cancer patients. *Proc Am Soc Clin Oncol* 23: 766a.

60. Anderson S, Brenner BM (1986). Effects of ageing on the renal glomerulus. *Am J Med* 80: 435–42.

61. Ten Tije AJ, Verweij J, Carducci MA, *et al.* (2005). Prospective evaluation of the pharmacokinetics and toxicity profile of docetaxel in the elderly. *J Clin Oncol* 23: 1070–7.

62. Pazdur R, Zimmer R, Rothenberg MI, *et al.* (1997). Age is a risk factor in irinotecan treatment of 5-FU-refractory colorectal cancer. *Proc Am Soc Clin Oncol* Abstr No. 921.

63. FDA Guideline for Industry: Studies in support of special populations. Available at: http://www.fda.gov/cder/guidance/iche7.pdf [last accessed August 2005]

64. Note for Guidance on Studies in support of special populations: Geriatrics (CPMP/ICH/379/95) Approved by CPMP September 1993. Available at: http://www.e-mea.eu.int/pdfs/human/ich/037995en.pdf [last accessed August 2005]

65. Aapro MS (2005). The frail are not always elderly. *J Clin Oncol* 23: 2121–2.

66. Baka S, Ashcroft L, Anderson H, *et al.* (2005). Randomised phase II study of two gemcitabine schedules for patients with impaired performance status (Karnofsky performance status ≤70) and advanced non-small-cell lung cancer. *J Clin Oncol* 23: 2136–44.

67. Bejetta E, Procopio G, Celio L, *et al.* (2005). Safety and efficacy of two different doses of capecitabine in the treatment of advanced breast cancer in women. *J Clin Oncol* 23: 2155–61.

68. FDA guidance: Food effect bioavailability and fed bioequivalence studies.. http://www.fda.gov/cder/guidance/5194fnl.pdf [last accessed August 2005]

69. Singh BN, Malhotra BK (2004). Effects of food on the clinical pharmacokinetics of anticancer agents: underlying mechanisms and implications for oral chemotherapy. *Clin Pharmacokinet* 43: 1127–56.

70. Valle M, Di Salle E, Jannuzzo MG, *et al.* (2005). A predictive model for exemestane pharmacokinetics/pharmacodynamics incorporating the effect of food and formulation. *Br J Clin Pharmacol* 59: 355–64.

71. Lancaster DL, Patel N, Lennard L, Lilleyman JS (2001). 6-Tioguanine in children with acute lymphoblastic leukaemia: influence of food on parent drug pharmacokinetics and 6-thioguanine nucleotide concentrations. *Br J Clin Pharmacol* 51: 531–9.

72. Rowinsky EK, Sol Lucas V, Hsieh A-L A, *et al.* (1996). The effects of food and divided dosing on the bioavailability of oral vinorebine. *Clin Cancer Pharmacol* 39: 9–16.

73. Reigner B, Verweij J, Dirix L, *et al.* (1998). Effect of food on the pharmacokinetics of capecitabine and its metabolites following oral administration in cancer patients. *Clin Cancer Res* 4: 941–8.

74. Damle B, Ravandi F, Kaul S, *et al.* (2001). Effect of food on the oral bioavailability of UFT and leucovorin in cancer patients. *Clin Cancer Res* 7: 517–23.

75. Herben VMM, Rosing H, ten Bokkel Huinink, *et al.* (1999). Oral topotecan: bioavailability and effect of food co-administration. *Br J Cancer* 80: 1380–6.

76. Swaisland H, Laight A, Stafford L, Jones H, Morris C, Dane A, Yates R (2001). Pharmacokinetics and tolerability of the orally active selective epidermal growth factor receptor tyrosine kinase inhibitor ZD1839 in healthy volunteers (2001). *Clin Pharmacokinet* 40: 297–306.

77. Rakhit A, Fettner S, Riek M, Davis S, Hamilton M, Frohna P, Abbas R (2003). Clinical pharmacokinetics of erlotinib in healthy subjects. *J Clin Oncol* 22: 149 Abstr. 596.

78. Beijnen JH, Schellens JHM (2004). Drug interactions in oncology. *Lancet Oncology* 5: 489–96.

79. Streetman DS, Bertino JS Jr, Nafziger AN (2000). Phenotyping of drug-metabolising enzymes in adults: a review of in-vivo cytochrome P450 phenotyping probes. *Pharmacogenetics* 10: 186–216.

80. Baker SD, Ten Tije AJ, Carducci MA, *et al.* (2004). Evaluation of CYP3A activity as a predictive covariate for docetaxel clearance. *J Clin Oncol* 22: 128s Abstr. 2006.

81. Yamamoto N, Tamura T, Murakami H, *et al.* (2005). Randomized pharmacokinetic and pharmacodynamic study of docetaxel: dosing based on body-surface area compared with individualized dosing based on cytochrome P450 activity estimated using a urinary metabolite of exogenous cortisol. *J Clin Oncol* 23: 1061–9.

82. FDA guidance for drug-drug interaction (1999). http://www.fda.gov/cder/guidance/2635fnl.pdf [last accessed August 2005]

83. Murray LS, Jodrell DI, Morrison JG, *et al.* (1998). The effect of cimetidine on the pharmacokinetics of epirubicin in patients with advanced breast cancer: preliminary evidence of a potentially common drug interaction. *Clin Oncol* 10: 35–8.

84. Dutreix C, Peng B, Mehring G, Hayes M, Capdeville R, Pokorny R, Seiberling M (2004). Pharmacokinetic interaction between ketoconazole and imatinib mesylate (Glivec) in healthy subjects. *Clin Cancer Pharmacol* 54: 290–4.

85. Van Kesteren Ch, De Vooght MM, Lopez-Lazaro L, *et al.* (2003). Yondelis (trabectedin, ET-743): the development of an anticancer agent of marine origin. *Anti-Cancer Drugs* 14: 487–502.

86. Rowinsky ER, Gilbert MR, McGuire WP, *et al.* (1991). Sequences of taxol and cisplatin: a phase I and pharmacokinetic study. *J Clin Oncol* 9: 1692–703.

87. Gianni L, Vigano L, Locatelli A, *et al.* (1997). Human pharmacokinetic characterization and in vitro study of the interaction between doxorubicin and paclitaxel in patients with breast cancer. *J Clin Oncol* 15: 1906–15.

Chapter 6

Statistical designs for first-in-man phase I cancer trials

Marc Buyse

6.1 Basic design requirements

The primary objective of first-in-man phase I trials is to define a recommended dose *safely* (i.e. with the smallest possible number of patients experiencing severe toxicities), *efficiently* (i.e. with the smallest possible total number of patients), and *reliably* (i.e. with high statistical confidence, which would generally require large numbers of patients). These three requirements are mutually contradictory, and phase I designs must find the best possible compromise between them. The safety requirement dominates the two others, as it is ethically imperative not to submit patients to undue toxicity, yet the very purpose of the phase I trial is to find a dose that has antitumour activity, which for many anticancer compounds is usually associated with acute systemic toxicity. The efficiency requirement mandates that the trial accrue few patients and use a reasonably rapid dose escalation scheme, otherwise many patients would potentially be exposed to non-toxic, but subtherapeutic doses. The reliability requirement means treating a sufficient number of patients at or near the recommended dose, otherwise this dose may be incorrectly chosen, or uncertainty about the true toxicity profile of the drug may be too high to develop it further. All of these considerations, which are essentially pragmatic and ethical, have a bearing on the statistical design of phase I trials.

For most designs considered in this chapter, toxicity will be the endpoint of interest. The purpose of these designs, except those appropriate for biological agents that do not have dose-limiting toxicities (see Section 6.10) is to identify dose levels at which significant toxicities are observed. As outlined in Chapter 3, the nature of these toxicities depends on the mechanism of action of the drug under investigation; however, the idea underlying the trial design is common to all drugs for which higher doses are associated with a higher probability of toxicity. The designs that are appropriate under these circumstances consist of escalating (and sometimes de-escalating) the dose until significant toxic events are observed.

6.2 Choice of doses: the 'modified Fibonacci' series

Prior to commencing a phase I trial, some information must be available, from preclinical experiments or other sources, about the range of doses that may potentially be tested. As discussed in Chapter 3, the minimum dose of interest is usually based on the toxicology of the most sensitive animal species (for instance, a common choice for the minimum dose is one-tenth the mouse-equivalent LD_{10}). The minimum dose will generally be the starting dose of the phase I trial. For some drugs, a maximum dose may be imposed by practical considerations such as drug availability or constraints in drug delivery, while for others no maximum is specified and the plan is 'open-ended'. The choice of the maximum planned dose is in fact less important than the choice of a minimum dose, as the trial will be likely to hit toxicities and terminate before the maximum dose is reached. Once minimum and maximum dose levels are determined, dose levels must be chosen in between these two. Historically, most phase I trials have used a spacing based on the so-called 'modified Fibonacci' series, in which the relative increase between successive dose levels is constant. This series is worth a short digression.

Leonardo Pisano Fibonacci (1175–1250), a mathematician who lived in Florence (Italy), is remembered for his celebrated series, which goes like this:

1, 1, 2, 3, 5, 8, 13, 21, 34, 55, 89, 144, 233, 377, 610, 987, ...

In Fibonacci's series, the first two terms are equal to 1, and thereafter each term of the series is equal to the sum of its two predecessors. This series is important because it appears with surprisingly high frequency in nature; it is in fact intrinsically associated with the growth of living organisms. The number of branches of a tree, the size of distinct compartments of a sea

Table 6.1 Ratio between successive terms in the original Fibonacci series, and in a 'modified Fibonacci' series

Fibonacci term	Ratio between successive terms	Modified Fibonacci term	Ratio between successive terms
1	–	1	–
2	2.0000	2	2.0000
3	1.5000	4	2.0000
5	1.6667	6	1.5000
8	1.6000	9	1.5000
13	1.6250	14	1.5556
21	1.6154	21	1.5000
34	1.6190	32	1.5238
55	1.6176	48	1.5000
89	1.6182	72	1.5000
144	1.6180	108	1.5000
233	1.6181	162	1.5000
377	1.6180	243	1.5000
610	1.6180	365	1.5021

shell, the size of petals of many flowers, all follow Fibonacci series. For the purposes of phase I dose escalation, the Fibonacci series is of interest because the ratio of any two successive terms of the series tends rapidly to a constant, as shown in Table 6.1.

In fact, the constant to which the ratio of successive terms asymptotically converges is nothing else than the golden number (≈ 1.618034), which has fascinated mathematicians, architects and artists for centuries. For the purposes of phase I designs, the Fibonacci series offers a very appealing dose escalation scheme, because successive dose levels increase in a geometric progression, i.e. in such a way that the *absolute* dose increases grow larger and larger while the *relative* dose increases are constant (each dose being about two-thirds larger than its predecessor) as shown in Table 6.1.

In practice, successive dose levels follow a Fibonacci series only in spirit. For instance, it could be appropriate to double the dose at low dose levels, and to increase it by only 50% beyond a certain threshold. Another common modification is to make the relative increments smaller (e.g. 33% or even 25% instead of 50%) at high doses. Moreover, the dose levels would be rounded off, such that for example a dose of 50 would be used instead of 48. Such dose escalation schemes would be said to follow a 'modified Fibonacci' series, an appellation that has been so abused that almost any scheme of dose escalation is now referred to as being a 'modified Fibonacci' series (Figure 6.1)

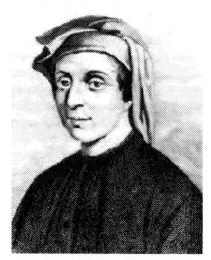
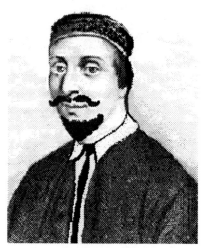

Leonardo Pisano Fibonacci   A modified Fibonacci
(1175 – 1250)   (20th century)

Figure 6.1 Fibonacci and ... a modified Fibonacci.

6.3 Dose–response relationship

Some of the phase I designs discussed below require, in addition to choosing dose levels, that a dose–response relationship be prespecified. This relationship, which may not be easy to determine before any data are available in humans, gives the probability of observing a dose-limiting toxicity (DLT) at each of the dose levels being tested. The relationship is usually assumed to be a monotonically increasing function, for which a given dose level has a probability of observing a DLT at least as high (but generally higher) than all of the lower dose levels. For instance, the line with solid circles in Figure 6.2 could describe a prespecified dose–response relationship for some new drug: the lowest dose level has a probability of only 5% of a DLT, the next dose a probability of 10%, the next dose a probability of just over 20%, etc. The other lines drawn in Figure 6.2 will be useful later in this chapter to discuss the continual reassessment method (CRM).

6.4 The 'classical' design

Many phase I clinical trials of cytotoxic agents are carried out using a standard or 'classical' design based on empirical considerations. This design finds its justification in the fact that the maximum tolerated dose (MTD) is usually defined as the dose at which one-third of the patients experience DLTs (should interest focus on some other proportion, say one-quarter or one-fifth, the

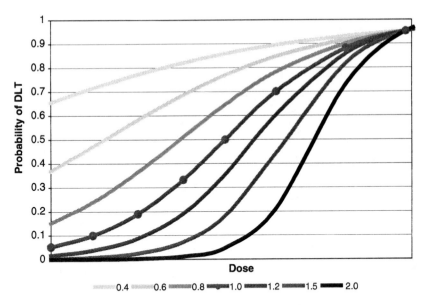

Figure 6.2 Probability of DLT (p) as a function of dose (d), for different values of parameter θ. The dose–response relationship is characterized by the logistic function $p = \exp(3 + \theta \times d)/[1 + \exp(3 + \theta \times d)]$.

design could be adapted accordingly). Note that the definition of MTD used in this book is not universal; refer to Table 3.6 in Chapter 3 to avoid confusion.

The design proceeds in cohorts of three patients, the first cohort being treated at the minimum dose of interest, and the next cohorts being treated at increasing dose levels as shown on the flowchart of Figure 6.3. The dose escalation stops as soon as at least two patients experience a DLT, either in the first cohort of three patients treated at that dose level, or in the two cohorts of three patients treated at that dose level. The recommended dose is usually defined as the dose level just below the level at which DLTs were observed in at least two patients. If, as is more likely, two DLTs were observed among six patients, then indeed the observed proportion of DLTs at the MTD is 33% (two of six). If, on the other hand, two DLTs were observed among three patients, then it is common to expand the cohort below by at least three patients, to ensure that there are fewer than two DLTs at that dose level. Some websites offer simple implementations of the classical design (see, for instance, reference [1]).

Although the classical design is still commonly used in phase I trials, it has some limitations:

a. too many patients tend to be treated at low doses, with virtually no chance of efficacy;

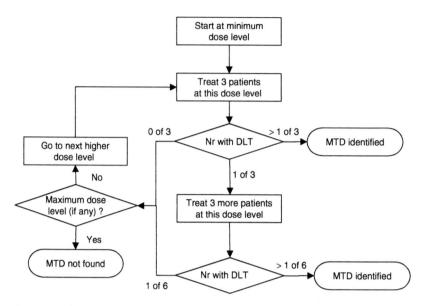

Figure 6.3 Flowchart for classical '3+3' dose escalation scheme. DLT, dose-limiting toxicity; MTD, maximum tolerated dose.

b. dose escalation may be too slow because of an excessive number of escalation steps, resulting in trials that take longer than needed to get to the MTD;
c. too few patients tend to be treated near the MTD, hence there may be substantial residual uncertainty about the dose recommended for further trials, which does raise ethical concerns. Indeed, if the recommended dose is chosen too low it may fail to have efficacy in phase II trials while if it is chosen too high it may put patients at unacceptable levels of risk in phase II trials;
d. no allowance is made for patient variability.

Some of these drawbacks are illustrated by the actual phase I trial of gemcitabine, as shown in Figure 6.4 [2]. The first DLT did not occur until the ninth dose level and the 27th patient. A total of 47 patients were treated at 13 dose levels, with at least three patients at each dose level, before the MTD could be determined.

6.5 Improvements to the 'classical' design

Ad hoc solutions have been proposed to address some the limitations of the classical design.

6.5.1 Accelerated titration

Simon *et al.* have shown through simulations based on a stochastic model fit to 20 phase I trials that 'accelerated titration' may result in substantial savings

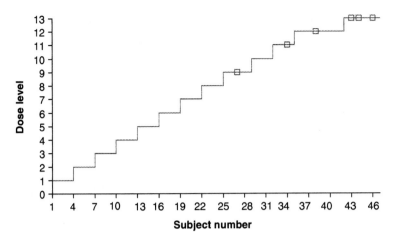

Figure 6.4 Dose escalation using the classical design (see reference [2]). Patients experiencing a dose-limiting toxicity are indicated by an open square.

in terms of number of patients treated at low doses as well as overall number of patients, at the expense of a slightly higher number of patients experiencing grade 3 or 4 toxicities [3]. They considered several schemes of accelerated titration, the general idea being to treat only one patient per dose level initially, and to increase the number of patients per cohort to three or to revert to a classical design as soon as the dose level is thought to have a high probability to be toxic, for instance when a DLT is observed in one patient, or grade 2 toxicities are observed in two patients. Variations include doubling dose steps initially, and introducing intrapatient dose escalation if only grade 0–1 toxicities were seen at the previous course.

6.5.2 Pharmacologically guided dose escalation

Another variation of the classical design makes use of pharmacokinetic data to guide in dose escalation [4,5]. Essentially, the approach assumes that dose-limiting toxicities can be predicted by plasma drug concentrations, and that the relationship between toxicity and plasma drug concentrations holds across species. The dose escalation proceeds as follows:

a. a target area under the curve is determined based on an appropriate animal model (say, one-tenth LD_{10} in mice);

b. pharmacokinetic data are collected on a first cohort of patients;

c. the dose is escalated rapidly in subsequent cohorts until the target area under the curve (or a predetermined proportion of the target area under the curve) is reached or dose-limiting toxicities occur;

d. thereafter, the dose escalation proceeds more slowly, as in the classical design.

6.5.3 Intrapatient dose escalation

As explained in Section 3.4.3.2 of Chapter 3, intrapatient dose escalation may be proposed on ethical grounds in order to increase the chance of an individual patient receiving a therapeutic dose at their second or third course even if they received a low dose at their first course. In the accelerated titration designs, the dose can be escalated if the worst toxicity was grade 0 or 1 in the previous course of that patient [3]. Although information obtained from intrapatient dose escalation could potentially be incorporated in the decision-making process, difficulties arise because

a. successive observations in a single patient are correlated (hence patients who do not experience a DLT during their first course are less likely to experience one during later courses);
b. the drug may have cumulative toxicities;
c. most patients cannot receive more than two courses, which induces a selection bias over the successive courses of treatment.

For all these reasons, there is little or no statistical advantage to using information from several dose levels in the same patient, as compared with decision-making based only on the first course of each patient. Results of trials using intra-patient dose escalation are also harder to present and interpret, because the same patient contributes information to several dose levels.

6.5.4 Patient choice of dose

To address the ethical dilemma of administering potentially low (inactive) doses, or potentially high (toxic) doses to patients who have failed all available therapies, some have suggested to let the patients choose among the possible dose levels [6]. It is unclear that such a patient choice, if fully and correctly informed, would in fact be more ethical than use of a well-defined scheme of dose escalation. It is clear, in contrast, that this approach has a large opportunity for selection bias, whereby the choice of dose primarily depends on the patients' condition, making the results of the trial hard to interpret and generalize.

6.5.5 Expanded cohort at recommended dose

It is often recommended, after DLTs have occurred, to treat an expanded cohort (say, of five to 10 additional patients) at the recommended dose to increase the confidence that this dose is indeed safe. A formal justification for the size of this additional cohort may sometimes be provided as outlined in Section 6.12 at the end of this chapter.

These *ad-hoc* solutions address some, but not all of the problems associated with the classical design, and therefore other designs have been proposed that will be discussed later in this chapter. There is, in fact, no formal statistical justification for the classical design. It is worrisome that this design does not guarantee that the dose recommended corresponds to any given percentile of the distribution function of the DLT probability [7]. Combined with the limitations outlined above, this fact has led to a large body of literature devoted to designs with better operating characteristics and a sounder statistical foundation.

6.6 Operating characteristics

Before turning to other designs, it may be useful to examine some of the 'operating characteristics' of the classical design, and of variations of it [8]. The operating characteristics include the probabilities of stopping at each of the dose levels (i.e. the probabilities of finding the correct dose, and the probabilities of recommending a dose that is either too low or too high), the expected number of patients in the whole trial (which is a random variable), the expected number of patients treated at each of the dose levels, the expected number of patients with toxicities overall and at each of the dose levels, and any other statistical quantity of interest. These operating characteristics can be either computed or obtained through simulation for various designs and for an assumed distribution of the probability of a DLT at each dose level.

For example, assume we wish to test seven increasing dose levels that have the dose–response relationship depicted by the unconnected dots in Figure 6.5. Note that dose level 4 has a probability of 33% of a DLT, and is therefore the target dose at which the trial should ideally stop. Figure 6.5 shows the cumulative probabilities of stopping (i.e. the probabilities of stopping at a dose or at any previous dose) for several designs based on the following stopping rules.

a. The ideal rule is one that stops exactly at dose level 4 (black line in Figure 6.5); this rule has a probability of zero of stopping at any dose other than dose level 4.

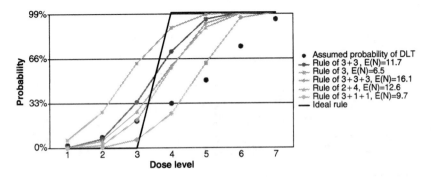

Figure 6.5 Cumulative probabilities of stopping for various rules. E(N) = expected number of patients.

b. A simple rule, which we call the 'rule of 3', is to stop as soon as at least one toxicity is observed among three patients (upper grey line in Figure 6.5). As might be expected, this rule is exceedingly conservative, and has an unacceptably high probability of stopping before dose level 4 is reached.

c. The 'rule of 3+3' used in the classical design (dark grey line in Figure 6.5). This rule, as outlined in Figure 6.3, mandates stopping as soon as at least two of six patients experience a DLT. It has a probability of 72% of stopping at dose level 4 or before. It has a probability of 37% of stopping exactly at dose level 4 (the target dose with 33% DLTs), 27% probability of stopping at dose level 3, and 24% probability of stopping at dose level 5, i.e. 88% probability of stopping at the target dose or one of the adjacent dose levels. It has 34% of stopping below the target dose, and 29% probability of stopping above the target dose. As the probabilities of stopping either too early or too late with this rule are not negligible, is it possible to improve on it? The expected sample size for this rule is equal to 11.7 patients.

d. One could think of adding a third cohort of three patients if two of six patients experienced a DLT at a certain dose level: this is the 'rule of 3+3+ 3'. This rule mandates stopping as soon as at least three of nine patients experience a DLT. Note that it is essential to use a prespecified rule to stop, unlike in Dagwood's cartoon (Figure 6.6)! This rule has lower probability than the classical rule of 3+3 of stopping earlier than dose level 4, but it has a larger expected sample size (16.1 as compared with 11.7 for the classical rule of 3+3). It also has larger probability of 'overshooting' and stopping at a dose level higher than 4.

e. One could also use a 'rule of 2+4', for which an additional cohort of four patients is added if one DLT is observed in a first cohort of two patients, with the same stopping criterion as for the classical rule of 3+3. Figure 6.5 shows that the probabilities of stopping for this rule are very close to those

BLONDIE

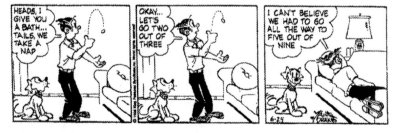

Figure 6.6 The dangers of using conditional tests to stop an experiment. © King Features Syndicate, Inc. All Rights reserved. Distributed by EM.TV Wavery B.v. -Rijswijk

for the rule of 3+3+3, but with a lower expected sample size (12.6 patients), which may make it more desirable.

f. Finally, one could use a 'rule of 3+1+1', also referred to as 'best of five' in the literature [7]. The flowchart for this rule is shown in Figure 6.7. It is more aggressive than the other rules, i.e. it will tend to stop at higher doses.

Most sensible rules have operating characteristics that are close to those of the classical rule of '3+3', but alternative rules may be better suited depending on the situation (e.g. more aggressive rules if the drug is not expected to be very toxic).

There is much experience with the classical design, and it has been shown to work reasonably well empirically, which is why it remains standard for many phase I clinical trials. Alternative designs that have a more solid statistical foundation are, however, worth exploring.

6.7 Continual reassessment method

The CRM, originally proposed by O'Quigley and colleagues in the early 1990s, is a statistical approach based on an assumed dose–response relationship,

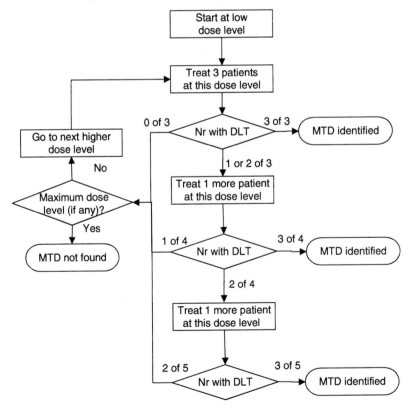

Figure 6.7 Flowchart for classical 'best of 5' (or '3+1+1') dose escalation scheme. DLT, dose-limiting toxicity; MTD, maximum tolerated dose.

which is described through a mathematical function linking the probability of a DLT and the dose level [9]. There is considerable freedom in the choice of a suitable mathematical function, the only two requirements being that:

a. The function should be monotonically increasing, i.e. such that the probability of a DLT at any dose level be at least equal to the probability at any lower dose levels.

b. The function should depend on only one 'parameter', which we will denote θ. The parameter is the quantity that determines the exact shape of the dose–response relationship, as illustrated in the following example.

One popular choice for the dose–response relationship is the logistic function, which is shown in Figure 6.2 for the following family of functions:

$$p = \exp(3 + \theta \times d)/[1 + \exp(3 + \theta \times d)]$$

where p is the probability of a DLT, d is the dose level, and θ is the parameter. Figure 6.2 shows that for small values of θ, the probability of a DLT increases very slowly at increasing dose levels, while for large values of θ, the increase is very sharp. Many other functions could be used to model the dose–response relationship, but the particular choice made here yields dose–response curves that seem plausible and have been studied in detail [10].

Besides the choice of a mathematical function to describe the dose–response relationship, the CRM also requires that an initial guess be available for the probabilities of DLT as a function of dose. Such a guess will generally be elicited from experts familiar with preclinical data, or clinical data on similar drugs. In the example of Figure 6.2, it is assumed that seven dose levels will be tested, with the following prior probabilities of DLT:

0.05 for dose level 1
0.10 for dose level 2
0.19 for dose level 3
0.33 for dose level 4 (target dose)
0.50 for dose level 5
0.70 for dose level 6
0.88 for dose level 7.

In this example, dose level 4 is the target MTD, i.e. the dose level for which 33% of the patients experience a DLT. These prior probabilities of a DLT fit the following model:

$$p = \exp(3 + d)/[1 + \exp(3 + d)],$$

which is one of the functions represented in Figure 6.2 (the function for which θ = 1). Thus, the value of θ, before any actual patient data have been observed, is equal to 1. A distribution is also specified for θ, for instance a flat distribution (if all values of θ are thought equally likely) or a normal distribution with mean 1 and a small variance (if it is thought very likely that θ is equal to, or close to, 1) or a normal distribution with mean 1 and a large variance (if the most likely value of θ is thought to be 1, but with other values for θ also likely). This is called a 'prior' distribution for θ.

The CRM then proceeds as follows:

a. The first patient is treated at the dose thought to be closest to the MTD (i.e. the dose where 33% of the patients experience a DLT). In our example, before any patient is treated, the MTD is thought to be dose level 4; hence the first patient should be treated at dose level 4.
b. This patient may or may not experience a DLT.
c. Having observed whether or not this patient experienced a DLT, the posterior distribution of parameter θ is calculated (using a so-called 'Bayesian' method). The mean of that posterior distribution yields an updated value of θ, which is in turn used to update the probabilities of a DLT at each dose level.
d. The process is repeated from step (a) for the next patient, until a prespecified condition is met, for instance that a certain number of patients be treated at the same dose level, at which point the trial may stop.

6.8 Improvements to the continual reassessment method

The CRM just described may be considered too aggressive, because the starting dose is the dose thought to be closest to the MTD and the dose can jump up by any number of levels at a time. Safety considerations have led several authors to propose the following modifications to the CRM [10–14]:

a. the first patient is treated at the lowest dose level based on animal toxicology (instead of the dose level thought to be closest to the MTD);
b. the dose may increase by only one level at a time;
c. at least two patients are treated at each dose level; and
d. an expanded cohort of patients is treated at the dose level just below the MTD, as this dose level would generally be the recommended dose level for phase II trials.

Obviously, if these constraints are adopted, the advantage of the CRM in terms of expected sample size is reduced. Figure 6.8 shows an example of dose escalation using a 'modified' CRM in which constraints a, b, and d above are adopted. The first three patients are treated at dose levels 1, 2, and 3, respectively, without a DLT. The fourth patient is treated at dose level 4 and experiences a DLT, upon which the dose is reduced to dose level 3 for the next three patients, none of whom experience a DLT. The dose is increased again to

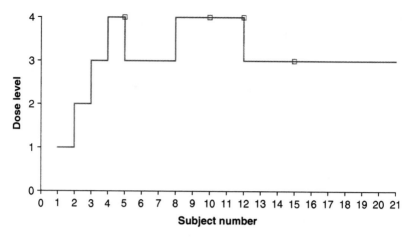

Figure 6.8 Dose escalation using the continual reassessment method. Patients experiencing a dose-limiting toxicity are indicated by an open square.

dose level 4, and back to dose level 3 after observation of two further DLTs. Dose level 3 is eventually found to be the recommended dose.

Simulation studies show that the CRM generally outperforms the classical design [15,16]. Although the CRM has met with some success, it has not been as popular as it could have been in view of its potential benefits. One reason for the limited use of the CRM or modified CRM may be the empirical observation that it does not always lead to more rapid study completion than the classical design, so that some investigators have questioned whether its use in the clinic was worth the effort [17]. Another reason for the limited use of the CRM may be that the method requires help from a statistician, or recourse to specialized software to carry out the calculations needed after treatment of every patient. Free availability of such software on the web could encourage wider use of the CRM (see, for instance, nice implementations of the CRM that can be downloaded from references 18 and 19).

Further refinements and extensions of the CRM have been described in the literature:

a. The CRM can use ordinal response (such as toxicity grade 1 through 4), rather than simple binary response (such as DLT grade 3 or 4).

b. The CRM can be extended to use two-parameter models, rather than the single parameter θ, to describe the dose–response relationship [20].

c. The CRM can be adapted for combination therapy. In this case, information available from phase I monotherapy trials of each component drug can be used to construct a prior distribution of the dose–response relationship for various doses of each drug [21].

d. The stratified CRM (or 'two-sample' CRM) allows for the population of patients to be subdivided into two or more groups with distinct risks of

DLT, a group of 'healthier' patients and a group of 'sicker' patients. The trial starts without making a distinction between the two strata, but the dose escalation becomes stratum-specific after observation of toxicities, such that the recommended dose may be different in the two strata [22].

e. The CRM may use likelihood estimation of θ, instead of the Bayesian approach described above [23]. Likelihood estimation does not require specification of a prior distribution for θ (which can be hard to do for clinicians and statisticians alike), nor the calculation of the posterior distribution for θ after observation of each patient. It is worth noting that the CRM is not intrinsically Bayesian, and it is a matter of taste or convenience as to which implementation is preferred.

f. The standard CRM pauses until each patient is observed long enough to have had an opportunity to develop a DLT. A modification using time-to-event information (TITE-CRM) allows continual enrolment of patients, assigning fractional weights to patients who have not experienced toxicity but have not yet completed the observation period [24].

6.9 Other statistically based designs

The CRM is not the only design based on a mathematical model [25]. Other designs have been proposed and compared with the CRM. Although there are situations in which they perform better than the CRM, it is unlikely that any design would be uniformly better in all situations, and differences in operating characteristics are usually modest.

6.9.1 Two-stage designs

The two-stage approach has been very influential and many phase I designs have used a first stage similar to that proposed originally by Storer [26]. The two stages proceed as follows: in the first stage, single patients are treated at increasing dose levels until a DLT is observed; in the second stage, cohorts of three to five patients are treated at various dose levels according to the number of DLTs observed. Specifically, a cohort is treated:

a. at the next higher dose level if no DLT was observed in the previous cohort;
b. at the same dose level if one DLT was observed in the previous cohort;
c. at the next lower dose level if more than one DLT was observed in the previous cohort.

The operating characteristics of this design are comparable with those of the CRM [7]. One interesting extension of this design has been proposed to allow the MTD to differ from the prespecified dose levels, which may be attractive if dose levels are far apart.

6.9.2 Up and down designs

These designs escalate or de-escalate the dose in successive cohorts of patients, in a partially randomized fashion. For instance, one design allocated treatment to each new patient as follows: if the last patient experienced a DLT, treat the next patient at the next lower dose level; otherwise, randomize the next patient to be treated either at the same dose level or at the next higher dose level. This is a fairly conservative design (as the dose is always reduced in case of a DLT). It can be shown that the design will eventually converge to the dose level that has 33% probability of DLT [27]. The properties of the up and down approach have been worked out for the general case where the target dose has any desired probability of DLT.

6.9.3 Escalation with overdose control

These designs use a Bayesian approach to constrain the proportion of patients who will receive a dose higher than the MTD [28]. Like the CRM, the method is adaptive in that it uses all information available to determine the next dose assignment. Its aim is to reach the MTD as fast as possible subject to the constraint that the predicted proportion of patients who receive a dose exceeding the MTD does not surpass a prespecified value. Simulations show that use of this method improves upon the classical approach in that fewer patients are treated at subtherapeutic levels and the MTD is estimated more accurately, and it improves upon the CRM in that fewer patients are treated at severely toxic levels.

6.9.4 Isotonic regression

The idea behind isotonic regression is to estimate the probabilities of toxicity at each dose level subject to the constraint that the dose–response relationship be monotonically increasing [29]. One instance where such an approach may be particularly advantageous is when two risk groups can be formed, in which case dose escalations in the two risk groups are linked through a two-way isotonic regression [30]. One very attractive feature of this approach is that it requires almost no assumptions or model and proceeds only on the basis of observed toxicity rates.

6.10 Dose escalation designs based on biological outcome measures

The primary goal of a phase I trial for a cytotoxic agent is to find the maximum dose that produces an acceptable level of toxicity in a low, pre-specified proportion of patients. In contrast, the goal of phase I trial designs for biological agents may be to find the minimum dose that produces a desirable biological outcome in a sufficiently large prespecified proportion of patients. For the purpose of this discussion, 'biological agents' refers to targeted non-cytotoxic drugs or agents that act though immunological mechanisms. The biological outcome of interest depends on the mode of action of the agent under consideration, and defining such an outcome may be the most challenging aspect of designing a relevant trial. For now, let us assume that there exists an assay that is feasible, reproducible, and with real-time results, to assess the biological effect of the agent. This assay may reflect changes in a target biomarker in the tumour or surrogate tissues, changes in imaging, or clinical manifestations of the agent's activity.

One could hypothesize a dose–response curve giving the probability of observing biological activity at each of the dose levels being tested just as was described for the probability of observing a DLT in Section 6.3. The dose of interest could be either the minimum biologically active dose, i.e. the lowest dose that produces the desired biological activity in a given proportion of patients, or the optimum biologically active dose, i.e. the dose that produces the desired biological activity in the largest proportion of patients (assuming that the dose–response relationship for biological activity is no longer monotonically increasing as was assumed for toxicity). The latter goal is more challenging and generally requires many more patients than are typically studied in phase I trials [31].

If we focus on identification of the minimum biologically active dose, designs similar to the classical design outlined in Section 6.4 can be entertained, and their operating characteristics calculated as in Section 6.6. Figure 6.9 shows a flowchart appropriate for the determination of the minimum biologically active dose. Note that this design, just as the design shown in Figure 6.3, is based on intuitively reasonable rules rather than on formally justifiable statistical criteria. This design is known as the '5/6 design', as it stops when biological activity is seen in five of six patients. Its characteristics, and those of other similar designs appropriate to detect biological activity, have been studied through simulation [32]. This design has 96% probability of escalating if the true proportion of patients with biological activity is 0.9, and 11% probability of escalating if the true proportion of patients with biological activity is 0.4. Two further refinements to this design may be needed in practice:

a. If the starting dose already achieves biological activity in five of six patients, then de-escalation rules can be used, for example: treat cohorts of three patients at decreasing dose levels until biological activity is seen in only 0 or 1 patient, then add three patients at the next higher dose level (unless it is

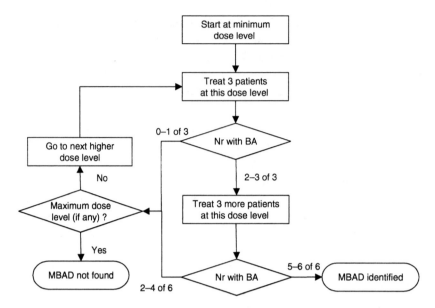

Figure 6.9 Flowchart for biologically based escalation scheme. BA, biological activity; MBAD, minimum biologically active dose.

the starting dose). The dose recommended is, just as in Figure 6.9, the dose for which biological activity is seen in at least five of six patients.

b. A maximum dose level can be prespecified to avoid trials that continue to escalate the dose even though the level of biological activity has reached a plateau under the target level.

The minimum biologically active dose should obviously be sought subject to a toxicity constraint, and therefore the design shown in Figure 6.9 must be used in conjunction with a stopping rule in case the MTD is reached at any of the doses under investigation for biological activity. This design could in fact be used in conjunction with one of the designs discussed above to identify the MTD. At each dose level, one looks for either biological activity or DLT, with the latter prevailing, in such a way that dose escalation stops as soon as the MTD is reached, in case the MTD were in fact lower than the minimum biologically active dose. As mentioned above, it may be difficult to identify an outcome that reliably reflects biological activity, and thus it may be appropriate to use an MTD-driven design to escalate to a maximum dose that is tolerable, with biological effect being a secondary outcome [33]. Under the assumption that the biological activity of the agent is monotonically increasing with dose, this approach would still provide the best chance of testing an appropriate dose of the drug in phase II or III clinical trials. When the outcome for biological activity is valid, however, biologically based escalation designs have the potential of recommending lower doses than would be obtained from MTD-driven designs.

6.11 Randomization and stratification

Phase I trials have seldom used randomization and stratification. Randomization can be considered not only to produce comparable groups, which is generally not required in phase I trials, but also to reduce the opportunity for selection bias whereby patients who enter the trial are selected differently depending on the dose level. For instance, healthier patients could be selected when the dose gets close to the MTD. The up and down design (Section 6.9.2) randomizes the next patient to be treated either at the same dose level or at the next higher dose level. Other randomized schemes could be considered, e.g. as part of a CRM design.

Stratification could also be useful when distinct subsets of patients are known to exist, e.g. 'healthier' patients versus 'sicker' patients. In this case, the stratified CRM (Section 6.8) or isotonic regression (Section 6.9.4) could be used to determine stratum-specific MTDs. Another situation that may become increasingly common is when a subset of patients express a target of interest, but the phase I trial does not have to be limited to that subset. Instead, patients could be stratified based on target expression.

6.12 Phase I/II trials

Even though the purpose of phase I trials is not to test for the antitumour activity of a new therapy, it is of interest to document any signs of activity, which may help in planning further trials with the therapy. Despite the small size of phase I trials, and the heterogeneity of patients treated in such trials, it may be advantageous to pre-specify the signs of activity that are expected, and to quantify the likelihood of observing such activity given the trial's sample size. If the trial has a provision for adding a cohort of patients at the recommended dose, it is of particular interest to look for activity in that expanded cohort of patients, which may for instance comprise 13 patients (three patients initially treated at that dose, plus an additional cohort of 10 patients). If that cohort is enriched or restricted to the patient types that are likely to respond to the agent, it may closely resemble a small phase II trial embedded in the phase I trial, and therefore similar statistical considerations as for phase II trials may be contemplated. It is debatable whether this approach is preferable to running an independent, definitive phase II trial with proper size and clear inclusion criteria. However, considerations of cost and speed may make this approach attractive, in which case it is important to outline explicit plans for it in the trial protocol. The boundary between phase I and II trials is particularly questionable in the development of targeted agents [34].

Assume that activity can be measured by a binary outcome (such as a response in measurable disease by RECIST (Response Evaluation Criteria in Solid Tumours) criteria, a response in a relevant tumour marker, the inhibition of a target, etc.), and call this outcome a 'response'.

6.12.1   No signs of activity

If no response has been seen among n patients treated at the recommended dose, there is 95% confidence that the true response rate does not exceed $1 - \sqrt[n]{0.05}$. More generally, if no sign of activity has been seen among n patients treated at the recommended dose, there is $(1 - c)$% confidence that the true response rate does not exceed $1 - \sqrt[n]{c}$. Table 6.2 shows the response rate that can be excluded with a given confidence if no response has been observed among n patients.

6.12.2   Some signs of activity

More promising is the situation in which some responses are seen among n patients treated at the recommended dose. As n is generally small, the confidence interval of the estimated response rate is too wide to be of much use (in other words, the true response rate is poorly estimated) [35]. Table 6.3

Table 6.2 Response rates that can be excluded with given confidence if no response is seen among n patients

n	95% confidence	90% confidence	80% confidence
10	26%	21%	15%
11	24%	19%	14%
12	23%	18%	13%
13	21%	17%	12%
14	20%	16%	11%
15	19%	15%	11%
16	18%	14%	10%
17	17%	13%	9%
18	16%	12%	9%
19	15%	12%	9%
20	14%	11%	8%
25	12%	9%	7%
30	10%	8%	6%
35	9%	7%	5%
40	8%	6%	4%

Table 6.3 Response rates that can be excluded with given confidence, as a function of the number of patients treated and the number of responses observed

No. of patients	No. of responses	With 90% confidence, the true response rate is	
		at least equal to	at most equal to
10	0	0%	21%
	1	0%	39%
	2	4%	51%
	3	9%	61%
	4	15%	70%
	5	22%	78%
	6	30%	85%
	7	39%	91%
	8	49%	96%
	9	61%	99%
	10	79%	100%
13	0	0%	16%
	1	0%	32%
	2	3%	41%
	3	7%	49%
	4	11%	57%
	5	17%	65%
	6	22%	71%
	7	29%	78%
	8	35%	83%
	9	43%	89%
	10	51%	93%
	11	59%	97%
	12	68%	100%
	13	84%	100%
16	0	0%	13%
	1	0%	26%
	2	2%	34%
	3	5%	42%
	4	9%	48%
	5	13%	55%
	6	18%	61%
	7	23%	67%
	8	28%	72%
	9	33%	77%
	10	39%	82%
	11	45%	87%
	12	52%	91%
	13	58%	95%
	14	66%	98%
	15	74%	100%
	16	87%	100%

provides the exact (binomial) confidence limits of the response rate for various numbers of patients and of responses that are likely to be seen in phase I trials. In practice, early signs of activity are important, but the confidence limits of the observed response rate are not.

In addition to the lack of precision of the estimated response rate, considerations of patient selection, stage of disease, and other known sources of heterogeneity will come into play when assessing the 'response rate' in a phase I trial, as the assessment of such responses is not the primary goal of the trial. Thus, in contrast to phase II trials in which responses are the primary outcome, responses observed in phase I trial are generally anecdotal and not subject to a rigorous statistical assessment, unless the trial protocol has a clear phase II section focused on assessment of the drug's activity.

References

1. http://biostats.upci.pitt.edu/biostats/ClinicalStudyDesign/Phase1Standard.html   [last accessed August 2005]

2. Abbruzzese JL, Grunewald R, Weeks EA, *et al.* (1991). A phase I clinical, plasma, and cellular pharmacology study of gemcitabine. *J Clin Oncol* 9: 491–8.

3. Simon R, Friedlin B, Rubinstein L, *et al.* (1997). Accelerated titration designs for phase I clinical trials in oncology. *J Natl Cancer Inst* 89: 1138–47.

4. Collins JM, Grieshaber CK, Chabner BA (1990). Pharmacologically guided phase I clinical trials based upon preclinical drug development. *J Natl Cancer Inst* 82: 1321–26.

5. Piantadosi S, Liu C (1996). Improved designs for dose escalation studies using pharmacokinetics measurements. *Stat Med* 15: 1605–18.

6. Ratain MJ, Mick R, Schilsky RL, Siegler M (1993). Statistical and ethical issues in the design and conduct of phase I and II clinical trials of new anticancer agents. *J Natl Cancer Inst* 85: 1637–43.

7. Storer BE (2001). An evaluation of phase I clinical trial designs in the continuous dose–response setting. *Stat Med* 20: 2399–408.

8. Reiner E, Paoletti X, O'Quigley J (1999). Operating characteristics of the standard phase I clinical trial design. *Comput Stat Data An* 30: 303–15.

9. O'Quigley J, Pepe M, Fisher L (1990). Continual reassessment method: a practical design for phase I clinical trials in cancer. *Biometrics* 46: 33–48.

10. Goodman SN, Zahurak ML, Piantadosi S (1995). Some practical improvements in the continual reassessment method for phase I studies. *Stat Med* 14: 1149–61.

11. Faries D (1994). Practical modification of the continual reassessment method for phase I cancer clinical trials. *J Biopharm Stat* 4: 147–64.

12. Möller S (1998). An extension of the continual reassessment method using a preliminary up and down design in a dose finding study in cancer patients, in order to investigate a greater range of doses. *Stat Med* 14: 911–22.

13. Piantadosi S, Fisher JD, Grossman S (1998). Practical implementation of a modified continual reassessment method for dose-finding trials. *Cancer Chemother Pharmacol* 41: 429–36.

14. Heyd JM, Carlin BP (1999). Adaptive design improvement in the continual reassessment method for phase I studies. *Stat Med* 18: 1307–21.

15. Chevret S (1993). The continual reassessment method in cancer phase I clinical trials. A simulation study. *Stat Med* 12: 1093–108.

16. Ahn C (1998). An evaluation of phase I cancer clinical trial designs. *Stat Med* 17: 1537–49.

17. Eckhardt S, Siu L, Clark G, *et al.* (1999) The continual reassessment method for dose escalation in phase I trials in San Antonio does not result in more rapid study completion. *Proc Am Soc Clin Oncol* 18: 163.

18. http: //www.cancerbiostats.onc.jhmi.edu/software.cfm [last accessed August 2005]

19. http: //biostatistics.mdanderson.org/SoftwareDownload [last accessed August 2005]

20. Braun TM (2002). The bivariate-continual reassessment method. Extending the CRM to phase I trials of two competing outcomes. *Control Clin Trials* 23: 240–56.

21. Kramar A, Lebecq A, Candalh E (1999). Continual reassessment methods in phase I trials of the combination of two drugs in oncology. *Stat Med* 18: 1849–64.

22. O'Quigley J, Shen LZ, Gamst A (1999). Two-sample continual reassessment method. *J Biopharm Stat* 9: 17–44.

23. O'Quigley J, Sloan LR (1996). Continual reassessment method: A likelihood approach. *Biometrics* 52: 673–84.

24. Muller J, McGinn C, Normolle D, *et al.* (2004). A phase I trial using the time-to-event continual reassessment strategy to escalate cisplatin with gemcitabine and radiation therapy for pancreatic cancer. *J Clin Oncol* 22: 238–43.

25. Storer BE (1998). Phase I Clinical Trials. In: *Encyclopedia of Biostatistics*. Wiley, New York.

26. Storer BE (1989). Design and analysis of phase I clinical trials. *Biometrics* 45: 925–37.

27. Durham SD, Flournoy N, Rosenberger WF (1997). A random walk rule for phase I clinical trials. *Biometrics* 53: 745–60.

28. Babb J, Rogatko A, Zacks S (1998). Cancer Phase I clinical trials: Efficient dose escalation with overdose control. *Stat Med* 17: 1103–20.

29. Leung D, Wang Y (2001). Isotonic designs for phase I trials. *Control Clin Trials* 22: 126–38.

30. Yuan Z, Chappell R (2004). Isotonic designs for phase I cancer clinical trials with multiple risk groups. *Clin Trials* 1: 499–508.

31. Korn EL, Arbuck SG, Pluda JM, *et al.* (2001) Clinical trial designs for cytostatic agents: are new approaches needed? *J Clin Oncol* 19: 265–72.

32. Hunsberger S, Rubinstein LV, Dancey J, Korn EL (2005). Dose escalation trial designs based on a molecularly targeted endpoint. *Stat Med* 24: 2171–81.

33. Korn EL (2004). Nontoxicity endpoints in phase I trial designs for targeted, non-cytotoxic agents. *J Natl Cancer Inst* 96: 997–8.

34. Collins JM (2000). Innovations in phase I trial design: where do we go next? *Clin Cancer Res* 6: 3801–2.

35. Christian MC, Korn EL (1994). The limited precision of phase I trials. *J Natl Cancer Inst* 86: 22.

Chapter 7

Writing the protocol

Elizabeth A. Eisenhauer

7.1 Introduction

A carefully conceived and written protocol document is essential for the conduct of any trial and the phase I trial is no exception. The rationale for the study, the background drug information, the population to be included, the selection of starting dose, how escalation will proceed and the endpoints that will be employed are all vital elements. Furthermore, description of how data will be analysed and decisions made regarding dose escalation and phase II dose recommendation must be included. This chapter will detail and offer examples of all these basic protocol elements for a phase I first-in-man trial. Where relevant, comments on how these elements should be modified for combination phase I trials will be included. Furthermore, Appendix III contains a sample generic protocol document that readers may find useful.

7.2 Outline of the protocol

Table 7.1 shows the major section headings normally found in a phase I protocol. There is no internationally accepted standard protocol template: there are many used that could be followed in writing a phase I protocol and the order of the elements and the exact section headings can vary between them. However, this table is representative of the organization found in many and lists the sections that ought to be included in any protocol. The description of sections that follow will be in the same order as is shown in the table. Individual investigators may wish to shift the order about, which is fine as long

Table 7.1 Elements of the phase I protocol document

Section	Description
Study schema	Summary of the essential elements of the study. This should be simple and logical and reflect the study objectives. It should include highlights of population, treatment plan and follow-up
Background and rationale	For the *disease* (if disease specific trial): description of standard treatment of disease and why the combination of the agents in the phase I trial is justified. Where will it lead?
	For the new *drug*: basic background information on its chemistry, preclinical efficacy, toxicology, pharmacology, and if appropriate, results of other clinical work
Objectives	Describes the primary and secondary objectives of the study
	The primary objective of phase I trial is to define the recommended dose of the new drug when given according to the protocol schedule
Patient population	Inclusion and exclusion criteria should be easily verifiable at the time of patient enrolment. Generally divided into major conceptual categories:
	Criteria regarding the patient status (e.g. performance status, organ function, non-pregnant, etc.)
	Criteria regarding the disease status (e.g. number of prior regimens, nature of prior treatment permitted, time since last treatment)
	Criteria specific to the drug: (e.g. able to swallow oral meds, minimum levels of special studies such as LVEF (Left Venticular Ejection Fraction))
	Criteria specific to the study (e.g. consent obtained for tissue biopsy)

Trial design	Define primary endpoint (usually DLT) Define starting dose Define DLT (or however else escalation will be limited), maximum tolerated dose (or maximum available dose), recommended phase II dose Describe escalation scheme, number of patients per dose level, how decisions about entry on to next level or expansion of dose levels will be determined. Indicate if patient entry on to cohorts will be randomized or assigned
Treatment	Treatment for individual patients. Premedication, postmedication. Retreatment and rules for dose modification
Trial procedures	Tests to be done prior to entry, during treatment, post treatment, and their frequency
Endpoints and evaluation criteria	Primary and secondary endpoints; criteria for evaluation to be used (e.g. CTCAE version 3.0 for toxic effects, RECIST criteria for objective response)
Statistical considerations	Review basic principles of trial design, and describe plans for analysis of clinical data, PK and correlative studies
Pharmacokinetics and correlative studies	Special samples (blood or tissue): how to collect, frequency of collection, how to process and ship
Serious adverse event reporting	What events must be reported and timelines/to whom
Data collection	Describe methods for data collection
Administrative issues	Trial responsibilities, documentation needed before starting, regulatory and ethical requirements. Quality assurance issues
Informed consent	Content must comply with Good Clinical Practice and other applicable regulations. See checklist in Table 7.10
Appendices	Appendices may include measurement scales to be used, more detailed information on laboratory analysis plans for special studies, calendar for case report form submission and reports

as the content remains the same. Content should include: background section on the disease(s) under study, and the drug(s) to be studied as well as information on the inclusion/exclusion criteria, design, treatment plan, study procedures and investigations, endpoints and their assessment, instructions for pharmacokinetics (PK) and other special studies, adverse event reporting, analysis plan, data collection procedures, and sections detailing investigator responsibilities and administrative issues.

7.3 Background information

7.3.1 First-in-man studies

For *first-in-man studies* of new agents, there is not a lengthy *disease*-background section generally included as it is usually the case that these trials enrol patients with a variety of tumour types. If not, and if entry is restricted to patients with only one tumour type, specific background information on that tumour should be included, as outlined below under 'combination phase I trials'.

In contrast, the *drug* background section of phase I first-in-man studies should be sufficiently explicit to justify the *choice of the drug, relevance of its target, starting dose,* and *schedule* to be studied. To be described in separate subsections are:

- *Chemical structure and physical properties of the agent.*
- *General remarks on why this agent is of interest.* For example, is it of novel structure or does it have new target? Is it an analogue of another active drug that overcomes resistance?
- *Description of the molecular target of the drug.* What is its relevance to cancer?; for example: Is it known to be prognostic? Does its inhibition and / or expression alter biological behaviour in preclinical systems? If the agent's target is unknown (and the drug has been selected from an empirical screen for antitumour activity), what studies to elucidate the drug mechanism and target have been undertaken and how are they interpreted?
- *Antitumour efficacy information.* Brief descriptions of the efficacy data that support the study of the agent in human trials must be found in this section. Include information from both *in vitro* and *in vivo* systems. Data on the effects on target vis-à-vis efficacy are important to include if known. Effects of schedule and route of administration should be described. A summary table of the data is useful here.
- *Animal toxicology.* Include the summary of key findings of single dose and repeat dose toxicology studies in two mammalian species. It is important to detail the effects of the toxicology studies that were undertaken using the clinical formulation and the schedule to be tested in patients in the protocol.
- *Preclinical pharmacology.* Provide summaries of the PK studies in animals. Information of importance is the expected half-life and key PK values that relate to efficacy (antitumour *in vivo* effects), target inhibition (which should link with efficacy) and toxicity. Data on protein binding, measured or theoretical effects of other drugs on metabolism and excretion should be

detailed here. If the drug is metabolized by common cytochrome P450 enzyme systems, which may have an impact on permitted concomitant medications, this needs to be highlighted. This section is especially important if there can be inferences made about recommended dose on the basis of PK. Linking a preclinical PK parameter (e.g. steady state above a minimum value for a minimum period of time) with information on *in vivo* efficacy and on inhibition of the molecular target(s) should be described here particularly if it will be used to justify a 'target' plasma level as an endpoint for dose escalation.

◆ *Clinical data.* If other phase I trials have been performed or are ongoing, summarize their results. If those trials are not yet complete, it is still helpful to have information on what the starting dose was and if any toxic effects have been seen up to the dose level for which there is information. If human pharmacology information is available that, too, is important to cite as it may help justify dosing intervals, among other things. Finally, if the drug to be studied is a member of a class that has been evaluated in humans in earlier studies, data from other trials are reasonable to summarize if they will help predict the likely clinical behaviour of the new drug. So for example, one might expect a new anti-sense oligodeoxynucleotide to have toxic effects reminiscent of other drugs of the same chemical structure, even if the target is different.

◆ *Summary and justification of starting dose and schedule.* The background information section should finish with a summary in which key aspects of the preclinical data are reviewed to justify the schedule selected for study and the starting dose in the trial. See Table 7.2 for an example of the steps to follow and the information required to justify the human starting dose. Note that in this example, the agent is an oral tablet, and the starting dose has been converted from mg/m^2 to a flat dose based on average body surface area of an adult ($1.7\,m^2$). This approach is often used when tablet sizes are fixed as precise surface area calculations are not possible.

7.3.2 Combination phase I trials

Combination phase I studies usually evaluate a new agent together with one or more other agents/therapies that are part of the standard of care. They may also be studies in which two or more investigational drugs are combined, though that is a less common scenario. Combination phase I trials are generally disease oriented, or confined to a subset of those conditions in which the 'standard' therapy is given. For example a trial of a new agent + docetaxel could enrol patients with any tumour type for which docetaxel is a

Table 7.2 Human starting dose: Sample justification with fictional agent LTK007

	Outcome	Comment
Mouse single dose oral LD10	1000 mg/kg	Using surface area conversion factor* of 3, this represents 3000 mg/m²
Mouse oral daily × 5 LD10	400 mg/kg daily × 5	This represents 1200 mg/m² Using conversion factor of 3
Dog oral × daily × 5: Toxic dose low	70 mg/kg daily × 5	This represents 1400 mg/m² Using conversion factor of 20
Planned human schedule	Daily × 5	Use the toxicology data of the daily administration in the most sensitive species to calculate human starting dose: in this case mouse
Starting dose	200 mg/day × 5 days (Divide into two equal doses = 100 mg b.i.d.)	1/10th the mouse equivalent LD10 (120 mg/m²) × average surface area of 1.7 = 204 mg flat dose Round to nearest 50 mg (tablet size) = 200 mg

*See conversion factors for commonly used species in Table 3.12, Chapter 3.

reasonable therapeutic option, provided they have not already received that agent. The background section in this type of protocol should include why this combination is of interest (e.g. preclinical synergy studies) as well as most of the other information listed above under first-in-man studies, with the addition of the single agent phase I results (and phase II or III results, if known) of the novel agent to be combined with standard therapy that help justify the combination under evaluation and the doses to be used. If two investigational agents are to be combined, justification of this approach based on appropriate combination animal efficacy and toxicology data must be given.

7.4 Study objectives

The objectives section of the protocol should be concise and divided into two parts: primary and secondary objectives.

The *primary objective* of phase I studies is usually stated as follows: 'To define the recommended dose of [*new agent*] when given in a [*specify route and schedule*]'. Clearly this statement needs modification if combination treatment is being evaluated. There, the primary objective is often stated as 'To determine the dose of [*new agent*] to be used when given in a [*schedule*] together with [*standard therapy*]'.

Secondary objectives list all of the ancillary outcomes that will be assessed. These can include all or some of the following, depending on the agent undergoing evaluation. The standard language usually goes as follows:

- To determine the toxic effects of the new agent and their reversibility, association with dose and PK measures.
- To determine the PK profile of the new agent.
- To measure the effect of the new drug on molecular measures of target effect in [*name tissue*] by [*name assay method*].
- To exploration the relationship between dose or PK measures with toxicity and with changes in molecular measures of target effect (PK–pharmacodynamic effects).
- To establish proof-of-principle for the new agent in inhibiting its target in human tissue.
- To assess preliminary evidence of antitumour effects in those patients with measurable disease by documentation of objective responses using standardized criteria

7.5 Study population

This section of the protocol defines clearly which subjects, usually patients, are to be entered into the study. Some prefer to list all criteria in terms of 'inclusion' criteria, whereas others elect to describe both inclusion and exclusion criteria separately. As noted in Chapter 3, in general first-in-man phase I trials nearly always enrol patients with a cancer diagnosis, although there are some circumstances in which healthy volunteers might be considered. Phase I studies that combine drugs or other cancer therapies with a new agent are always conducted in cancer patients.

- *Example: a first-in-man trial with healthy volunteers as subjects.* For example, a new aromatase inhibitor (anti-oestrogen), intended ultimately for study in breast cancer patients, may undergo a dose-seeking trial in healthy female subjects before it is evaluated in cancer patients. This type of agent is not usually dosed to toxicity; rather measures of plasma oestrogens serve as a surrogate for adequacy of dosing. This type of study is a reasonably safe undertaking for short-term treatment of healthy, non-pregnant subjects. In this example, the inclusion criteria should specify the age range and menopausal status of patients.
- *Example: a first-in-man trial with cancer patients as subjects.* A new oral agent targeted to cyclin-dependent kinases is entering the clinic (fictionally named: LTK007). This agent produces myelosuppression (primarily

neutropenia) and diarrhoea in animal toxicology testing. In the trial, patients with advanced or metastatic solid tumours, incurable with standard measures, are to be entered. The primary endpoint of the trial will be treatment-related toxic effects and secondary endpoints will include assessment of PK, tumour response, and effects on downstream measures of cell cycle in serial tumour biopsies. In this example, patients must have recovered from toxic effects of earlier treatment, be able to swallow oral medications, have baseline chemistry and haematology values within the normal range, and have tumour lesions accessible for repeated biopsies.

Table 7.3 outlines, in the form of a checklist, the major headings to consider in inclusion and exclusion criteria.

7.6 Study design

The design section provides the 'meat' of how the trial will run. Indicate the starting dose (and again state briefly why, reiterating key points from the end of the Background section), how many patients per dose level will be entered and how long they will be followed to assess dose-limiting events, what observation(s) will limit or permit dose escalation, and when and how patients will be enrolled on to the next dose level. It is sometimes a useful strategy to permit an extra patient to be entered on to a dose level in the instance when the cycle-length is very long. In that way, if one of three patients drops out early for disease progression, there is already a patient in place to replace them. If this suggestion is implemented, it must, of course, be included in the protocol as part of the design plan.

This part of the protocol must also describe how the recommended phase II dose will be determined. Note that even if the *plan* is to make dose recommendations and escalation decisions on the basis of *non*-toxicity measures, the protocol must contain a section describing how dose escalation will take into account toxic effects seen in patients. Even those drugs thought to have limited likelihood of significant toxicity, must have protocols written to assure patient safety is considered in making dose escalation and dose recommendation determinations. This section must clearly define the terms to be used in the protocol: maximum administered or maximum tolerated dose, dose-limiting criteria and so on. See Table 3.6 in Chapter 3 for terminology. The highlighted terms found there are used in this book.

Table 7.4 and the addendum to this chapter give subject headings and a worked example, respectively, of a design section with the fictitious cyclin-dependent kinase inhibitor, LTK007, mentioned earlier. This section may also

Table 7.3 Major headings for inclusion and exclusion criteria

			Example	Timing
Inclusion	Tumour type		Solid tumours	
	Disease extent		Incurable by standard therapy. Must have evidence of disease clinically or radiographically (disease identified only by serum marker is not allowed)	
	Prior therapy	Chemotherapy	Up to 3 prior chemotherapy regimens	≥4 weeks since last dose
		Radiation therapy	Permitted Must have recovered from toxicity	≥4 weeks since last fraction, unless palliative low dose
		Surgery	Permitted	≥4 weeks since last major surgery
		Hormone therapy	Permitted	
	Age		≥18 years	
	Performance status		ECOG performance status 0, 1, or 2	Within 7 days prior to study
	Haematology		Absolute granulocyte count $\geq 1.5 \times 10^9/l$ Absolute platelet count $\geq 100 \times 10^9/l$	
	Biochemistry		AST (Aspartate aminotransferase) $<2 \times$ upper limit of normal (ULN) Serum bilirubin <ULN Serum creatinine <ULN	
	Cardiac		Left ventricular ejection fraction (by MUGA scan or echocardiogram)	
	Pregnancy test	In women of childbearing potential	Serum pregnancy test negative	
	Consent		Written Informed consent prior to patient entry. Consent form used	

(Continued)

Table 7.3 *Continued*

		Example	Timing
Inclusion (cont'd)		must be approved by the appropriate ethical committee.	
	Availability for follow-up	Patients must be available and willing to undergo study procedures at the treating centre	
Exclusion	Concomitant therapy	Patients undergoing simultaneous therapy with other anticancer agents: standard or investigational	
	Allergy	Patients with any prior allergy to the class of medication to be given	
	Serious illness	Patients with concurrent serious medical illness such as congestive heart failure, active serious infection, etc.	
	Able to take medication	Patients must be able to swallow the oral investigational agent under study	

Table 7.4 Design section (see worked example in Addendum to this chapter)

(a) Subject headings

1. Starting dose/route: What is it and how is it justified?

2. Dose escalation: What are the planned dose escalation steps? A table is most useful. Remember to include a −1 dose level as the starting dose may be too high! Also include reference to allow intermediate dose levels

3. Methods:

How will dose escalation proceed? What is minimum number of patients per dose level? How will patients be entered on each dose level (assigned or randomized). On what basis (end-points) will dose escalation, reduction, expansion take place? How long will each cohort be followed before decisions about next step (to expand, escalate, reduce) is taken? Who will make decisions? When/how will patients be replaced if they do not complete the required observation period? Will intrapatient dose escalation be allowed?

4. Definitions:

Define the following for your protocol

- ◆ *Maximum administered dose (MAD)* (or maximum tolerated dose; MTD)
- ◆ *Dose-limiting toxicity* (applicable when toxic effects *is planned* to limit escalation) *or*
- ◆ *Dose-limiting pharmacokinetic measures*: (applicable when pharmacokinetic measure such as steady-state concentration *is planned* to limit escalation) *or*
- ◆ *Dose-limiting biologic measures:* (applicable when molecular measurement of drug effect *is planned* to limit escalation)
- ◆ *Recommended phase II dose*: how the recommended dose will be established. Note here if there is a planned expansion of this dose level to gain further information on its safety or other parameters; *this step is highly recommended for all trials.*

describe how long patients should receive therapy and what conditions would lead to discontinuation of study drug (e.g. progression, toxicity), but this is more commonly found in the treatment section below.

7.7 Treatment

This part of the protocol document describes in detail the treatment to be given to each patient. Although the dose level will be assigned when the patient enters the study, the premedication, postmedication, and dose adjustments must be outlined. What is written must be consistent with the design section and the definition of dose-limiting toxicity: that is, adverse events that would be considered *dose limiting* in the Design section must lead to *dose reduction or discontinuation* in the Treatment section. The converse need not always apply; that is, events leading to dose reduction may not always be considered dose limiting, but this should be well thought through. The inability to deliver drug (particularly in the first cycle or treatment period) because of toxic effects requiring dose reduction, may mean that the dose being administered is too high. Internal consistency between the dose reduction plan and the definition(s) of dose-limiting toxicity is important.

The number of cycles (or total treatment duration) allowed, and rules for stopping treatment (maximum number of cycles, adverse events, and/or disease progression) must be described. Dose reduction steps should, ideally, be the same as the dose levels. That is, patients requiring a dose reduction in a cycle should be treated at a lower dose level (dose levels same as in the Design section), rather than simply with a percentage decrease in dose. Table 7.5 gives an example.

Although many cancer drugs were historically dosed in 'cycles' of therapy, i.e. a treatment period followed by a rest and observation period, some new agents, particularly oral drugs, are being given continuously. In the first phase I trial of such agents, consideration can be given to having the duration of therapy in the entire trial or in the first dose levels of the trial be a finite period (e.g. 7 days) rather than administer continuous drug treatment from the first patient treated. This is done in order to assure there are no surprises in cumulative toxic effects or pharmacological measures, etc. There are several examples of some drugs that are now given continuously in phase II and III trials where the first phase I trial used an interrupted schedule (e.g. 7 days on/7 days off) until safety was established and PK understood. This approach is empirical, however, and if toxicology supports continuous daily dosing, there is no requirement to consider shorter periods of treatment in the first human trial.

Another issue with continuous dosing regimens, be they intravenous (e.g. weekly treatment) or oral (e.g. daily treatment) is how to, or even if to, define a

Table 7.5 Examples: dose adjustment
Haematological adverse events (for an intravenous agent)

	Nadir counts			
	Absolute granulocytes (× 10^9/l)		**Platelets (× 10^9/l)**	**Dose drug next cycle**
Day 1 dose adjustments	≥0.5	AND	≥25	No change
	<0.5 for <5 days	AND	≥25	No change
	<0.5 for ≥5 days or neutropenic infection or febrile neutropenia	OR	<25 or thrombocytopenic bleeding	reduce 1 dose level
	Treatment day counts			
	Absolute granulocytes (× 10^9/l)		**Platelets (× 10^9/l)**	**Dose drug this cycle**
	≥1.5	AND	≥100	Treat on time; no change in dose
	<1.5	OR	<100	Hold until recovery. Adjust dose level according to nadir counts as above. If no recovery after 2 weeks, patient should be removed from protocol therapy

Another example for chronic oral dosing

Grade of event	Management/next dose
≤ grade 1	Symptomatic—no change in dose
Grade 2	Hold until ≤ grade 1—resume at same dose
Grade 3	Hold* until < grade 2—resume at 1 dose level lower if indicated†
Grade 4	Off protocol therapy

*Patients requiring a delay of > 2 weeks should go off protocol therapy.
†Patients requiring > 2 dose reductions should go off protocol therapy.

'cycle' or 'treatment period'. The advantage of arbitrarily defining a cycle as, for example, a 4-week period of therapy, is that the concept is well ingrained and it defines periods of time around which investigations can be conducted. It is clear that this is an artificial concept in this setting, so it is up to investigators and sponsors whether they take this approach.

Another practical issue is how to handle dose reductions in the setting of a split dose treatment. Treating a patient on days 1, 8, and 15 of a 28-day cycle is an example: here, in order to preserve the planned dosing intervals in the face of toxicity, usually dose reductions on days 8 and 15 are advised and, if toxicity prohibits restarting treatment on day 1 of the next cycle, it is delayed until recovery and the dose for all days on that cycle adjusted depending on the magnitude and nature of the toxic effects incurred.

7.8 Trial procedures

This protocol section describes the tests to be done before entry, as well as during and after treatment. Those to be done before entry must be consistent with the inclusion/exclusion criteria. If for example, a minimum creatinine level is required for patient entry, then serum creatinine must be one of the specified pre-study tests. The converse need not be true; not all baseline tests must be matched to an entry criterion. Thus, radiological studies may be required at baseline to document any measurable disease even though the presence of measurable disease is not an eligibility criterion. Pretreatment and on-treatment investigations are usually summarized in a table, an example of which is found in Table 7.6. Poststudy testing is usually quite abbreviated in phase I trials: generally a patient is brought back for assessment 4 weeks after completing therapy and thereafter follow-up ceases, except to report late toxic effects.

7.9 Endpoints

As noted, toxic effects (adverse events) are one of the most important phase I trial endpoints as they represent the primary endpoint in many cases. Even if not a primary endpoint, assessment of adverse events is an essential component of first-in-man and combination phase I trials. Other important trial endpoints include objective response, measures of PK, measures of molecular effects of drug in normal or tumour tissue (including proof of concept studies), and functional imaging studies of drug effects. This section of the protocol should describe the standard criteria that will be used to document the major trial measurements. If measures are being studied for which there are no reference standards (often the case when investigational molecular measures or functional imaging studies are undertaken), the methods to be used to categorize or quantify these measures should be recorded here, or in a methodology appendix.

7.9.1 Adverse events

Regardless of whether toxicity is the primary endpoint of the phase I trial, assessment of toxic effects, or more properly, adverse events, is of paramount importance. For new agents, the description of drug-related adverse events begins in the first-in-man phase I trial; however, because of the small sample

Table 7.6 Example: pretreatment and on-treatment investigations table

Required investigations	Pre-study timing	*Indicate*	*frequency*	*on study*	*here*
Physical Physical exam Blood pressure, heart rate					
Haematology CBC and differential Coagulation studies: PTT, INR					
Biochemistry AST, bilirubin, creatinine, alkaline phosphatase, albumin, calcium Electrolytes (Na+, K+, Cl−)					
Radiology* CT scan chest and abdomen Other imaging studies as indicated clinically					
Other investigations Serum marker studies 24-hour urine collection					
Special investigations Blood sampling for pharmacokinetic assays Skin biopsies for special translational studies *Adverse events* Assessed using CTCAE version 3.0					

*Patients with a CR or PR should have scans repeated after 4 weeks to confirm response.

size of these studies the listing of toxic effects may not be complete and will undoubtedly be broadened as the drug moves to later phases of investigation. Furthermore, it may not be clear when adverse events take place whether or not they are truly drug related unless they have been predicted by animal studies. Those events comprised of subjective symptoms (e.g. nausea, fatigue, myalgia) cannot be predicted by animal studies and may be disease-related so particular care is needed in writing the protocol to make it clear that *all* adverse events must be documented so that, with time and more complete dose-level information, there will be an opportunity to sift through the data to identify what seem most likely to be drug related. This requirement to record adverse events means that there must be a standard set of criteria used to describe and grade them, that the date of onset relative to treatment must be captured, and that an investigator-declared relationship of the event to study treatment should also be recorded.

7.9.2 Standard toxicity criteria

'Toxicity criteria' describe adverse events in categories and grades with grade 0 meaning 'normal' or 'none' and grade 4 meaning life-threatening toxicity. Although the WHO criteria were created first [1] these have been supplanted in most cancer settings by the Common Toxicity Criteria (CTC) developed by the US National Cancer Institute. The original version of the CTC contained 49 toxicity terms grouped into 18 categories. Modifications have added new terms to categorize new effects of treatment and to allow for more comprehensive reporting. In 1998 version 2.0 of the CTC was launched and in 2003 version 3.0 of the criteria (now called Common Terminology Criteria for Adverse Events or CTCAE) was launched (see link to this document in Appendix I). This version contains over 200 adverse event terms (no longer called 'toxicities') grouped into 28 categories. Included as adverse event terms are toxic effects of treatment, symptoms of disease or other medical events as well as objective findings (such as chemistry and haematology results). A phase I protocol should require patients to have a *baseline assessment* to document symptoms or residual toxic effects from previous treatment and then periodic assessments of toxicity over the course of the therapy. In general, toxicity is recorded as the worst grade for each effect for each patient in each reporting interval. In phase I trials, the summary report should include a description of toxic effects by *dose level* by either patient, or cycle, or both.

7.9.3 Response criteria

Although objective tumour response is not the primary outcome of phase I trials, it is often a secondary outcome measure. *Tumour response* refers to the description of objective change in measured tumour lesions during the course of therapy. As for toxic effects, criteria for response in solid tumours were first developed in the 1970s to standardize the description of clinical trial outcomes. The World Health Organization Criteria were the most commonly utilized for many years [1], but because many academic groups and pharmaceutical firms had developed their own interpretations of the non-explicit aspects of these criteria and had adapted them for their own use, they were no longer a common standard and this led to confusion in interpretation of trial results [2]. In response to these problems, an International Working Party was formed in the mid-1990s to standardize and simplify response criteria. New criteria, known as the RECIST criteria (*Response Evaluation Criteria in Solid Tumors*), were published in 2000 [3]. Like earlier sets of criteria, RECIST response assessment requires baseline measurement of malignant lesions and then periodic re-evaluations to determine the maximal degree of shrinkage (if any) or growth of the overall tumour burden. Unlike earlier criteria in which tumour assessments were based on the mathematical sum of products of bidimensional measurable lesions, the RECIST criteria define measurable disease on the basis of only a single diameter and determine the tumour burden by summing the longest diameters of measurable lesions. This switch was based on both theoretical considerations as well as actual data and simplifies the process of response calculation. Like the WHO criteria before it, RECIST defines four main response categories: complete response, partial response, stable diseased, and progressive disease (see Table 7.7 for definitions). The protocol section describing assessment of objective response must comply with these guidelines. The US National Cancer Institute's Cancer Therapy Evaluation Program (CTEP) has developed a protocol section to incorporate in trials that employ RECIST as a tool for investigators (see web link in Appendix I). The text found at this source may be 'cut and pasted' into the protocol document's section on Endpoints when RECIST criteria are used.

Given the nature of the patient population in most phase I trials, solid tumour response criteria are the most likely to be employed to assess this secondary endpoint, but there are also standard criteria for non-Hodgkin's lymphoma [4], acute myeloid leukaemia [5], malignant glioma [6], and for tumour marker response such as PSA and CA-125 [7,8]. If the phase I population is confined to one tumour type in which RECIST are not appropriate criteria, the relevant response criteria should be used. Table 7.8 supplies a quick reference list of criteria for reporting response in various circumstances.

Objective response is generally utilized as a primary endpoint only in phase II studies where it can provide an objective measure from which decisions can be taken regarding further study of the drug or regimen. However, it is often a secondary endpoint in phase I trials: in first-in-man studies the observation of responses in even a few patients may help direct future development decisions for the drug. In combination phase I trials, the use of known active therapies in conjunction with a new drug implies that responses are expected and in these trials sometimes documentation of response is sufficiently important to what might happen next with the combination that patient entry is, in fact, restricted to those in whom measurable disease is present so that response can be assessed in all patients.

Table 7.7 Response definitions by RECIST criteria [3]

Target lesions	Non-target lesions	New lesions	Overall best response	Best response for this category also requires
CR	CR	No	CR	≥4 weeks confirmation
CR	Non-CR/non-PD	No	PR	≥4 weeks confirmation
PR	Non-PD	No	PR	≥4 weeks confirmation
SD	Non-PD	No	SD	Documented at least once ≥4 wks. from baseline
PD	Any	Yes or No	PD	No prior SD, PR, or CR
Any	PD*	Yes or No	PD	No prior SD, PR, or CR
Any	Any	Yes	PD	No prior SD, PR, or CR

*In exceptional circumstances, unequivocal progression in non-target lesions may be accepted as disease progression.

Note: Patients with a global deterioration of health status requiring discontinuation of treatment without objective evidence of disease progression at that time should be reported as 'symptomatic deterioration'. Every effort should be made to document the objective progression even after discontinuation of treatment.

Reproduced with permission.

Table 7.8 Selected standard response criteria

Site	Standard response criteria	Reference number
Solid tumours	RECIST: Therasse P, J Natl Cancer Institute, 2000	[3]
	WHO: Miller AB, Cancer, 1981	[1]
Non-Hodgkin's lymphomas	Cheson BD, J Clin Oncol, 1999	[4]
Acute myeloid leukaemia	Cheson BD, J Clin Oncol, 2003	[5]
Brain tumours	Macdonald DR, J Clin Oncol, 1990	[6]
CA125 response (ovarian cancer)	GCIG criteria: Rustin GJ, J Natl Cancer Inst, 2004	[8]
PSA response criteria (prostate cancer)	Bubley GJ, J Clin Oncol, 1999	[7]

7.9.4 Other endpoints

Other measures used in phase I trials, such as those for laboratory measures of target effect, PK, and functional imaging, are described in the relevant protocol sections for those tests where both methodology and endpoints should be detailed.

7.10 Statistical considerations: design and analysis

This section reiterates the major features of the trial design and indicates how the clinical data from the trial will be tabulated and analysed. Any statistical tests to be done on the clinical, PK, or correlative assay data should be described here. In general, formal statistical comparisons between dose groups are discouraged as in the typical phase I trial, these are small cohorts and non-randomized. However, within patient comparisons of data such as before/after biopsy results, or PK assessment at two different time points, may be more formally compared. It is preferred that if formal testing is to be done, this should be confined to one or two variables, and be prespecified in the protocol. Statistical tests should not be applied *post-hoc* once results are reviewed to avoid problems of multiple comparisons and data-driven analysis. If the phase I trial is one in which there is randomization between dose levels (such as in phase Ib trials conducted after the first-in-man study is completed), comparisons between dose groups is permitted, but it must be remembered that the cohort size must be large enough to allow adequate power to undertake such comparisons. Once again, such comparisons, if planned, should be described prospectively in this protocol section.

7.11 Pharmacokinetics

This important section of the protocol describes the measurement of PK (the study of drug absorption, distribution, metabolism, and/or excretion). Chapter 9 describes the principles of PK evaluation in great detail. Here we consider the information that must be supplied in the protocol:

7.11.1 Sample collection

Although information on sample collection should appear in the overall table of study tests, in this protocol section a more detailed set of sampling instructions should be provided. Details of how much blood is to be taken, in what type of tube or container, at what intervals before and after drug administration, and how it is to be handled, processed, and stored should be explicitly stated. Be sure that it is clear what 'time Zero' is for the table describing PK collection. Information on where the samples are to be shipped should be clearly indicated.

7.11.2 Pharmacokinetic assay methods

If necessary, the methods for PK analysis can be added in this section, attached as an appendix, or simply referred to if previously published.

7.11.3 Pharmacokinetic data analysis

The methods for analysis of the data should be described here, including the modelling to be used and how summary information by dose level will be generated.

7.12 Correlative or translational studies

Many phase I studies will incorporate special assays in normal tissue (e.g. peripheral blood mononuclear cells, skin, buccal mucosa) or in fresh tumour tissue. The purpose of the assays may vary and should be clearly stated in the preamble to this section. For example, it may be the case that measures undertaken will be used to determine the effect of drug on downstream measures of target inhibition. Alternatively the results of such test may be intended as 'proof-of-concept' or 'proof-of-principle': i.e. indicate that, at least in some patients, the drug is having its intended molecular target effect (e.g. inhibition of tyrosine kinase phosphorylation). Following the statement of purpose, this section of the protocol must detail the procedures to be undertaken:

7.12.1 Tissue sampling

Describe the type of tissue (e.g. peripheral blood mononuclear cells, buccal mucosa, tumour), how it is to be biopsied or sampled, including the type of biopsy permitted (e.g. fine needle aspirate, core biopsy, open biopsy), how much tissue is to be taken (for blood samples, the volume and type of tube), how it is to be processed, fixed, and stored. Clear labelling and shipping instructions should be provided. The frequency of sampling should also be addressed. If a separate consent form is needed, that should be clearly indicated (see example in Appendix III).

7.12.2 Assay methods

Describe the assay method to be used and in which lab it will be undertaken. Options may include assays that are immunohistochemically based, those that quantify protein or gene expression, those that are functional and more. Indicate here what the controls will be (usually reference tissues of known characteristics) and how results will be quantified, if applicable. Sources of critical reagents such as antibodies, gene array chips, etc. should be specified. Furthermore, references should be supplied, if available, for the assay development and validation. If the assay was used in the preclinical assessment of the drug, that is important to note, as it will be of interest to contrast the clinical results with those predicted from animal models.

7.12.3 Assay results and analysis

The plan of analysis should be described. How will summary data be presented? How will relationships between dose, PK variables, and assay output be described? Will within-patient results be displayed (e.g. before/after treatment). How will these be described? Is there an a priori critical level or change in expression of a key marker that will be sought?

7.13 Serious adverse events

'Serious' adverse events are those that require hospitalization (or prolong existing hospitalization), lead to death or disability. The criteria for an event to be labelled serious are found in Table 7.9. These are transcribed from the International Conference on Harmonization (ICH) and may be subject to slight modification in various jurisdictions. Serious adverse events usually require special reporting mechanisms; and those that are deemed to be drug-related and unexpected (serious unexpected adverse drug reactions) must be reported in strict timelines to the relevant government regulatory authority and the ethics committee responsible(s) for a trial. Expected events are those that have been seen in clinical trials in the past and are recorded in the Investigator Brochure (and should thus be in the consent form). As first-in-man

Table 7.9 ICH Definition of serious for adverse event reporting*

A serious adverse event is any untoward medical occurrence that:	Comments
Results in death	
Is life threatening	The term 'life-threatening' in the definition of serious refers to an event in which the patient was at risk of death at the time of the event; it does *not* refer to an event which hypothetically might have caused death if it were more severe
Requires inpatient hospitalization or prolongation of existing hospitalization	
Results in persistent or significant disability/incapacity	
Is a congenital abnormality/birth defect	
Other important medical events	Medical and scientific judgement should be exercised in deciding whether expedited reporting is appropriate in other situations, such as important medical events that may not be immediately life-threatening or result in death or hospitalization but may jeopardize the patients or may require intervention to prevent one of the other outcomes listed in definition. These should also usually be considered serious (e.g. intensive emergency room treatment for bronchospasm; blood dyscrasias, or convulsions)

*From ICH Harmonized Tripartite Guideline: Clinical Safety Data Management: Definitions and Standards for Expedited Reporting E2A. See Appendix I.

phase I trials are administering a new drug for the first time, any serious event is, by definition, 'unexpected' as there is no clinical experience with the agent. All protocols must have a section detailing what the definition of serious adverse events and serious adverse drug reactions are and how/to whom to report them. Many cancer trial protocols are written in a way so as to exclude from the 'serious' definition those hospitalizations that are scheduled for trial-related procedures or for terminal cancer care after progressive disease.

7.14 Data collection

This section will describe the process of data collection; for example, on case report forms, or by electronic data capture. The frequency and type of data collection may be included in a table in this section or as a protocol appendix. Methods for collating data and programs used to compile and analyse it for reporting purposes can also be described.

7.15 Administrative issues

This section describes important practical and quality control information:

7.15.1 Trial sponsorship

Indicate who has legal responsibility for the overall conduct of the study: i.e. who is the trial sponsor (see also Chapter 8).

7.15.2 Pre-trial documentation

List the documents required before the/any institution may begin to enrol patients in the study. At a minimum these must include full ethical approval of the final protocol and consent form(s) by a properly constituted committee, approval of the protocol by the relevant government authority, collection of the investigator statements and curriculum vitae as required by regulations. Confidentiality and other agreements, such as contractual arrangements, will also need to be in place (see Chapter 8 for details).

7.15.3 Investigator responsibilities

Usually these are taken from GCP but should be articulated here. Other types of trial personnel should be described if appropriate.

7.15.4 Ethics process

The protocol must indicate the nature of ethics review required for the protocol and amendments as well as how the ethics committee should be constituted. Compliance with relevant local and national standards is a must.

7.15.5 Patient entry

Practical information about how patients will be entered (e.g. via telephone registration, web-based process or other) are to be described here.

7.15.6 Quality control

Measures that will be used to assure the accuracy of the clinical data collection are detailed in this section. On-site monitoring plans, audits, central review of any data, etc. should be indicated.

7.16 Consent form

A sample consent form should be part of any multicentre protocol as it will be modified according to local criteria for ethical committee review. If the study is a single centre trial, the consent form included in this section of the protocol will be the version that will be submitted for ethical review. The consent form should use simple language to describe the purpose of the study and the measures and treatments that will be undertaken. If possible, it should be available in all the language(s) of the patients who will be enrolled. If this is not the case, and a translator is needed for the informed consent process, the form (and medical record) for the patient should document this and include the signature of the translator. Check with the relevant ethics committee responsible for a checklist of items that must be included. Table 7.10 lists the elements of a consent form as stipulated by GCP (Appendix I contains direct web links to GCP and other ICH documents). Depending on the local requirements, extra research investigations such as tumour biopsy studies may be part of the main study consent form or separate documents. If such special studies are *required* to be undertaken in all patients enrolled in the trial, it makes most sense to include the relevant details in the main trial consent document. When such studies are optional, some institutions ask that there be a separate consent form so patients can decide independently if they wish to take part. The advantage of this latter approach is that the processes and consents for the study and any optional substudies are clearly demarcated. The disadvantage if that if there are two consent forms, some ethics committees require that both contain all the required ICH-GCP elements, meaning there is a great deal of redundancy in the second form, as it repeats much of the same information found in the first.

7.17 Appendices

Protocol appendices may contain a variety of items that don't 'fit' easily elsewhere. For example, toxicity and response criteria can appear as appendices as can performance status definitions. Case report form submission

Table 7.10 Checklist for Informed Consent Document (ICH Good Clinical Practice)

Element	Comments for phase I (note: ICH refers to 'subjects'; this table has substituted 'patients')
The trial involves research	The opening statement should be an acknowledgement of the patient's illness and state of disease 'I understand I have a cancer that is no longer curable with standard treatments' and give the background about the new agent, why it is being tested (it has shown promise in studies of animal cancers) and, for first-in-man studies, acknowledge it has never before been given to patients with cancer.
The purpose of the trial	The purpose is to define the recommended dose of the new agent, document its toxic effects, and other purposes as defined by goals of the protocol.
What are the trial 'treatments'	Caution regarding use of the word 'treatment' since it implies efficacy. 'Investigational Agent' or 'Investigational Drug' are preferred. Consent form must be clear that the dose will be increased during the course of the study, so the dose for each new patient is assigned when they go on the trial. The form should indicate what will determine how high the dose goes (toxicity or something else).
Trial procedures to be followed; including all invasive procedures.	Sometimes a separate page showing the schema or list of tests is helpful to the patient.
Patient's responsibilities	The consent form should state that the patient understands he/she must return to the treating centre to undergo assessments and tests as described.
Those aspects of the trial that are experimental.	The drug itself is experimental.
The foreseeable risks or inconveniences	For first-in-man studies, the list of possible effects comes from the toxicology. It is also useful to include a statement that 'other serious unforeseen effects besides those listed may result from treatment, since this is the first time this drug has been given to humans'. State what will happen in event of toxicity (decrease or discontinue drug) in general terms. Include a statement that patients will be informed of new serious or frequent toxic effects that arise during the course of the trial.
The reasonably expected benefits	Benefit cannot be promised, or implied as likely, in a first-in-man study. It is reasonable to state that the possibility of benefit may exist, but it is unlikely and unknown if it will occur. If a figure is needed, the overall rate of tumour regression (usually temporary) in trials such as this is about 5%.

(Continued)

Table 7.10 *Continued*

Element	Comments for phase I (note: ICH refers to 'subjects'; this table has substituted 'patients')
The alternative treatments available to the patient	State what they are. If applicable, include a statement that no further active cancer therapy is an option.
The compensation and/or treatment for trial-related injury.	State here if the patient's care will/will not be covered in the event of adverse events requiring treatment. State if other 'compensation' for injury is available
Payment to the subject	Although healthy volunteers are often reimbursed, patients are not.
Anticipated expenses	Patients should be made aware if participating in the trial means extra costs such as travel, parking, hotel stays, meals etc. and if those costs are covered in any way.
Voluntary participation	Participation is entirely voluntary and patients may withdraw, without penalty or loss of benefits to which they are otherwise entitled, at any time.
Access to records	State who will see information concerning their case (on forms) and who may review their medical records (e.g. pharmaceutical company, government auditor), and that such individuals/groups observe strict confidentiality.
Confidentiality	Records on the patients will be kept confidential. In any publication, their identity will not be revealed.
New information	New information arising which might be relevant to the patient's decision to continue therapy will be made available: in phase I trials this generally means new toxicity information.
Contacts	Who to contact for further information, for discussion of the rights of trial subjects, in event of injury.
Study duration	When/how/why will study drug be stopped. How long will the study and the follow-up be.
Number of patients planned for the trial	Estimate numbers needed to finalize dose recommendation.

schedule, a telephone/contact list and the consent form itself may also all appear as appendices. In general the appendices should contain 'reference' items to facilitate the study conduct, but should not contain the critical elements without which the study could not be completed.

References

1. Miller AB , Hoogstraten B, Staquet M, Winkler A (1981). Reporting results of cancer treatment. *Cancer* 47: 207–14.
2. Baar J, Tannock I (1989). Analyzing the same data in two ways: a demonstration model to illustrate the reporting and misreporting of clinical trials. *J Clin Oncol* 7: 969–78.
3. Therasse P, Arbuck SG, Eisenhauer EA, *et al.* (2000). New guidelines to evaluate the response to treatment in solid tumors (RECIST Guidelines). *J Natl Cancer Inst* 92: 205–16.
4. Cheson BD, Horning SJ, Coiffier B, *et al.* (1999). Report of an international workshop to standardize response criteria for non-Hodgkin's lymphomas. NCI Sponsored International Working Group. *J Clin Oncol* 17: 1244–53.
5. Cheson B, Bennett JM, Kopecky KJ, *et al.* (2003). Revised recommendations of the International Working Group for diagnosis, standardization of response criteria, treatment outcomes, and reporting standards for therapeutic trials in acute myeloid leukemia. *J Clin Oncol* 15: 4642–9.
6. Macdonald DR, Cascino TL, Schold SC Jr, Cairncross JG (1990). Response criteria for phase II studies of supratentorial malignant glioma. *J Clin Oncol* 8: 1277–80.
7. Bubley GJ, Carducci M, Dahut W, *et al.* (1999). Eligibility and response guidelines for phase II trials in androgen-independent prostate cancer: recommendations form the prostate specific antigen working group. *J Clin Oncol* 17: 3461–7.
8. Rustin GJ, Quinn M, Thigpen T, *et al.* (2004). Re: new guidelines to evaluate response to treatment in solid tumors (ovarian cancer). *J Natl Cancer Inst* 96: 487–8.

Addendum Design section: worked example with fictional agent LTK007

Starting dose

The starting dose of LTK007 will be 100 mg p.o. b.i.d. × 5 days every 28 days. (LTH = Licensed to Kill.) This dose is based on animal toxicology (see Protocol Section XX) and represents one-tenth the mouse equivalent LD10 (MELD10) dosage in the daily oral schedule.

Dose escalation

The dose of LTK007 will be escalated in increments according to the dose escalation scheme outlined in the following table.

Dose level	Dose of LTK007 given orally, twice daily × 5 days every 28 days (total daily dose)	Minimum no. of patients
−1	75 mg b.i.d. (150 mg total)	−
1 (starting)	100 mg b.i.d. (200 mg total)	3
2	200 mg b.i.d. (400 mg total)	3
3	400 mg b.i.d. (800 mg total) Continue to double dose until grade 2 toxicity related to drug is seen at level 'n', then begin escalation as shown below. Round calculated dose to nearest 50 mg	3
$n + 1$	$1.4 \times n$	3
$n + 2$	$1.4 \times n + 1$ Continue escalating at $1.4 \times$ preceding dose until MTD	3 etc.

Intermediate dose levels or further splitting of the total dose into t.i.d. or q.i.d. dosing may occur dependent on emerging safety information and/or pharmacokinetic data if available.

Methods

The rate of subject entry and escalation to the next dose level will depend upon assessment of the safety profile of patients entered at the previous dose level. Toxicity will be evaluated according to the NCI Common Terminology Criteria for Adverse Events (CTCAE), Version 3.0 (see Appendix IIIa).

A minimum of three patients will be entered on each dose level. All three will be followed for one completed cycle of therapy (28 days) and subsequent enrolment of new cohorts will be based on the toxicity assessment in that first cycle and the documentation of any dose-limiting toxicities (for definitions see below). The investigator and subinvestigators will review all the data of each cohort together by teleconference with the study sponsor before making a decision regarding the next steps to be taken.

Intrapatient dose escalation is permitted as described below.

Definitions

Maximum tolerated dose

1. *If none of three patients exhibit dose-limiting toxicity (DLT) at this dose level:*

    ♦ dose escalation to the *next* dose level may begin in a *new* cohort of patients

- patients enrolled on the *previous* dose level who are still receiving therapy may now undergo intrapatient dose escalation to *this* dose level provided they have experienced no drug-related toxicity grade 2 or more.

2. *If one of three patients exhibit DLT at this dose level:*
   - expand dose level to a total of six patients
   - if no further DLT events seen, dose escalation to the *next* dose level may begin in a *new* cohort of patients and patients enrolled on the *previous* dose level who are still receiving therapy may now undergo intrapatient escalation to *this* dose level provided they have experienced no drug-related toxicity grade 2 or more
   - if one or more further DLT events are seen (i.e. two or more of six patients), this dose level will be considered the MTD.

3. *If two of three patients exhibit DLT:*
   - This dose level will be considered the MTD.

Before opening the next higher dose level all toxic effects at the preceding dose level will be reviewed and expansion or escalation will be undertaken as appropriate. Conference calls between investigators and sponsor will be organized.

Dose-limiting toxicity

Toxicity will be graded using CTCAE version 3.0 (see Appendix XX). Any DLT must be a toxicity that is considered related to study drug. DLT is defined as follows.

During cycle 1

1. *Haematological*
   - absolute granulocyte count (AGC) $< 0.5 \times 10^9/l$
   - febrile neutropenia (ANC $< 1.0 \times 10^9/l$ with fever $> 38.5°C$)
   - platelets $< 25 \times 10^9/l$
   - bleeding due to thrombocytopenia

2. *Non-haematological*
   - diarrhoea $\geq$ grade 3 despite use of antidiarrhoeal medication
   - rash $\geq$ grade 3 (or grade 2 if it is medically concerning or unacceptable to the patient)
   - other grade 3 organ effects thought to be treatment related
   - missing >2 doses of treatment for toxicity reasons.

Recommended phase II dose

As described above, the MTD is that dose in which two of three or two of six patients experience DLT.

Normally *one dose level below* that dose will be considered the recommended phase II dose. If the MTD is seen at the starting dose level, then dose level '−1' will be the recommended dose.

If clinically appropriate, intermediate dose levels may be studied to assure that the recommended dose is the highest tolerable. Further, if pharmacokinetic data suggests that saturable absorption of drug is occurring on a b.i.d. oral administration level, further dose splitting to t.i.d. or q.i.d. schedules may be considered if DLT has not been seen.

Up to a total of 10 patients may be treated at the recommended dose to ensure information on the safety profile at that dose is complete.

Patient replacement

Three patients within a dose level must be observed for one cycle (28 days) before accrual to the next higher dose level may begin. If a patient is withdrawn from the study prior to completing 5 days of therapy and a further 17 days of follow-up without experiencing a DLT prior to withdrawal, an additional patient may be added to that dose level. Patients missing two or more doses due to toxicity will not be replaced as these patients will be considered to have experienced a DLT

Chapter 8

Before you begin

Elizabeth A. Eisenhauer

8.1 Introduction

There are many administrative and organizational steps that must be undertaken before a phase I trial may begin. An extremely important step for *all*
investigators is to become familiar with the document on Good Clinical
Practice (GCP) [1], developed by the International Conference on Harmonization (ICH) and adopted by the regulatory authorities in the United States,
European Union, Japan, Canada, and many other international jurisdictions.
This comprehensive document details the responsibilities of investigator and
sponsor in conducting clinical trials, provides guidance on Ethics Review
Board composition, responsibilities and function, outlines templates for content of the protocol and consent form, and the documents that must be on file
before, during, and after the trial. Although GCP was developed for use as an
Industry Guidance document, in fact it is being applied to academic studies
more and more. In some countries *all* trials of drugs, whether investigational
or marketed, whether sponsored by industry or academic investigator, must be
conducted according to GCP standards if used in an investigational setting.

8.2 Regulatory filing

Each country or region has a process that must be undertaken before a
trial can begin. For any individual study, compliance with these processes is
an absolute requirement. Although this book cannot supply an exhaustive
list of what must be done, in general, documentation about the drug, its

Table 8.1 Summary of regulatory submissions for first-in-man phase I trials

	United States	European Union Member States
Name of submission	Investigational New Drug (IND) application*	Clinical Trials Authorisation (CTA)
Who may sponsor?	Investigator ('sponsor-investigator'), individual, academic institution or organization, pharmaceutical company, or other organization	Individual, company, institution, or organization
Forms	FDA 1571 form†: cover sheet with sponsor details, and other information about the application	Sponsor must first register trial and obtain unique number from EudraCT, a database of all interventional clinical trials of medicinal products.‡ The CTA application form must then be completed and accompany the submission§
Table of contents	Required	
General information /cover letter	Introductory statement and general investigational plan *for the drug* (generally 2–3 pages)	Cover letter¶, which should introduce the submission, cite the EudraCT number and should draw attention to the fact that it is the first administration of a substance to humans.
Study information	Protocol document(s) (may file more than one trial protocol with initial submission)	Protocol document
Investigator information	FDA 1572 form and CV (to be submitted to the sponsor, and incorporated into IND application)	Required by some member states
Drug information	Investigator's Brochure Chemistry, manufacturing and control Pharmacology and Toxicology Previous human experience	Investigator's Brochure Investigational Medicinal Product Dossier (IMPD)—Full IMPD for first-in-man trial
Other	Additional information or other relevant information is requested by FDA	Copy of ethics committee opinion in the member state concerned, when available. Insurance and indemnification information: member state specific

*For FDA IND application details see http://www.access.gpo.gov/nara/cfr/waisidx_00/21cfr312_00. html and see also: http://www.fda.gov/cder/guidance/clin2.pdf
†For FDA forms see: http://www.fda.gov/opacom/morechoices/fdaforms/cder.html
‡To get a EudraCT number see: http://eudract.emea.eu.int
§To get information on application form and process: https://eudract.emea.eu.int/eudract/index.do
¶Specific information required by *individual members states* to be found at: http://eudract. emea.eu.int/docs/Detailed%20guidance%20CTA%20.pdf
Website references were all last accessed August 2005.

formulation, toxicology, and non-clinical efficacy along with the protocol itself and other information must be submitted by the study's sponsor to the relevant government authority for review and authorization (see section on Sponsor below). This submission is referred to as an Investigational New Drug application (IND application) in the United States and is made to the Food and Drug Administration (FDA). In member states of the European Union, the submission is called a request for a Clinical Trials Authorization (CTA) made to the relevant national authorities. In Canada it is a Clinical Trials Application (CTA) submitted to the appropriate department in Health Canada. Usually a minimum time must elapse for the review to take place and there may be questions about aspects of the submission that are sent back to the sponsor for clarification before the submission is cleared and the trial can proceed. Some of the information required for the non-clinical aspects of the submission is described in Chapter 2, and the remainder of the content required for US and EU submissions is summarized in Table 8.1. Note, however, that regulations regarding content are *not* static so it is important to consult with local government authorities prior to beginning a submission process. There are a few common terms and requirements that merit comment.

8.2.1 Investigator

The trial investigator (or 'principal investigator' in the parlance of some regions) has the ultimate responsibility for the correct conduct of the trial at the local institutional level. This includes shepherding the protocol through the required initial and annual review committees at the institution, preparation for study activation, the identification of eligible patients, subject recruitment and proper informed consent process, the administration of trial treatments and arrangement of investigations according to the protocol plan, the medical care of patients on the trial, appropriate storage and handling of investigational agents, data collection, record keeping, and preparation for any required audits, and on site monitoring. The investigator must be appropriately qualified to manage the patients who are to be enrolled as well as appropriately educated with respect to the study plan and the investigational agent to be used. Furthermore, the investigator must have sufficient *time* to perform the required functions. He/she may delegate some of the tasks to qualified personnel, such as co-investigators (or sub-investigators), nurses, data managers, and pharmacists, but those individuals must be adequately schooled in the particulars of the trial. GCP indicates that the investigator should maintain a written record of the individuals to whom significant trial-related duties have been delegated. As noted earlier, all investigators should

Table 8.2 *Selected* investigator responsibilities*

Major area of responsibility	Selected subsections	Comments
Investigator qualifications and agreements	Investigator must have appropriate education and training to conduct the study and supply CV	
	Investigator must be familiar with the appropriate use of the investigational agent	
	Investigator must comply with GCP (!)	
	Investigator must maintain a list of qualified persons to whom trial related activities must be delegated	Delegation should be documented in writing on site. SOPs should indicate how this is done and how those delegated to are trained
Adequate resources	Investigator must show that he/she can recruit the required number of patients and also show he/she has sufficient time and appropriate facilities to conduct the study	
Medical care of trial subjects	Investigator must provide adequate care during the study and for any adverse events	It is important to ensure that referring physicians and hospitals are aware the patient is on a trial. Should adverse events arise that require admission to hospital, this should be done, if at all possible, under the investigator's care
Communication with IRB/IEC	Investigator must have written approval from the appropriate institutional ethics committee before the trial begins	
	Investigator must supply the Investigator's Brochure to the committee and all required documents during the trial	
Compliance with the protocol	Investigator must follow the trial as written in the protocol, and obtain approval of ethics committee before implementing an amendment	Deviations allowed for immediate hazard

Investigational product	Investigator is responsible for appropriate handling, storage and dispensing of investigational product	Normally this responsibility is delegated to a qualified pharmacist
Randomization procedures and unblinding	The investigator should follow the trial procedures in accordance with the protocol	For phase I trials, this means patient registration before treatment begins and treatment at assigned dose
Informed consent	Investigator must comply with relevant regulations and adhere to ethical principles Consent form content is described (see Table 7.10 in Chapter 7)	Informed consent includes not only written information but also a discussion with the patient. The discussion may be shared with a designated person
Records and reports	Investigator responsible for data collection and its accuracy in comparison with source documents. Case report form changes must be dated and initialled. Trial documents should be maintained as required by GCP section 8	Again, this is usually delegated to a qualified nurse or data manager
Progress reports	Investigator responsible for reporting as needed to Institution/ethics committee, and sponsor especially on issues that change trial conduct or risk to patients/subjects	
Premature termination or suspension	Investigator must inform trial subjects and required authorities/ethics committee	
Final report	Investigator responsible for final report, if required by regulatory authorities	

*Content of Table 8.2 is abbreviated from ICH GCP (E6) Section 4. See Appendix I for web reference.

review and abide by the GCP document as they perform their duties: it is not something that is appended to a protocol to simply add weight! It contains important information about investigator responsibilities (See summary of duties of the investigator in Table 8.2).

On a practical note, the investigator should ensure that she/he has appropriate medical insurance that will cover untoward events that might arise in the course of a phase I trial. Malpractice coverage varies: most insurers cover activities associated with professional practice, including those of an investigator on an approved (by regulatory authorities and ethical committee) phase I trial. Finally, many pharmaceutical sponsors require the investigator to sign a statement regarding his/her conflict of interest with respect to the company and the product under study.

8.2.2 Sponsor

The trial sponsor is the individual or organization that assumes *legal responsibility* for the conduct of the trial according to the regulations and guidelines in place for that country or region. Thus, the sponsor must assure the trial is conducted according to principles of GCP where this is the accepted standard. That means ensuring that investigators are qualified to conduct the study, that they are adequately informed about the trial procedures and have the time and resources to conduct it, etc. The sponsor must also ensure that ethical review by appropriately constituted ethical committees takes place before the study begins and patients receive investigational treatment. In addition, the sponsor must undertake measures to make certain that data quality is maintained as the trial proceeds by review of source documents and other processes, and must ensure that serious, unexpected adverse drug reactions are reported appropriately to all required individuals and bodies. It is important to note that the sponsor is not always a pharmaceutical firm; individual investigators, institutions, and academic research groups may sponsor studies, but if doing so, must understand and undertake the relevant sponsor duties. Table 8.3 shows a selected list of duties as described by ICH GCP. Note in particular the need for appropriate insurance coverage: if required by the relevant regulatory authority, the sponsor should provide insurance for patients and should indemnify investigators and institutions against claims arising from the trial by patients and others.

8.2.3 Protocol

The *final* protocol document including all appendices is a standard part of all regulatory submissions.

Table 8.3 *Selected* sponsor responsibilities*

Item	Sponsor responsibility
Quality assurance (QA) and Quality Control (QC)	Written standard operating procedures (SOPs) for QA and QC to assure conduct of trial and data recorded are in compliance with protocol and are accurate and reliable
Trial design	Sponsor must utilize qualified individuals (physicians, biostatisticians, clinical pharmacologists, etc.) for design, data collection, and analysis of the study
Trial management	Sponsor should utilize appropriately qualified individuals to supervise conduct of the trial, to handle and verify data and to analyse data. There are special rules for electronic data handling. An Independent Data Monitoring Committee (IDMC) may advise the sponsor, but should have written SOPs and maintain records of meetings Each subject to be identified by an unambiguous subject identification code.
	Retain sponsor-specific documents for time periods described in GCP
Investigator selection	Sponsor is responsible for selecting the investigators/institutions qualified to perform the study. They must agree to conduct the trial in compliance with GCP
Compensation to subjects and investigators	If required by local regulatory authority, the Sponsor should provide insurance or should indemnify the investigators/institutions against claims arising from the trial, except for claims that arise from malpractice or negligence
Financing	Financial aspects of the trial should be documented in an agreement between the sponsor and the investigators/institutions
Regulatory authority submission/notification	Before initiating the trial, the sponsor must seek and obtain the required regulatory approval or permission (as required by the relevant authorities)
Confirmation of Review by Ethics Committee (IRB/REB/IEC)	The sponsor must obtain from the investigator/institutions, a copy of the initial and ongoing ethical approvals of the protocol as well as the name and address of the committee, and a statement that it is organized and operates according to GCP and applicable laws. Information must also be supplied on any conditions associated with approval or withdrawals or suspensions of the trial by the ethical committee
Information on investigational products	Sponsor must assure sufficient efficacy and safety data available to justify the proposed trial and must update the Investigator's Brochure with any significant new information
Manufacturing, labelling, packaging	Sponsor must ensure the product is manufactured according to GMP, what the acceptable storage conditions are (and inform those who must know), that the packaging and labelling is acceptable and compliant with local regulations

(Continued)

Table 8.3 *Continued*

Item	Sponsor responsibility
Supplying investigational agent	Sponsor is responsible for ensuring investigational drug supply to the institution(s) in the trial and for the procedures that the investigator/institution should follow for receiving, tracking, dispensing, and handling the drug
Record access	Sponsor should ensure access to source documents for monitoring, audits, and regulatory inspection
Safety information	Sponsor is responsible for ongoing safety evaluation of the investigational products and must notify the institution(s) and regulatory authorities of findings that could adversely affect safety or impact conduct of the trial
Adverse drug reaction reporting	Sponsor is responsible for expedited reporting to regulatory authority(ies), investigators/institutions, ethics committee(s), of serious, unexpected, adverse drug reactions (*adverse drug reactions are adverse events that are thought to be drug-related*)
Monitoring	Sponsor should ensure the trial is adequately monitored to verify that reported data are accurate and complete and that the trial is being conducted in compliance with GCP and regulatory requirements. The sponsor should determine the nature and extent of monitoring necessary to accomplish this
Audit	The sponsor is responsible for performing audits as part of QA to evaluate compliance with the protocol, SOPs, GCP, and other requirements
Early termination	The sponsor must notify investigators/institutions, their ethics committees, regulatory authorities if the trial is stopped early, and offer the reasons
Clinical study reports	The sponsor must prepare final or ongoing reports as required

*See ICH Good Clinical Practice for **detailed description. See Appendix I for web reference.**

8.2.4 Investigator's Brochure

The Investigator's Brochure (also called the Clinical Brochure; the Investigator Drug Brochure) is a summary document of the drug under study. It includes information on the physical, chemical, and pharmaceutical properties of the new drug, data on preclinical studies [pharmacology, including efficacy, toxicology, and pharmacokinetics (PK)] and on any clinical studies that have been conducted. For phase I first-in-man trials this latter section will be incomplete of course, but as clinical data emerges, the Investigator Brochure is updated, often on an annual basis. Table 2.5 found in Chapter 2 describes the recommended table of contents listing for an Investigator's Brochure as outlined by ICH.

8.2.5 Other documents

Each country or region has compiled lists of documents and forms that must be completed to file the appropriate submission to local authorities for review. Table 8.1 and Appendix I of this book provide some useful links to access this information in various countries/regions.

8.3 Contract

It is almost always the case that phase I trials of new cancer drugs will be conducted through partnerships: either between academic collaborators or between academic investigators and pharmaceutical industry, both large and small. Investigator/institution–industry partnerships are the most common. Regardless of the nature of the collaborations, they are usually (for academic partnerships) or always (for industry partnerships) formalized by a letter of agreement or contract. As most academics are not trained in contract law, this process may seem somewhat overwhelming to the novice as contracts are generally pages long and utilize language that is unfamiliar. Investigators must ensure that their institution's legal or contracts officer has an opportunity to review the agreement as it is being developed, but the investigator cannot pass on all responsibility to her/his institution, as much of the contract will be about what the investigator has *agreed to deliver*, and that is something only the she/he can attest to. Key elements to keep in mind when reviewing a contract are summarized in Table 8.4, and include: responsibilities of company and investigator/institution, intellectual property considerations, indemnification arrangements, access to trial data, publication restrictions, payment amounts, and schedule. Freedom to publish, even if results are not as 'positive' as expected is key. It is reasonable to expect the company to have rights to review and co-author publications if they have contributed to the data and content, but they should not be able to unduly delay or block publication on

Table 8.4 Important contract elements

Element	Comment
Trial responsibilities	Ensure that the contract makes it clear who is responsible for which aspects of the trial. This may be best accomplished by an appendix to the contract that details which of company, investigator, and/or institution is responsible for the various aspects of the trial such as developing the protocol, case report forms, ethics review, regulatory review, database development, trial report, pharmacokinetic analyses. Many such appendices also include expected timelines
Sponsor	The contract must be clear on which party is the legal sponsor. The sponsor must file any regulatory documents and will have responsibility for overall trial conduct, SAE reporting etc. as outlined in Table 8.3
Intellectual property (IP)	The contract must specify who has rights to any discoveries or inventions that arise as a result of the research. Clear language should specify who has IP rights (it could be more than one party) and how information about inventions made will be disclosed and if investigators and/or institution have any negotiating rights or options
Ownership	The contract must identify who 'owns' the data that result from the trial. If the investigator(s) do not own the data, the contract must indicate that they have access to the data for teaching and publication. If the investigator will hold the database, the contract must specify if, when and how the data will be transferred to other parties. If tissue samples are collected for research, the contract should indicate which party will store samples and which has decision-making authority regarding their use
Publications	The contract must specify who has the right to publish the data. **It should be clear that the trial data WILL be published.** Timelines should be included for review of draft publications or presentations (usually 10 days for abstracts or presentations and 30 days for manuscripts). (If the company will publish part of the report, the investigator(s) must be given reciprocal reviewing rights). Delays beyond that should be allowed for confidentiality or IP reasons only, and should be limited in length. The company should not have the right to block submission if it disagrees with the investigator's interpretation of results. Generally, although not in the contract, most such disagreements are easily dealt with by open and honest communication between parties
Confidentiality	The contract will contain reference to what written or other materials supplied by the sponsor to the investigator are to be regarded as confidential and with whom they may be shared. If there is a separate confidentiality agreement that has been signed, care must be taken to make sure that the contract and the confidentiality agreement are concordant. Care should be taken to avoid listing the research/study results as being 'confidential'. **If this is done, it may serve to block the ability to publish results**
Indemnification and Insurance	The contract will specify how the parties will bear responsibilities for each other in the case of legal action taken by patients or others. In general, the investigator/institution must be responsible for their own acts of negligence. The insurance and

indemnification to be held by the sponsor and manufacturer need to be clearly stated. Which party will take responsibility for events that arise from protocol treatment-related outcomes (provided the protocol is followed as written) and for events directly related to drug product should be indicated: some countries require detailed information on this to be submitted to the regulatory/competent authority when the Clinical Trials Authorization is requested. Care should be taken that investigators are not being asked to indemnify other parties for actions that they cannot supervise or be responsible for. Finding appropriate language in this section of the contract and obtaining the required insurance coverage may be a source of prolonged negotiation

Termination	The contract should specify who, and under what conditions, can stop the study. Most concern is raised when business decisions alone lead to trial termination. The contract should be clear about what consultations must take place before the trial is closed prematurely. Some institutions will not sign contracts that allow the sponsor to prematurely terminate the study for non-scientific or non-safety reasons
Consistency	Make sure the protocol document and the contract/appendices are consistent with respect to such things as SAE reporting responsibilities, accrual expectations, roles and responsibilities
Payments	The contract should specify amount and timing of any funding arrangement. Generally individual investigators should not receive personal compensation, rather funding should be made to an institutional account
Signatures	Investigators are not generally considered 'legal entities'. The investigator's institution must sign the contract as well. The investigator's signature can attest to the fact that the investigator agrees with the content of the contract, but it is the institutional signature that counts

the basis of a disagreement on the interpretation of results. If the investigator or an academic group is not holding the trial database, the opportunity for trial investigators to access the database to query it or to understand analysis outputs is also crucial and should be accommodated in the contract under most circumstances. Recent major journals have cited this latter issue as a critical one in developing a publication that is credible [2] and many journals now require the first author to attest to the completeness and accuracy of the reported data in a manuscript submission.

8.4 Protocol review

Every trial must receive *ethical committee* approval before opening for patient enrolment. The Ethics Committee, also called Institutional Review Board (IRB), Independent Ethics Committee (IEC), Research Ethics Board (REB), and other monikers, has the responsibility of safeguarding the rights, safety, and well-being of trial subjects. To do so, it must conduct an independent review of a number of trial documents and other information including: the protocol, consent form, any other material to be used by or given to patients, investigator qualifications, subject recruitment procedures as well as the Investigator Brochure (or similar background information on the drug as appropriate), and information about any payment that will be made to patients. The committee must also be responsible for *ongoing* review of submitted serious adverse events, trial amendments, and ensure the continued conduct of the trial is appropriate by an annual approval process. Various regulations dictate the complement of ethics committee members required for review at each step. All initial ethics reviews must be done by the 'full' (as defined in guidelines) committee and other reviews may be full committee or expedited depending on the nature of the material and the local regulations. Countries vary regarding how IRB/IEC membership and procedures are codified: in some it is subject to governmental regulation and in others it is subject to guidelines only. Table 8.5 outlines IRB/IEC composition and function as per ICH GCP guidelines. Essentially, all institutions at which phase I cancer trials are conducted will have an appropriately constituted ethical committee and process already in place. The investigator's responsibility with respect to this process is to ensure the committee has all the relevant documents and forms submitted prior to the study start and throughout the trial, including submission of safety reports and serious adverse events reports as required. It is also important that the protocol document that the ethics committee reviews is the *same* (i.e. final) version as that submitted for approval by the regulatory authority. The investigator is also responsible for addressing the committee's questions or concerns in a timely way.

Table 8.5 Investigational Review Board/Institutional Ethics Committee (IRB/IEC) composition/function*

IRB/IEC composition	At least five members
	At least one member whose primary area of interest is in a non-scientific area
	At least one member independent of institution/trial site
Functions	Written operating procedures of functions, including definition of a quorum for decision making
	Written records and minutes in compliance with GCP and regulatory requirements
Decisions	Decision of the IRB/IEC should be made at announced meetings at which at least a quorum is present
Participants	The investigator may provide input, but should not participate in deliberations or the vote/opinion of the IRB/IEC
Responsibilities	Major responsibility is to safeguard the rights, safety and well-being of trial subjects
	Trial: IRB/IEC must review protocol, amendments, informed consent form(s), subject recruitment procedures, Investigator's Brochure, and other safety information, as well as information about payment/compensation to subjects
	Investigator(s) review: review investigator CV and other documents to assess his/her qualifications for performing the trial
	Trial review: initial review prior to trial activation, as well as ongoing (continuing) review of each active trial at least once per year. Further, ongoing safety review or serious unexpected adverse drug reactions
	Outcome of IRB/IEC decision may be categorized as:
	◆ approval
	◆ modifications required prior to approval
	◆ disapproval
	◆ termination/suspension of prior approval

*This summary is condensed from ICH Guideline E6: Good Clinical Practice Section 3. Please note that there may be additional, or more stringent requirements, for composition and function within individual countries or regions. See Appendix I for web reference for GCP.

In addition to ethical committee review, other institutional or sponsor review committees are now commonplace: examples include institutional scientific review (by colleagues of the investigator for example), resource utilization, pharmacy, and nursing reviews. In most institutions there is a standard sequence through which a new trial protocol must pass: those institutions that are most efficient often conduct reviews in parallel. Some have observed that the speed of passage through the various layers required to officially open a new trial for accrual is related to the energy and enthusiasm the investigator has for the study; rapid responses to questions raised by various review bodies enable the protocol to move quickly to approval. Institutions or investigators with very poor track records in study activation timelines will lose opportunities for future studies.

8.5 Trial registration

Recently, editors of major medical journals have made it a requirement that clinical trials must be registered in an acceptable public registry prior to treatment of the first patient in order to be published once they are completed [3,4]. This effort is to ensure that the public is aware of all trials that are being performed, not only those that are published because they have favourable outcomes. It is hoped this endeavour will reduce publication bias. Although registration for phase I trials may not always be mandatory, it is recommended that investigators involved in phase I trials should ensure that their trial is registered on such a database before enrolling patients. Failure to do could result in difficulty publishing the results when the trial is completed.

8.6 Setting up the project

Although it may seem that once a protocol is finalized, all the various approvals required are completed, and all the relevant clinicians have been made aware that the trial is approved that it is ready to begin, this is not the case; there remain a number of practical aspects to setting up a successful phase I project in the institution in which it is to be carried out.

8.6.1 Nursing and data management

Many institutions have specialized cancer research nurses and these individuals are in some respects the most important team members. Well trained research nurses may undertake a number of trial-related tasks under the investigator's supervision and delegation (remember that the investigator must officially delegate these tasks!), including screening patients for eligibility and initial discussion of the trial with potential subjects, treatment administration, assessment of adverse effects, blood or tissue collection, preparation and shipping samples for PK and special studies, and case report form (CRF) completion (to name a few). Because of their vital role, it is recommended that the primary study research nurse have the opportunity to review the protocol while it is still in draft form: she/he may identify practical issues regarding patient treatment or monitoring that are best addressed by changes to the protocol document before it is finalized. Beyond this, it is essential that research nurses, data managers (if applicable), investigators, and other team members (see below) meet *before* the trial is open in their institution to 'walk through' the protocol, educate personnel about the trial procedures and treatment plan as well as how to complete data collection forms (CRFs).

If a pharmaceutical company is sponsoring the trial, they often organize such face-to-face meetings themselves. Who will be responsible for drawing and spinning blood after hours? Who will make the lab and radiology bookings to comply with the protocol calendar? And who will ensure that all results of those tests are available and seen by the investigator as soon as they are available? Experienced nurses often develop trial activation checklists for such practical organizational matters to use in their own institution (see example in Appendix III).

Research nurses or, in some institutions, data managers, are also responsible for maintaining all required trial files and organizing ethics committee and other internal committee submissions (e.g. some institutions have resource or pharmacy committees that protocols must pass through before they can begin). Whoever is responsible for this aspect of the trial coordination, ideally they should have a set of written standard procedures to describe how trial organization is managed. GCP includes a section on 'essential trial documents', which provides an overview of the files that the investigator and sponsor must maintain to enable evaluation of the trial quality and conduct by external reviewers (see section 8.0 of the GCP).

Standard operating procedures (SOPs) are detailed written instructions to achieve uniformity in the performance of trial-related procedures. Institutions participating in clinical trials need to have SOPs for key trial activities, such as Ethics committee processes, patient recruitment, registration (or randomization) procedures, adverse event reporting, delegation of study responsibilities, and CRF completion. A sample list of SOPs that should be created to facilitate institutional compliance with GCP is found in Appendix III.

CRF completion by either nurses or data managers must also be taught: if the data collection forms are not familiar, reviewing them prior to usage is important. Similar education is required for remote electronic data capture processes. Knowing who to call if questions arise when data are being entered on the form or computer screen is also important as it may be some weeks between the educational experience and when data submission is first taking place. Furthermore, it is important to understand that the CRF content must be traced to 'source' documents in case of audit. That means that the medical record, flow sheets, pharmacy records, prescription copies, and/or clinic notes must contain the information recorded on the CRF.

8.6.2 Pharmacy

Before beginning a phase I trial, the research pharmacist must review the drug information in the protocol and Investigator's Brochure. In addition, the pharmacy must have adequate, secure facilities to store and prepare drug as per protocol. All trials of investigational drugs require that a log of receipt/dispensing be maintained and the pharmacy must employ appropriately trained personnel for this quality control aspect of the study. Details of disposal or destruction of empty vials or their return to the sponsor must also be tracked.

Generally, the sponsor that is supplying drug will need to know the name/address of the pharmacist who will be responsible for receiving shipments. The drug shipment will not take place until all required approvals for the protocol are completed. Shipments are accompanied by a trial-specific drug log, an acknowledgement form to send back to indicate the drug arrived safely, and usually information on how to reorder drug when supplies are low (it is important for pharmacist to keep an eye on this as drug may take several days to arrive). *Use of investigational supply of drug for non-trial patients is strictly prohibited.*

As some protocols require extensive pre- and post-therapy administration of fluids or supportive care medications, some pharmacists prepare a pre-typed order sheet or computer order entry screen so that not only the trial medication but all co-medications and fluids are prescribed correctly. The pharmacist must pay special attention to drug reconstitution protocols and information on special bags or tubing that may be required to be sure these are available when the trial opens as not all may be supplied. In case there is no pharmaceutical sponsor, a sample drug log is provided in Appendix III.

8.6.3 Sample processing, packaging, shipping

As almost all phase I trials involve sending blood or tissue specimens to specialized research facilities for PK or other assays, there must be clear instructions in the protocol or appendices about how to procure the sample, into what type of container or fixative it is to be taken, how it is to be processed (e.g. centrifugation within how long after sample is drawn at what speed and at what temperature), how the final sample is to be labelled and stored, and, finally, to whom it is to be shipped. A patient-specific log sheet to record when PK or pharmacodynamic samples are taken is important to track what is due and when. In general, tubes and labels are supplied by sponsoring pharmaceutical companies but this may not always be the case, particularly for sample shipping on academic trials where the shipment is to a research laboratory. In these cases, the receiving laboratory must provide detailed information on what, how, and when to send specimens. The trial institution will need to make up labels and be sure it has the correct packaging (e.g. dry ice, etc.) and shipping forms (e.g. courier forms, custom forms) to transport specimens containing biological materials correctly and safely. Most laboratories ask that the sending institution ship only on certain weekdays to ensure that samples can be received during normal working hours. Furthermore, the receiving facility should be notified *before* the sample is shipped so that they are aware it is on its way. All of these aspects of the trial must be sorted out before the first patient is seen and the pre-trial meeting serves as the best time to do this.

8.6.4 Treatment delivery

Some protocols require long-term infusions or frequent visits for treatment. The investigator and their team must ensure there are outpatient or inpatient beds available to conduct the trial. Many clinics have a co-ordinator for bed space; this individual is the one with whom these aspects of trial set up are to be co-ordinated. If patient samples are to be obtained 'after hours' of operation, the logistics of doing this must be addressed before the first patient is enrolled.

8.6.5 Funding

Developing a budget for the trial is part of the process of negotiating the contract, or for academic funded studies, making the grant application. In general, funding is needed to support those costs over and above usual medical care: research nurse time, pharmacist time, data manager time, special equipment, special laboratory assays, and special imaging studies. Institutions/countries vary as to whether extra funding for blood tests done in the hospital laboratory, routine radiological studies and physician's visits required by the protocol are costed into the trial budget or are paid through the usual health care insurance channels. Similarly, physician fees may not be charged if patient care is covered by national or other insurance. If the institution conducting the trial is also responsible for data collection, cleaning, analysis, and report generation, and is the sponsor of the trial, funding to cover the personnel costs associated with overall trial management and analysis are also required. Institutional rules regarding indirect costs/overhead payments must be factored into the budget. In general, *direct* physician payment or incentives for recruitment other than reimbursement for medical visits or procedures should *not* be part of remuneration for clinical trials as this creates a significant conflict of interest. To assure that trial funding is handled appropriately, all payments should be made to an institutional or departmental account, not into a physician's personal bank account. A sample format for a phase I budget is provided in Appendix III.

8.7 Summary

The background work required to get a completed protocol activated is substantial. Although the setting of this chapter is phase I studies, most of what has been written applies to all clinical trial protocols. An efficient and well-oiled 'machine' for trial start-up, along with adequate numbers of well-qualified personnel add substantial quality to the trial conduct and make the entire process much more efficient.

References

1. International Conference on Harmonization Guideline (E6) on Good Clinical Practice may be found at: http://www.ich.org (direct link for pdf version is: http://www.ich.org/MediaServer.jser?@_ID=482&@_MODE=GLB [last accessed August 2005]
2. Davidoff F, DeAngelis CD, Drazen JM, *et al.* (2001). Sponsorship, authorship, and accountability. *N Engl J Med* **345**: 825–6.
3. De Angelis CD, Drazen JM, Frizelle FA, *et al.*; International Committee of Medical Journal Editors (2004). Clinical trial registration: a statement from the International Committee of Medical Journal Editors. *CMAJ* **171**: 606–7.
4. De Angelis CD, Drazen JM, Frizelle FA, *et al.*; International Committee of Medical Journal Editors (2005). Is this clinical trial fully registered? A statement from the International Committee of Medical Journal Editors. *CMAJ* **172**: 1700–2.

Chapter 9

Practical aspects of pharmacokinetics and pharmacodynamics

Chris Twelves

9.1 Introduction

Pharmacology studies are an integral part of early clinical trials and contribute vital information for the subsequent development of a drug. Pharmacokinetic (PK) studies may, somewhat simplistically, be defined as describing 'what the body does to a drug', whereas pharmacodynamic (PD) studies describe 'what a drug does to the body'. Historically, in the development of antiproliferative cytotoxics, the main focus has been on PK. In the modern era, with more rationally designed, targeted therapies, PD studies are increasingly important.

Clinical pharmacology studies are planned and carried out in the context of information gained in preclinical evaluation. *In vivo* preclinical PK indicate how a drug may be handled in man and can suggest the minimum plasma values or 'target' PK exposure that may determine whether a potentially therapeutic dose level has been achieved. Likewise, PD markers indicating that a drug has inhibited its target can only be meaningfully incorporated in clinical trials if they have been fully evaluated in preclinical models.

Pharmacology studies add considerable time and expense to early trials, so why are they so important? In the first instance, plasma PK provides a description of the general behaviour of a drug and answers clinically import-ant questions: How much drug is there in the blood? Are concentrations achieved that are active in preclinical models? For how long is drug present? How is the drug metabolized and eliminated from the body? As dose is increased in the phase I trial are the PK linear? i.e. is there a proportionate

in drug exposure. This information may influence how the phase I
conducted. Pharmacokinetically guided dose escalation, where dose
ents are specifically directed towards a target PK exposure based on that
which is associated with toxicity in preclinical models [1], has not found
widespread acceptance. However, some trials of non-cytotoxic agents or
biological therapies, such as that of the anti-epidermal growth factor receptor
monoclonal antibody cetuximab, have used PK data to define the dose for
further studies; this and other examples of phase I trials that used PK to
establish the recommended dose are shown in Table 3.9 found in Chapter 3.
More often, however, PK data inform decisions regarding by what route and
how frequently a drug is administered or even that a drug should not be
developed further, if potentially therapeutic plasma concentrations cannot be
achieved. It may also be possible to identify the factors accounting for variability in how a drug is handled by different individuals. Causes of this
interindividual variability include organ impairment, drug interactions, or
genetic polymorphisms in drug metabolizing enzymes.

PD studies may indicate whether a drug is having its desired effect. A
descriptive approach asks simply whether the tumour shrinks, whereas a
mechanistic approach seeks to identify molecular endpoints. This may involve
sampling tumour or surrogate 'normal' tissue and measuring the effect of a
drug on a specific molecular target or pathway and relating this to the
intended biological effect such as inhibition of cell proliferation. Alternatively,
functional or molecular imaging techniques such as magnetic resonance
imaging/spectroscopy, or positron emission tomography may detect biochemical or functional changes induced by a novel compound. Where the effects of
a drug (either efficacy or toxicity) can be measured, correlations may be
sought with plasma or tissue drug levels. These PK–PD relationships may
again influence the choice of dose or schedule for subsequent trials.

PK and PD analyses require considerable technical expertise, but the clinician
plays a key role, first in recognizing the need to incorporate such studies and then
in ensuring that the additional studies are practical and clinically relevant.

- First, a decision has to be made as to what it is appropriate and feasible to
  measure in a particular population of patients, how many measurements
  are needed and when should they be made. For example, collection of blood
  samples overnight is easy to include in a protocol but difficult in practice.
  Likewise, multiple tumour biopsies may be intellectually attractive to the
  investigator but less appealing to a patient with advanced cancer.
- Next, the clinical investigator requires a method and a collaborator, or
  team, to perform the PK or PD studies and to analyse the results. It is

pointless agreeing to participate in a trial incorporating PK or PD studies if a centre does not have the human and other resources, or skills necessary.

♦ It is important to ask if the results of these studies will be believed and utilized appropriately. The assay or imaging technique needs to be validated, increasingly to specific standards with detailed quality control and standard operating procedures (SOPs) covering sample handling, assay reproducibility, sensitivity, and specificity. These practicalities may not be a priority to clinical investigators, but are vital if decisions on subsequent drug development will be based on the outcome of these laboratory investigations. Moreover, regulatory authorities do recognize the importance of quality control, so these issues are not optional when translational data are to be included in licensing applications.

♦ Finally, although most phase I trials do quite appropriately include pharmacological studies, it is not possible to incorporate all studies in all trials. It may, therefore, be best to address certain questions in specific cohorts within a phase I trial or in a separate study. For example, a biochemical signal may be sought to demonstrate 'proof-of-concept', i.e. that a drug is hitting the desired target, but not to determine dose escalation; under those circumstances, tumour biopsies may best be obtained in the expanded cohort treated at the recommended dose.

9.2 Pharmacokinetics

9.2.1 Principles of pharmacokinetics

It is beyond the scope of this book to teach PK, which is covered in detail in many texts [2]. It is, however, useful to review briefly the terms and principles that investigators will come across when writing or reviewing a protocol.

PK is the study of drug absorption, distribution, metabolism, and excretion (often referred to as 'ADME'). These factors are usually characterized by taking a series of timed blood samples, measuring the concentration of parent compound and relevant metabolites, then plotting a curve of concentration (typically on a logarithmic scale) versus time. This was done manually in the past but straightforward computer programs now perform this task. After intravenous (i.v.) administration, there is usually an initial rapid fall in plasma concentration as the drug distributes into the tissues. Later, the fall in plasma concentration is slower as the drug is eliminated. The more samples that are taken over a longer period of time, the greater the accuracy of the picture of a drug's fate. This must, however, be balanced against the practicalities of taking and processing the samples. Although most PK studies are of drug and metabolite levels in blood, measurements can also be made in other fluids (urine, ascites, cerebrospinal fluid) or solid tissues (normal or tumour).

The fundamental parameters that describe a drug's behaviour are: area under the concentration–time curve (AUC), peak plasma concentration (C_{max}), total plasma clearance (CL), volume of distribution (V_D), and terminal half-life ($t_{1/2}$).

As the term suggests, AUC represents the size of the area below the curve when a series of drug concentrations are plotted versus time. AUC reflects total drug exposure and is determined by the dose and clearance of a drug. The AUC can be calculated simply, without deriving a PK model; a more sophisticated approach is to fit the concentration–time data to a PK model and derive AUC from the model. The AUC can be calculated up to the final sample time point (AUC_t), or the concentration–time curve can be extrapolated to infinity (AUC_{inf}). In both cases, but especially where there is considerable extrapolation, the final component of the AUC will be influenced heavily by the later concentration time points, usually low values where any inaccuracy in measuring drug levels may have a disproportionate impact on apparent drug exposure. Therefore, although late samples some days after drug administration are inconvenient for the patient, they are often an important part of the PK study. AUC, as an expression of total drug exposure, is often studied in relation to efficacy or toxicity. In some cases, where a drug has to be above a threshold concentration for activity, the observation of AUC above that threshold or the time that the drug concentration surpasses the PK threshold may be used for such correlative studies.

CL reflects the rate at which a drug is removed from the plasma as it distributes into the tissues, is metabolized and then eliminated. It reflects the volume of plasma (blood, etc.) 'cleared' of drug per unit time (e.g. ml/min or l/h). There is an inverse relationship between CL and AUC (AUC = dose/CL). CL often varies widely between individuals treated at a given dose, so understanding the reasons behind differences in CL is important in explaining variability in drug exposure between patients.

The terminal half-life ($t_{1/2}$) represents the time for drug concentration to fall by half over the final part of the concentration–time curve when drug elimination is the dominant process. Terminal half-life determines the time to eliminate drug; after 4–5 half-lives, a drug will effectively have been fully eliminated. Terminal half-life may also determine the schedule of drug administration; to achieve adequate exposure a drug with a short terminal half-life may be best given over successive days or by prolonged infusion.

Other PK parameters include the maximum plasma drug concentration (C_{max}) and volume of distribution (V_D). C_{max} may correlate with drug effects, especially toxicity. The time to reach C_{max} (known as T_{max}) varies according to mode of administration, being short after bolus injection and longer after infusion or with oral drugs. V_D is less straightforward as it does not represent a physiological volume. Rather, V_D relates plasma concentration to the total amount of drug in the body. A drug that is retained in the vascular compartment would have a V_D of that compartment. By contrast, a drug that distributed and was concentrated in the tissues, with very low plasma concentrations, might have an apparent V_D greater than the total body volume of water. V_D can be used to determine loading doses if it is important to rapidly achieve and then maintain drug concentrations above a certain threshold value. V_D depends on molecular weight, lipid solubility, and binding to tissues and plasma proteins.

9.2.2 Sample collection and processing

The protocol should specify how and when samples are to be collected, the volume to be sampled, how the sample should then be handled prior to storage, and how it should be stored prior to shipping for analysis [3].

The procedure for sampling should be carefully described. Blood will usually be collected from an indwelling cannula or catheter in a vein of the arm contralateral to that through which the drug was administered if the i.v. route is used. It is important to establish that the cannula, syringes, and tubes in which the sample is collected, processed, and stored are compatible with the investigational agent; highly reactive molecules may adhere to materials, invalidating assay results. If patency of the cannula is to be maintained with a heparin flush, a volume representing the 'dead space' of the cannula should be taken and discarded before each PK sample is collected.

Sampling schedules will differ when PK are being studied in other tissues. Estimation of urinary concentrations may be relevant for compounds that are excreted by the kidneys. Although simple in theory, urine collection can be difficult in practice. Specific containers are required, with the appropriate preservatives. Calculating the total amount of drug or metabolite eliminated in the urine requires voiding the bladder and discarding that urine at the start ($t = 0$), and knowledge of the total volume of urine subsequently passed. There is, however, always the risk that a patient will inadvertently fail to collect all their urine. Alternatively, urine may be collected over blocks of time collecting all urine passed, either over a series of 4-hour periods or 0–4, then 4–8, and 8–24 hours following drug administration. Simply collecting 'spot samples', i.e. a limited volume of urine at specific times is easier but yields less information. Repeated sampling of ascites or cerebrospinal fluid is impractical, so spot samples in these instances may be useful to establish whether a drug penetrates a particular compartment. Measurement of drug levels in solid tissues is addressed below.

It is impossible to overstate the importance of identifying designated staff, appropriately trained, for PK sample collection and processing. The usual model is to employ research nurses for this purpose. Relying on medical staff with other clinical commitments increases the likelihood that samples will not be taken or handled appropriately. It is very easy to leave a sample in the centrifuge if another patient becomes unwell. Worse than missing data are misleading data. Incorrect recording of when a sample was taken, or failing to process the sample in a timely manner, can generate spurious estimates of drug concentrations.

The patient consent form or information sheet must describe the sampling procedure, and any associated risks or additional demands on the patient. It may, however, be appropriate to describe the maximum number of samples and total volume of blood to be taken, along with the period over which they may be collected, rather than exact timing and volume of each sample. This can allow adjustment of sampling times, and the number of samples collected, within the limits specified in the patient information sheet without the need for protocol amendments as additional information becomes available from patients treated early in the trial.

9.2.2.1 Timing of samples

Early in the development of a new agent a comprehensive PK profile will usually be required, comprising 10–20 samples during drug administration and the 24–72 hours thereafter. It is important that samples are collected at the specified times, and even more important that the *actual* as well as planned sampling time is recorded. This is facilitated by a detailed work sheet, specifying the planned sample times, and with spaces to record when the samples were actually taken. Another important aid is a digital timer(s).

The sampling schedule is determined first by the route and mode of administration. After a bolus or short i.v. infusion samples might be collected pre-dose, at the end of infusion, 10, 20, 30, and 45 minutes after the end of infusion, then at 1, 2, 4, 6, 8, 10, 24, 48, and perhaps 72 hours. Where a prolonged infusion is utilized, an additional two or three samples would usually be taken during the infusion. Likewise, with oral drugs, samples would be timed to identify the T_{max} and C_{max} following absorption, as well as the subsequent periods of distribution and elimination. Preliminary PK data from preclinical or earlier clinical studies may assist in planning the sampling schedule. When a drug has an especially rapid fall in initial plasma levels, greater emphasis may be placed on early time points. By contrast, if the elimination half-life is long, accurate determination of the later phase of the concentration–time curve through additional time points would be appropriate. For drugs given with the aim of maintaining effective plasma concentrations over a period of weeks or months, the priority is to define steady state or minimum drug concentrations. This can be done by collecting samples prior to each treatment, in addition to defining the single dose PK described above.

Practical issues and attention to detail are important. The timing of early samples, within the first 15 minutes, can be especially difficult. A small error, of perhaps 30 seconds, can have a major effect on the calculated PK parameters. Indeed, collection of a sample from the cannula may take up to 60 seconds and it may not be clear whether the 'start' or 'stop' time is that which should be recorded. The specific needs of sample processing (centrifugation, separation, freezing) may also determine how close together early samples can be collected or handled by a single person. In studies of drug combinations, where the PK of more than one agent is being studied, it is important that the timing of samples is matched if this is possible. For example, previous studies of drug X may have utilized initial sampling times of 5, 15, 30, and 45 minutes, whereas those for drug Y used 10, 20, 30, and 40 minutes. In a combination study it is neither feasible nor sensible to collect samples at all of these time points. Rather, the investigator should discuss with the pharmacokineticist which combination of a limited number of samples provide the most information for both agents.

9.2.2.2 Sample processing

The specific details of sample handling and storage will be determined by the nature of the PK study and investigational agent. For example, are drug levels to be measured in serum or plasma, is total or free drug to be assayed? These questions will influence processing of the sample, so the procedures must be specified in the protocol, and/or a separate working document that can be kept by the research nurse, and is available where the sample collection and processing are being undertaken.

In general, blood samples are taken into prepared tubes; these are often heparinized, but any additives must be specified. The samples are usually placed on ice, then centrifuged before separating the plasma, which is then divided into aliquots to be frozen at $-20°C$ or $-70°C$. The samples are subsequently transferred to the designated laboratory for analysis.

Again, practical issues are of paramount importance. Labelling of the tubes at all times is vital; an unlabelled tube is at best useless and a wrongly labelled sample can generate incorrect and misleading data. It is important to use labels that retain their adhesiveness when frozen. Furthermore, the print or ink used on these labels should not be water-soluble. Protocols may specify that the sample is to be centrifuged immediately; this is difficult if a specialized centrifuge must be used that is located in another department or building. The speed and time of centrifugation should be specified, as should the need (or otherwise) for a chilled centrifuge. In some cases, red blood cells rather than plasma will be needed; again, the investigator must be clear that they have the necessary resources to separate the samples as directed. The sample is usually divided into two or more aliquots in order that the analysis can be done on one aliquot keeping the other in reserve should there be problems with the assay and a need to repeat the measurement. The investigator must have access to appropriate storage conditions on site. Typically this will be in a −70°C freezer, but freezing may damage some samples so it is important to check the protocol. A careful record should be kept of where and when samples were stored. Procedures should be in place to monitor freezer temperatures, with alarms set to go off should the freezer fail and with personnel identified who can be contacted outside working hours in that eventuality.

The final stage in sample handling will usually be ensuring the transfer of samples to an analytical laboratory. This may be done by a local collaborator or a commercial courier. Either way, it is important to identify who will collect the samples, when this will happen and how they are to be handled. Samples will often need to be transferred frozen, so it must be clear at what temperature they are to be maintained, who will provide the dry ice, flasks, and other equipment required. It is equally important that the recipient laboratory has clearly defined procedures to record receipt of the samples and their transfer to storage. It can be helpful to alert the analytical laboratory that samples are due to be sent before they are dispatched so that the necessary arrangements can be made for their receipt. At a simple level, if samples are collected from the hospital on a Friday and arrive at the laboratory the following day when no one is present to receive them, the data are lost. Similarly, there must be procedures at both the hospital and analytical laboratory to locate the person responsible for the samples, and arrangements in place for someone else to act as replacement in the event of holidays or sickness. Finally, with many trials now being international, when the study is being planned it is important to be clear about cross-border transfer of biological samples, or personal patient information, and to acquire the appropriate documentation.

9.2.3 Assay methods

The quality of PK data is dependent on the standard of the analysis. Detailed texts describe the increasingly sophisticated bioanalytical methods that are now available. This section aims to provide the clinical investigator with sufficient insight into bioanalysis to understand the basic terminology and procedures involved, and to interpret the data.

At its simplest, there are three stages to bioanalysis. First, the sample must be 'cleaned' up and the drug(s) of interest extracted. The drug and its metabolites need then to be separated from each other and any remaining contaminants. Finally, the compounds of interest must be detected and quantified. Analytical techniques are becoming more and more sensitive and increasingly these processes are being automated.

High-pressure liquid chromatography (HPLC) is the classical method for sample separation. Other techniques may be used, such as gas chromatography for volatile compounds. Historically, the separated peaks were detected and quantified based on their fluorescence or absorption of ultraviolet or visible light, and these techniques may still be used to analyse compounds that cannot be ionized efficiently for mass spectroscopic (MS) detection. MS is, however, increasingly the method of choice for detection, being highly sensitive, rapid, and efficient.

9.2.3.1 Sample extraction and separation

Both gas chromatography and HPLC linked to traditional ultraviolet or fluorescence detection techniques require quite complex sample preparation and extraction. Liquid–liquid extraction exploits differences in solubility to selectively localize analytes in one solute (or liquid phase) while other material distributes to the other liquid phase. Solid phase extraction utilizes carefully selected cartridges containing the stationary phase with specific physico-chemical characteristics through which the solvent bearing the analytes is passed; the analytes retained in the solid phase are then washed off and collected.

HPLC separation can also be linked to MS detection. Because MS itself provides further selection beyond HPLC separation, requirements for sample preparation are generally less rigorous. Protein precipitation, in which an organic solvent such as acetronitrile is added to the sample to precipitate out the proteins, is quick, simple, and broadly applicable for MS analysis.

Whatever the means of sample preparation, in most cases the next stage is HPLC separation. This comprises a column or series of columns packed with solid phase that has specific physico-chemical properties so it interacts with the analyte. A 'C-18 column' is widely used, and a solvent containing the analytes is passed through the column under pressure. The solvent and contaminants pass through, while the analytes are retained by the column then eluted off under pressure and collected. Differences in the interactions between several analytes of interest and the solid phase lead them to be eluted off the column more or less rapidly. Hence, there is temporal separation of the peaks subsequently detected, distinguishing each chemical entity.

9.2.3.2 Detection

Having separated out the analytes of interest they need now to be identified and quantified. HPLC separation (abbreviated to liquid chromatography or LC) followed by MS detection, commonly known as LC/MS/MS, is increasingly the method of choice. Typically, the eluants from the HPLC column are introduced into the ion source of a mass spectrometer, generating ions. A first mass analyser passes these ions as a beam having the mass-to-charge ratio of the analyte(s) into a chamber where they collide with an inert gas. The ions fragment, and a second mass analyser passes a beam with pre-set mass-to-charge ratio corresponding to that of the ion fragment towards a detector. This LC/MS/MS system, comprising three key elements, is termed a triple quadrupole. It is more specific than single-stage LC/MS, which utilizes a single MS and no collision chamber.

Other detection techniques such as ultraviolet and fluorescence are well established, but now used less widely because LC/MS/MS offers substantial advantages in terms of simpler sample preparation and greater speed with enhanced specificity and sensitivity.

Irrespective of the assay procedure, standard curves are prepared by analysing known concentrations of the compounds of interest and plotting the signal strength, e.g. peak height, versus these known concentrations. The signal of each of the compounds detected in the clinical sample is then compared with the standard curve to determine its concentration. Quality control samples are included in each assay run.

9.2.3.3 Method development and validation

By definition, the initial doses of a new agent in first-in-man phase I studies are low, with correspondingly low plasma drug levels. Assays need, therefore, to be highly sensitive as well as specific and reproducible. The requirements of Good Clinical Laboratory Practice (GCLP) are also highly demanding, so it may take a great deal of time to establish an assay of sufficient quality for use in an early clinical trial (see below). It is important, that method development and validation begin many months in advance of patient entry to the trial.

Guidelines have been published for method validation [4], and acceptable limits for assay performance defined. A detailed review of these guidelines is outside the scope of this text, but important assay parameters include: extraction efficiency, accuracy, precision, specificity, sensitivity, and reproducibility.

The stability of the analyte, under different conditions (frozen room temperature, after thawing and re-freezing) and for varying periods, is also evaluated. Once all the validation parameters have been determined, a final report is required describing the bioanalytical methods and a complete set of SOPs should be prepared detailing each step of the analysis.

9.2.3.4 Good Clinical Laboratory Practice

Good Clinical Practice represents the international standard for the design, conduct, and reporting of clinical trials. The principles of Good Clinical Practice are incorporated as document E6 of the internationally accepted International Conference of Harmonization guidelines [5]. Implementation of the European Union Clinical Trials directive [6] further defined standards and requirements for the clinical conduct of trials in the European Union member states. All these guidelines are, however, vague with regard to the analysis of samples within those trials. Preclinical pharmacology studies are covered by guidelines on Good Laboratory Practice [7], but they do not pertain to studies on clinical material in clinical trials. Nevertheless, in some countries the principles of Good Laboratory Practice have been applied to the analysis of clinical samples.

Phase I trials and associated PK analyses have often been carried out at academic centres without the infrastructure for Good Laboratory Practice-like quality control. Recognizing, however, the need to be seen to perform analytical work to the appropriate standards, SOPs were increasingly introduced as a means of demonstrating quality standards. More recently, rising levels of regulation, along with the desire of academic centres and groups to be integrated into the drug development process, have led to the concept of GCLP that seeks to provide a framework for sample analyses within clinical trials. It applies those principles of Good Laboratory Practice that are relevant in the setting of a clinical trial, while adhering to the principles of Good Clinical Practice.

GCLP defines standards and requirements across a broad range of activities [8]:

- roles and responsibilities of laboratory staff
- facilities for the trial, waste disposal and archiving
- SOPs for the work performed
- the analytical plan
- processing and tracking of trial materials
- conduct of the work, including requirements for computer systems
- reporting results
- quality control
- independent quality audit

- storage and retention of records
- confidentiality.

In the UK the charity Cancer Research UK is leading an initiative to introduce GCLP. The British Association of Research Quality Assurance runs courses and produces documents on GCLP.

A more detailed review of GCLP is not appropriate here, but investigators need to be aware of the increasing need to apply these principles to the analysis of samples from early trials. Where laboratory studies are one of the primary aims of a study, or may be included in a regulatory submission, GCLP will be increasingly important. On the other hand, GCLP would not be a requirement where the assays are considered secondary, not impacting directly on the conduct of the trial or its outcome, and not anticipated to be part of a regulatory submission. It is important, therefore, that the investigator be clear why assays are being performed so that the appropriate level of quality control or GCLP can be applied.

More and more, GCLP will affect in which laboratories PK analysis can be undertaken, the time to set up and validate the assay, how long it will take to generate a laboratory report and the overall cost of laboratory studies. From a practical perspective, these developments are helpful insofar as they underpin and validate laboratory data, provided the requirements do not become so stringent as to obstruct the analysis of clinical samples.

9.2.4 Data analysis

Concentration–time (C × T) data are first plotted for each patient, using a linear scale for time and logarithmic scale for drug and, where appropriate, metabolite concentrations. Figure 9.1 is an example of how this might be shown in a study report. In this figure, taken from a phase I report of 17-allylamino, 17-demethoxygeldanamycin (17-AAG), C × T data for the drug and its metabolite are displayed for several patients treated at the highest dose level [9].

9.2.4.1 Compartmental and non-compartmental analyses

There are two general approaches to PK data analysis, compartmental and non-compartmental analysis.

Non-compartmental analysis is the more straightforward. Such analyses generate the basic PK parameters described above, without the need for devising a model or making extensive assumptions about the data. Although these analyses can be done manually, by 'curve stripping', in practice PK programmes perform the same function more rapidly. The main limitation of non-compartmental analyses is the restricted scope for modelling or

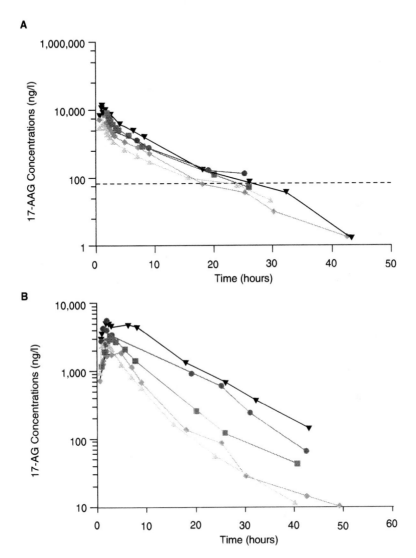

Figure 9.1 (A) Plasma concentration × time curves of 17-allylamino, 17-demethoxygeldanamycin in patients at 450 mg/m^2. The dotted line represents the mean IC$_{50}$ of the NCI 60 *in vitro* tumour cell line panel. (B) Plasma concentrations of the metabolite 17-amino, 17-demethoxygeldanamycin. From Banerji *et al.* (2005) *J Clin Oncol* **23**: 4152–61. Reprinted with permission from the American Society of Clinical Oncology.

simulating the data. In the context of early clinical trials, non-compartmental analyses is, therefore, widely applicable when the initial requirement is to define basic parameters.

In contrast, compartmental analysis is more complex, requires expertise in the handling of PK data, but is potentially more informative. A series of compartments are defined, between which the drug and metabolites pass. In a simple model a central compartment is defined, essentially the blood or plasma into which drug first distributes. It then distributes into one or more peripheral compartments, representing extravascular tissues and organs. The compartments are 'virtual' rather than physiological, and the number of compartments can be increased depending on the complexity of the model. This more sophisticated approach can help in understanding how a drug is handled. For example, a non-compartmental analysis may identify the fact that a drug has non-linear kinetics, e.g. there is a disproportionate rise in AUC in a phase I trial as dose is increased; a compartmental analysis can identify how and where the drug is distributed, explaining the cause of this non-linearity. Figure 9.2 provides an example of the application of this approach to the analysis of the PK of paclitaxel [10]. In this figure the authors illustrate the model they developed to describe the non-linear disposition of this drug.

Several programs for PK models are available, including PCNONLIN (SCI Software, Lexington, KY, USA), ADAPT II (Biomedical Simulations Resource, University of Southern California, Los Angeles, CA, USA), and WinNonLin (Pharsight Corp., Mountain View, CA, USA). The PK of E7070 provides a good illustration of the use of such models [11].

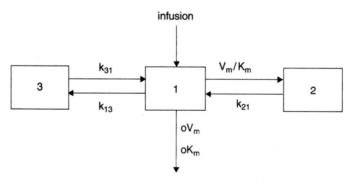

Figure 9.2 Representation of three-compartment model developed to described paclitaxel disposition. Reprinted from Kearns *et al.* (2005) *Semin Oncol* **22** (3 Suppl. 6): 16–23, with permission from Elsevier.

9.2.4.2 Population pharmacokinetics and limited sampling techniques

These terms come up quite frequently when discussing early clinical trials and drug development. Both represent more advanced approaches to the use of PK data. Whereas the approaches described earlier in this chapter use large numbers of samples from a small group of patients to define the kinetics of a drug in each individual, population PK and limited sampling strategies seek to gain more information from fewer blood samples in a large population. They are often based on preliminary data obtained in phase I trials and applied to later phase trials.

Population PK use modelling to describe how a drug is handled *across a population* rather than in a series of individuals. NONMEM (non-linear mixed effect modelling) is the best known population PK software program, but it requires highly specialized operators [12]. A NONMEM analysis uses fewer samples, collected from a large number of patients at differing (but accurately recorded) time points, and the data are analysed for the population. Both the interindividual variability and the residual random variability can be estimated and the influence of factors such as age and organ impairment can be investigated systematically. The use of population PK in drug development has been reviewed [13]. One of the best illustrations of how population PK can be used is the effect of liver dysfunction on docetaxel kinetics and toxicity [14].

A limited sampling strategy is one that allows PK data to be calculated *for an individual* based on only a few carefully timed samples. This makes PK studies possible in phase III trials where the collection of a full data set of 15–20 blood samples would usually not be feasible. Hence, although limited sampling strategies may be based on data from phase I trials, they are usually implemented in later phase trials. The most straightforward approach to developing a limited sampling strategy is to collect a conventional data set for a population and then define the PK parameter of interest, usually AUC. Stepwise linear regression is then undertaken on a subpopulation, the 'training set', with AUC the dependent variable and each of the individual time points independent variables [15]. Alternatively, a compartmental model can be fitted and the optimal sampling package of ADAPT II [16] used, or a population approach using NONMEM may be implemented [17].

9.3 Pharmacodynamics

PD endpoints assess *the effects of a drug on the body*. Although the focus of much recent interest due to the introduction of new targeted therapies, we should remember that traditionally phase I trials of cytotoxics include PD assessments in the form of monitoring blood counts to reflect toxicity to the bone marrow. Even with the increasing importance of targeted therapies, clinical findings may still be PD endpoints as with the dose-related skin rash typical of epidermal growth factor receptor inhibitors [18]. Similarly, the hypertension associated with inhibitors of vascular endothelial growth factor and its receptor reflects known mechanisms of action [19]. In both cases, however, the clinical finding was validated by correlation with inhibition of the target or downstream molecular measures in biopsy or imaging studies. With many targeted therapies a clinical PD endpoint has not been identified. Accordingly, there is increasing emphasis on molecular and functional changes, measured either in tissue samples or by imaging techniques, that measure target inhibition.

9.3.1 Principles of pharmacodynamics

PD markers can be used in different ways within an early clinical trial, usually of a novel biological or targeted therapy. While planning the study, it is important to establish why and how PD studies are to be incorporated.

- *To define dose escalation.* Here the measurement of PD effects are incorporated into the trial as a primary endpoint so they can be used to assess the magnitude of a biological effect and its relationship to the dose of drug administered. Hence, it is necessary to study PDs, using a fully validated assay, on all patients at each dose level, with clear implications for conduct of the trial. Indeed, where there is considerable between-patient variability in the magnitude of that PD effect, it may be necessary to treat more patients than usual at each dose level in an attempt to figure out differences in biological effects.
- *To define the recommended dose.* Again, the PD measurements are a primary endpoint. If there is no expectation or intention to escalate dose until a formal maximum tolerated dose is reached, it may be necessary to make detailed PD assessments at all dose levels to define the recommended dose. Alternatively, the maximum dose administered may be based on toxicity or by having achieved a specific PK threshold. In that case, detailed PD studies may be carried out at the top dose level and perhaps a second, lower dose at which there was either evidence of activity or potentially effective exposure was achieved. This can establish whether or not maximal dosing is required to achieve the biologically effective dose.
- *To provide 'proof-of-concept'.* This is a quite different situation, with PD studies aiming simply to establish that the drug has its expected or designed molecular effect. Although this can be done by conducting the PD studies in all patients as part of the phase I trial, this has disadvantages.

PD studies are often costly and time-consuming, and invasive procedures such as tumour biopsies may delay trial recruitment. In this context PD studies may be a secondary rather than a primary endpoint, and may only be required in a subset of patients (e.g. those treated at the recommended dose, or those treated at a centre with access to specialized functional imaging equipment). It is, however, important to clearly specify which patients will be studied. If complex imaging or invasive biopsy studies are 'optional' there is a likelihood that they will not be carried out so where they are important, PD studies should be mandatory.

♦ *To explore novel markers.* When a new drug enters the clinic, the target may not be fully defined, or a validated assay demonstrating target inhibition may not yet have been developed. The phase I trial is a unique opportunity to learn how a drug is acting over a range of doses, even where this information will not directly influence the conduct of the trial. Under these circumstances 'exploratory' or 'experimental' PD studies, carried out in a systematic manner can be valuable in their own right.

The above aims may, however, overlap. A proof-of-concept study may confirm that a dose is biologically effective, and the use of PD markers to guide dose escalation and determine their recommended dose may provide *de facto* evidence of proof-of-concept. Likewise, an exploratory study may identify markers that are incorporated at a later stage of the trial or in a subsequent study. In some circumstances, a separate PD study may be conducted once the first-in-man study is complete. A proof-of-concept study may then be carried out at the recommended dose. Where the optimal biological dose has not been fully defined, PD effects may be studied at two different doses (e.g. the maximum tolerated dose and a lower, well tolerated dose). It is not yet clear to what extent a positive 'signal' from PD studies can provide the rationale for a larger, randomized trial. This is relevant because, whereas achieving a pre-defined response rate in a phase II trial traditionally provides that rationale for cytotoxics, objective responses may not be anticipated for at least some biological agents so an alternative signal is needed.

Issues specific to tissue biopsies and functional imaging are discussed below. Several general points are, however, worth making. First, it is important that preclinical studies (and perhaps as well previous clinical studies of related compounds) have defined the appropriate target, PD marker and desired biological outcome. This will often take the form of demonstrating dose-dependent changes in a signalling pathway in tumours that respond to the drug in preclinical models. However, despite the emphasis on rational development of targeted therapies, drugs will often have more than one target or biological effect. It is also possible that the antitumour activity that has been observed preclinically may not be mediated by the inhibition of the putative target. This is illustrated by the development of sorafenib, which was first thought to be a 'specific' inhibitor of raf-1 kinase [20]. Subsequently, sorafenib was found to act on several other kinases [21] inhibition of which may mediate its activity in some tumours. Under these circumstances, using a PD marker, either to provide proof-of-concept or to guide conduct of the study, may be positively misleading. It is important therefore, to be rigorous when selecting a PD marker but also to interpret the laboratory data cautiously and be flexible in conducting the clinical trial.

It is also important to define how the clinically relevant biological effect is best measured. Obviously, this depends on the drug and its target, but whether this takes the form of tissue biopsy or imaging, the PD assay must be validated and a clear protocol must be developed. Where the PD marker is the *primary* endpoint and fundamental to the conduct and outcome of the trial, the same principles of GCLP apply as were described above. It is necessary not only to define what is measured and how, but also the size of the biological effect that is considered 'desirable' or to reflect adequate target inhibition, and in what proportion of patients. In the absence of clinical data from related drugs, this will often mean extrapolating from good quality preclinical experiments.

Related to this is the question of how many patients are needed for adequate evaluation of the PD marker. Intuitively, we might anticipate that incorporating a PD marker within an early trial would make the study more efficient and reduce the number of patients required. In the longer-term, such studies almost certainly will streamline the development process, but in a phase I trial *more* patients may be required than when the primary endpoint is determined by toxicity. For a trial to show a dose–response in target inhibition from 40% at one dose level to 90% inhibition at a higher dose, 17 evaluable patients would need to be treated at each level [22].

The biopsy or assay procedures must be described adequately in the Patient Information Sheet (PIS) and/or informed consent document. It should be clear whether or not consenting to the PD study is a prerequisite of trial participation. A single PIS covering the clinical and PD aspects of the study will usually suffice where it is not possible to opt out of the PD study. In some cases one PIS may be adequate even if it is possible to participate only in the clinical study; this does, however, require that it be clear to the patient what they are consenting to. In other cases a separate PIS may be needed for the PD studies. Investigators may be guided by experience in their own institution or seek guidance from their local ethics committee.

Finally, it is important to establish that each trial centre has the resources for PD studies. Genuinely close links between the clinic and the PD laboratory are vital. Laboratory scientists must be directly involved in writing the protocol and acknowledged as authors and co-investigators. It is equally important that the imaging or molecular pharmacology teams are involved in a timely manner. Even more so than with PK studies, novel PD assays or imaging procedures may take many months to set up and validate, where necessary, to GCLP standards. Without the closest involvement of non-clinical scientists, PD studies are doomed to failure.

9.3.2 Tissue biopsies

When developing targeted therapies, taking tissue samples to establish whether a drug is modulating the desired target is logical, desirable but not straightforward. Even when preclinical experiments have defined the target and an assay has been established, important questions remain: Which tissue and how much? When should it be taken? How should it be handled or processed? How are the data to be analysed and interpreted?

9.3.2.1 Sample collection

Ideally, all patients should be included and target inhibition should be measured in the tumour, comparing samples before and after treatment. In addition, more than one baseline sample may be required to assess normal variability, and several at different times during and after treatment to determine the onset of target inhibition, the maximal effect and recovery to baseline. Each sample should also be sufficiently large that repeat measurements can be made and tissue stored for future use. To do this across all dose levels in a phase I trial will usually be impractical as it would limit the study to patients with multiple tumour deposits accessible for repeat biopsy, and many would not consent to multiple biopsies. It is, therefore, necessary to clearly establish the reasons for doing the PD studies, to define the relevant patient group and then develop a scheme that is both scientifically sound and clinically feasible.

More often than not, tumour biopsies will yield the most relevant information, but they are also usually the most challenging. The exception is leukaemia, where tumour cells are easily available. Although tumour biopsies are also relatively straightforward in patients with superficial melanoma, head and neck cancer, cervical cancer, or women with soft tissue metastases from breast cancer, other sites are less accessible. Nevertheless, repeat liver biopsies can also be safe and feasible [23,24]; examples of phase I trials incorporating serial molecular tissue measurements are shown in Table 3.8

in Chapter 3 [18,25–27]. The patient population must, however, be selected carefully, taking into account the key PD question(s), the study drug, and target under evaluation. It may be appropriate to mandate tumour biopsies from patients with specific tumour types only after certain toxicities occur indicating a potentially clinically relevant dose is being administered, once a target PK exposure is achieved, or after a PD signal has been seen in other surrogate tissues.

Because they are more easily accessible, normal tissues are attractive as 'surrogates' to measure cellular changes in molecular effects. It is a prerequisite of using such tissues that the appropriateness of the tissue in question and validity of the assay be confirmed first in preclinical models. The surrogate tissue should express the target in animals, and exhibit either a dose-related or pharmacokinetically related inhibition of the target that parallels target inhibition seen *in vivo* in tumours. The most convenient surrogate tissue is peripheral blood mononuclear cells, which can be sampled easily and frequently; buccal mucosa and skin are also easily accessible.

Preclinical data will guide the initial timing of samples; these may change as initial clinical data become available, but it is important that a degree of consistency be maintained throughout the study in order that the data can be meaningfully interpreted. Practical issues are also important, multiple time points being feasible for peripheral blood mononuclear cells or buccal smears but not for more invasive procedures. The question of how much tissue to sample is again determined by the needs of the assay and the feasibility of the procedure. At one extreme a large volume of tissue may be available by surgical excision of a tumour; the opposite is true where tissue is obtained by fine needle aspiration or even percutaneous biopsy. The smaller the biopsy, the greater the risk of sampling error (the tissue may not be representative of the tumour, it may be necrotic or may not even contain malignant material). Whatever the circumstances, the amount of tissue required should be clearly specified; 'as much as you can get' is not acceptable!

All aspects of sample collection, processing, storage, and transport must be described clearly in the study protocol. This will be along the lines described above for PK sampling, but for PD samples additional information may also be important. For example, from which skin surface should a skin biopsy be taken, and to what depth? How should the mouth be prepared before obtaining a buccal smear?

It is unusual for a statistical power calculation to be used to determine the number of patients to be sampled. This is understandable given our limited knowledge regarding target expression and its variability in different patients or tumours, and the optimal level or duration of target inhibition. Such uncertainty is, however, unsatisfactory if a PD marker is the primary end-point. Nevertheless, PD studies can define biological activity, as with the aromatase inhibitor anastrozole where six to eight patients were enrolled per dose level and peripheral blood oestradiol levels were the endpoint [28].

9.3.2.2 Tissue-based pharmacodynamic assays

The first question is what to measure and how. This may be fairly straightfor-ward when measuring cellular drug levels to demonstrate, for example, that a delivery system does generate drug preferentially in tumour tissue. More often, PD studies involve measuring inhibition of the specific target of a new drug. Important questions include whether the level of protein expres-sion, its phosphorylation status or downstream changes in cell signalling should be the PD endpoint. Preclinical studies will guide the decision as to what is measured, but practical aspects such as how robust or repeatable the assay is, how much tissue is needed and the condition or processing of that tissue are also important. Where several assays are undertaken, the one that constitutes the 'primary' endpoint should be defined upfront.

A range of assays is available to measure PD endpoints in plasma, normal tissue, and tumour samples. These include ELISA, immunohistochemistry, Northern and Western blotting, gene expression arrays and real-time poly-merase chain reaction. In the setting of drug development, most assays are refined and developed for a specific target by the academic or pharmaceutical company that generated the new molecule, and are not validated to GCLP. If the PD measurements are a primary endpoint of the trial, the assay should be validated to GCLP, which is time consuming and expensive. The principles and implications of GCLP were described with respect to PK assays in Section 9.2.3.4 and the same considerations apply to PD assays. Even where the PD endpoints are secondary or exploratory, aspects such as test-to-test reprodu-cibility should be assessed along with practical issues such as the effect of storage and extremes of heat. It is also necessary to define who will interpret the data and according to which criteria, i.e. what will constitute a 'positive' result. These questions are clearly defined for clinical toxicities and radio-logical tumour response, but much more difficult for PD assays.

Development and validation of the assay must be completed and the SOPs written before the trial opens.

9.3.3 Functional/molecular imaging studies

Imaging has long been central to anticancer drug development as a means of defining the extent of disease and monitoring response to treatment. In this context clear guidelines have been developed, the most widely used being is the RECIST criteria for response assessment [29]. More recently, functional or molecular imaging has been developed as a relatively non-invasive means of assessing *in vivo* the effect of new agents on both malignant and normal tissues [30]. In the USA, the National Cancer Institute has established several In Vivo Cellular and Molecular Imaging Centres; Cancer Research UK has established the Pharmacodynamic/Pharmacokinetic Technologies Advisory Committee that reviews the use of these approaches in hypothesis driven early clinical trials; Cancer Research UK also supports a PET research group at the Wolfson Molecular Imaging Centre in Manchester.

Functional imaging methods include dynamic contrast enhanced magnetic resonance imaging (DCE-MRI), positron emission tomography (PET), functional (or dynamic) computerized tomographic (CT) scanning, and ultrasound (US). Functional imaging has been used to study drug distribution, changes in tumour metabolism, and alterations in blood flow. Functional imaging is very attractive in certain situations, but this remains an evolving and often complex area of research. The feasibility of functional imaging is clear, but there are major challenges around standardization of data acquisition and analysis between centres. In many cases it also remains unclear to what extent changes detected by molecular imaging reflect altered tumour biology and ultimately changes in clinical outcome.

As with other PK and PD studies, the first step in functional imaging studies is to define the appropriate endpoint. This will be determined by the mode of action of the investigational agent and preclinical data. An endpoint that is clinically relevant and linked to tumour response would be preferred but this may only be apparent with hindsight. It is also important to define ahead of the trial not only the key endpoints but also the criteria defining an 'effect' or biological response. This threshold will vary with each drug and be determined in part by what is judged significant from preclinical or earlier clinical studies. It is also determined, however, by the reproducibility or otherwise of the technique. As described below, there are many sources of variability in functional imaging studies. It may, therefore, be necessary to study 10–15 patients at a single dose level to be confident of identifying the effect of a drug using these studies. The need to image 30 or more patients mandates either that multiple institutions be involved in the study or that the data be acquired over a longer period than would be usually be necessary to explore an expanded cohort in a phase I trial. Where multiple sites are used, the issue of consistency between institutions is crucial.

The majority of functional imaging studies have focused on angiogenesis inhibitors and vascular targeting agents, assessing tumour blood flow and perfusion, but there is potential to apply these approaches more widely. The range of functional imaging techniques, each with its own strengths and weaknesses, is described briefly below. From a practical point of view, perhaps the most important action for an investigator is to seek out and talk to the functional imaging team as early as possible when planning a clinical trial. A dialogue with them should identify what should be imaged, how, and when. It is also important to define the technical capabilities and manpower of the functional imaging team, because such studies may be limited locally by the absence of specific equipment, lack of funds, or access to the equipment. Long before the trial opens, the functional imaging team will need to define the protocol for data acquisition and processing, match this to the protocol in use at other sites if this is a multicentre study, and establish the reproducibility of the measurements.

9.3.3.1 Magnetic resonance

MR technology is best known as a means to image the size and structure of tumours, and define their relationship with adjacent tissues. It has been refined to offer several new means to measure PD endpoints. An important advantage of MR imaging and spectroscopy is that, because there is no ionizing radiation involved, serial examinations do not raise the safety issues linked to PET and CT.

It is beyond the scope of this chapter to describe in detail the techniques involved or the clinical data that are emerging, so only limited examples will be quoted.

- DCE-MRI uses changes in the site and intensity of signal after i.v. injection of the standard low molecular weight paramagnetic contrast agent gadolinium-DTPA to generate information on tumour perfusion, vessel density and permeability, and blood volume. DCE-MRI has acted as a biomarker for anti-angiogenic agents such as PTK787/ZK222584 [31]. Permeability to larger particles, and an estimate of blood volume, can be obtained using larger molecular weight contrast agents such as ferric oxide, that are retained in the vascular space to a greater extent.
- Diffusion weighted MRI uses changes in the rate and diffusion of water molecules to study alterations in the tumour microenvironment that may predict subsequent response to anticancer treatment.
- Blood oxygenation level dependent (BOLD) ^{1}H MRI exploits the paramagnetic properties of deoxyhaemoglobin to demonstrate vessel density, as well as the volume, flow, and oxygenation of blood in those vessels.
- Magnetic resonance spectroscopy (MRS) utilizes the same principles as MRI, but a high field strength (>1.5 tesla) magnet is required, as is additional hardware and software. Whereas MRI uses the ^{1}H signal to

produce an image, with MRS the data are used to generate a biochemical spectrum of specific metabolites. MRS is applicable only to atoms with particular properties, such as ^{1}H, ^{31}P, and ^{19}F, and has low sensitivity. Nevertheless, ^{31}P-MRS can provide information about the pH, bioenergetics, and membrane phospholipids in a selected region of interest that may again be an early indication of response to therapy [32]. In addition, there is the potential to study the tissue PK of drugs using MRS, but this is limited by the nuclei visible to MRS and its low sensitivity. ^{19}F-MRS has, however, been used to study the tissue PK of 5-fluorouracil [33].

9.3.3.2 Positron emission tomography

PET uses radio-labelled positron-emitting isotopes to show where a compound is, how much is present, and what effect it has. It is sensitive and quantitative, but special localization is less good than. A further issue is that facilities are needed to generate the labelled compound, and that isotopic label then has a limited half-life over which PET data can be acquired. PET is quite demanding for the patient, a perfusion scan taking about 3 hours in all, with the need for arterial cannulation and exposure to ionizing radiation.

♦ [^{18}F]-fluorodeoxyglucose (^{18}F-FDG) PET is used diagnostically to characterize potential tumour masses because of the avidity with which they take up glucose and for staging purposes. It has also been used to demonstrate the rapid metabolic response of gastrointestinal stromal tumours to imatinib that occurs long before any change in size [34]. These observations have encouraged as yet unproven hopes that [^{18}F]-FDG PET may identify patients benefiting from a cytostatic agent without having an objective radiological response.

♦ Other metabolic probes have also been used. Thymidine uptake relates to DNA synthesis and [^{11}C]thymidine PET has been used to monitor changes in tumour proliferation and inhibition of the enzyme thymidylate synthase [35].

♦ Tumour perfusion can be studied by [^{15}O]-H$_2$O PET and blood volume by [^{15}O]-CO PET. A potential limitation is the short half life of ^{15}O, and there may be contamination of data in the region of interest by signal from adjacent areas.

♦ Tissue PK can be studied by injecting and imaging the radio-labelled compound. In a study of the experimental cytotoxic XR5000, conventional PK studies showed that potentially therapeutic blood levels were achieved. PET studies showed drug distributed into tumours, but there was also significant uptake into other tissues, and at the maximum tolerated dose saturation of tumour XR5000 uptake was not achieved [36].

9.3.3.3 Dynamic computed tomography and ultrasound

Dynamic CT is a more straightforward technique that can be incorporated into standard CT examinations to measure tissue perfusion, blood volume, capillary permeability, and microvessel density. The attractions of dynamic CT include the fact that it is widely available and quantification is less complex than for DCE-MRI. Dynamic CT methodology is as yet less well developed than DCE-MRI and fewer clinical data are available. Recent developments in US, including microbubble contrast agents, make it possible now to study much smaller vessels than was previously possible, although limited tissue penetration may restrict its use to cutaneous studies.

9.3.4 Data analysis

The analysis of data from PD studies in tissue samples is complex, at least in part because of the wide range of assays that are employed. The issues in relation to functional imaging are, however, still more difficult. A start has been made, with specific recommendations for assessing antiangiogenic and antivascular therapeutic effects by MRI [37] and [^{18}F]-fluorodeoxyglucose PET to measure tumour responses [38]. Nevertheless, there remains a need to standardize further the acquisition, analysis, and reporting of data, so that comparisons can be made between centres and trials.

Reproducibility and quantification are major issues in functional imaging studies. For example, if the day-to-day variability in a parameter is 25%, it will not be possible to say whether a drug causing a fall of 20% is biologically active. Moreover, reproducibility will differ not only depending on what imaging technique and parameter are being used but also which tissue is being studied. The reproducibility of DCE-MRI is better in the brain than in the thorax and upper abdomen, which are affected by motion artefacts induced by respiration and the cardiac contraction. The importance of reproducibility was illustrated when liver metastases were studied by DCE-MRI over an 8-hour period, and the coefficient of variability was 11%; under these circumstances a 15% change in K_{trans} would be required to show drug activity [39].

The question of quantification is important whether functional imaging is used to provide proof-of-concept, to determine dose or in an exploratory manner [40]. Jayson *et al.* detected an impressive median decrease of 44% in first-pass permeability (K_{fp}) using DCE-MRI in patients receiving the anti-vascular endothelial growth factor monoclonal antibody HuMV833. However, the heterogeneity of this response was such that, using conventional cohorts of three patients, it was difficult to distinguish the PD effects at different dose levels [41]. A more accurate assessment of the number of patients to be treated can be made if the degree of change in an imaging endpoint that is deemed 'significant' is defined *a priori* and the reproducibility of the technique is understood. For PET, the standard deviation of the difference between repeat measurements is reported to be about 10% for both the standardized uptake value (SUV) and rate constant for uptake of FDG into tissue (K1). With DCE-MRI a coefficient of variation of 20% is quoted for measurements of K_{trans}, a measure of vascular permeability per unit volume. Using these figures, it is estimated that 10–15 patients would need to be imaged to measure a change in 15% with some statistical accuracy. In the context of a phase I trial, it is impractical to employ multiple cohorts of this size, all undergoing relatively complex imaging. It is, therefore, likely that a more conventional trial design will often be used to demonstrate tolerability and define a maximum dose level. Two or three cohorts can then be expanded, perhaps one at the maximum safe dose and a second at the lowest dose showing consistent but minor toxicity; an intermediate dose may be evaluated depending on results from the initial imaging studies.

Tumour heterogeneity, both between and within patients, is also a major issue for functional imaging studies in a hypothesis driven early trial; this is in marked contrast to the relative consistency of recording toxicity to normal tissues in a conventional phase I study. With high resolution techniques, a specific region of interest is selected. The region of interest may be selected empirically, leading to an area with a particularly 'bright' but unrepresentative signal being selected. Likewise selecting a different image slice or region of interest for sequential studies will introduce further variability. Limiting the imaging studies to patients with a particular tumour type that is well suited to the imaging modality may also be considered as a means of improving the consistency of data, but this can slow down recruitment.

Where multiple study sites are involved, the question of uniformity between sites is crucial. Imaging systems from different manufacturers may not be compatible, and even where the same equipment is used, research groups often devise their own data acquisition and analysis programs. More complex algorithms may generate additional biological data but are also more difficult to standardize. A single patient preparation and imaging protocol, with a single database analysed in a uniform manner is vital if the data are to be meaningfully interpreted. The concept of GCLP is only now being extended to functional imaging, but the concepts discussed previously in relation to PK and other laboratory analyses will become more and more relevant.

9.4 Pharmacokinetic–pharmacodynamic relationships

Relationships should be sought between drug exposure (i.e. PK) and markers of activity, be they clinical (usually toxicity) or novel (PD). Interestingly, most publications do not present PK–PD correlations; rather, a correlation is first shown between dose and PK (C_{max}, AUC or steady-state concentrations), then relationships between dose and activity are explored. Although less scientific-ally sound, this approach does reflect clinical practice where drug exposure is expressed in terms of dose rather than PK.

Modelling of PK–PD relationships in relation to toxicity is applied in an increasing proportion of phase I trials. A recent review of the place of such modelling in phase I trials described situations where modelling was or was not likely to be valuable and discussed issues of practical implementation [42]. One issue in phase I trials is that most patients are treated at relatively low dose levels with a low incidence of drug-related toxicity. Significant toxicities tend, therefore, to be grouped together at the higher dose levels or (exposures) which may distort PK–PD analyses. Such approaches are widely used through all stages of drug development; reviews specific to PK–PD modelling in the clinical development of docetaxel [43] and capecitabine [44] have recently been published.

The simplest analyses investigate the relationship between drug exposure and adverse effects by, for example, plotting dose versus AUC or C_{max}, and highlighting those patients with grade 3 or 4 or dose-limiting toxicity. Alter-natively, mean AUC or C_{max} may be compared in those patients with and those without significant toxicity. More sophisticated mathematical models have been devised to investigate in more detail the relationship between PK parameters, and the PD effect. These relationships have been best described in relation to antiproliferative cytotoxics and myelosuppression. The modified Hill equation, or E_{max} model, describes a sigmoidal relationship between a PK parameter, in most cases overall exposure as reflected by AUC, and 'effect' expressed as a percentage change. For example:

$$\% \text{ change in endpoint} = 100\% \times C^h / [C^h + EC_{50})^h]$$

where C is the PK parameter, h is the Hill constant that describes the shape of the sigmoid relationship, and EC_{50} is the value of C that achieves a 50% maximal effect. Applying the Hill model to the relationship between AUC and myelosuppression:

$$\% \text{ fall in neutrophils} = 100\% \times AUC^h / [AUC^h + EC_{50})^h]$$

Other PK parameters such as C_{max} or steady-state concentration (C_{ss}) can also be modelled in this way. Modelling relationships is, however, more difficult for non-haematological toxicity where evaluation is more subjective and the categories represent non-continuous variables. In such cases, a logistic regression model may be used to relate the PK parameter to toxicity expressed on the conventional CTC grading system. Correlations between PK and tumour response have also been difficult to establish, partly because anti-cancer drugs are often used in combination and also because response is usually only manifest after several cycles of treatment, whereas in most cases kinetics are studied during cycle 1 only. Appropriate statistical support is important to ensure that the analysis of data is conducted appropriately.

The quantification of both tissue-based endpoints and functional imaging is a continuing challenge. A distinction can be drawn between two of the settings in which PD data are collected, i.e. to provide proof-of-concept or to identify the recommended dose. In the first setting, PD markers have proved effective in many studies in demonstrating proof-of-concept. This is valuable, and certainly strengthens the case for further development of an agent. It is not, however, the same as proof of clinical efficacy because the link between PD markers and patient benefit is often unproven. This link can usually only be confirmed retrospectively when phase III trials give clinical validation of the endpoint. The second setting, using PD data to select dose, is a greater challenge. In the majority of cases, both tissue-based and imaging studies more convincingly show a threshold dose or concentration of study drug above which a target is seen to be inhibited, than a clear dose–response curve that plateaus above a certain level of drug exposure. With functional imaging studies, one of the difficulties is that large numbers of patients may need to be studied at each dose level and doing this throughout dose escalation is unlikely to be feasible.

PK–clinical PD correlations have been reviewed [45]; selected examples of such studies are shown in Table 9.1 [11,14,46–48]. Recent examples of how tissue drug levels influence the development of a drug and some PK–laboratory correlations are shown in Table 9.2 [49–53]. Selected examples of the several dynamic imaging studies using both DCE-MR and $[^{15}O]H_2O$ PET were shown in Table 3.10 in Chapter 3 [54–57]. Studies with the vascular endothelial growth factor receptor tyrosine kinase inhibitor valatanib (PTK787/ZK222584) were especially interesting [31,58]. As shown in Figure 9.3, the clear fall in Ki across the dose range shown using DCE-MRI gave proof-of-concept. Even though the cohort sizes were too small to discriminate clearly between PD effects at different dose levels, modelling of the imaging data supported a dose of >1000 mg for further study. The subsequent phase III trial in metastatic colorectal cancer did not, however, achieve its primary endpoint [59]. One possible explanation for these disappointing results is that the schedule of valatanib may not have been optimal to achieve consistent drug exposure, a PK rather than PD issue. Interestingly, trials with combretastatin A4 phosphate using both DCE-MRI [56,57] and PET [60] gave

Table 9.1 Selected pharmacokinetic–clinical pharmacodynamic relationships

Drug	Analyses	Results	Reference
Indisulam	NONMEM analysis of pharmacokinetic data from phase I trials	Model predicted severity and duration of neutropenia and thrombocytopenia Schedule-dependent differences in kinetics of haematological precursor	van Kesteren et al. (2005) [11]
Irinotecan	Semi-physiological compartmental model Patients studied in phase I SN38 glucuronidation rates studied	Biliary index (SN38/SN38 glucuronide) concentration ratio correlated with diarrhoea Clinical significance uncertain	Gupta et al. (1994) [46]
Docetaxel	Limited sampling of patients from 24 phase II studies Bayesian population pharmacokinetic/pharmacodynamic analysis	Docetaxel clearance predicted severe/febrile neutropenia Cumulative dose predicted time onset of fluid retention Patients with elevated liver enzymes had reduced docetaxel clearance	Bruno et al. (1998) [14]
Paclitaxel	Relationships to toxicity and efficacy sought Patients received either 135 or 175 mg/m² as a 1- or 3-h i.v. infusion in a phase III study	No significant correlation between AUC and toxicity However, exposure above threshold paclitaxel concentration correlated with changes in neutrophil count	Huizing et al. (1993) [47]
Topotecan	Pharmacokinetics compared between treatment arms Data from 4 phase I studies using 4 different schedules of oral topotecan	Correlations found between AUC of topotecan lactone and myelosuppression	Gerrits et al. (1999) [48]

NONMEM, non-linear mixed effect modelling.

Table 9.2 Selected pharmacokinetic–laboratory pharmacodynamic relationships

Drug	Analyses	Results	Reference
Capecitabine (oral 5-FU pro-drug)	Specific study after phase I completed and recommended dose established Patients received capecitabine before surgery Tissue levels of 5-FU measured in plasma, tumour, and normal tissue	Levels of 5-FU more than 20-fold higher in tumour compared with plasma Levels of 5-FU more than 3-fold greater in colorectal tumours than adjacent normal mucosa Development continued	Schuller et al. (2000) [47]
MAG-CPT (i.v. polymer bound camptothecin)	Ten patients scheduled for colorectal cancer surgery Received MAG-CPT 1, 3, or 7 days before surgery Mag-bound and free CPT levels measured	No evidence of selective delivery to tumours Polymer delivery programme discontinued	Sarapa et al. (2003) [50]
Erlotinib (oral EGFR inhibitor)	Within phase I study, patients had biopsy of normal skin at baseline and at day 21 of treatment Expression and activation of EGFR, and downstream markers (ERK, p27)	28 patients studied Using IHC phospho-EGFR expression fell and p27 expression rose on treatment, but not dose-related	Malik et al. (2003) [51]
Gefitinib (oral EGFR inhibitor)	65 patients studied in phase I trials before treatment and at day 28	Thinning of stratum corneum and other histological changes in epidermis Phosphorylation of EGFR lower, but p27[KIP1] higher, on gefitinib Biochemical effects not dose-related, but seen at doses well below maximum tolerated dose	Albanell et al. (2002) [52]
CCI-779 (mTOR inhibitor)	Peripheral blood mononuclear cells studied from healthy volunteers and patients p70[s6] assayed by immunoblot	p70[s6] kinase activity across 10-fold range of doses Inhibition of p70[s6] at 24 h correlated with time to progression	Peralba et al. (2003) [53]

EGFR, epidermal growth factor receptor; CPT, camptothecin; 5-FU, 5-fluorouracil; IHC, immunohistochemistry

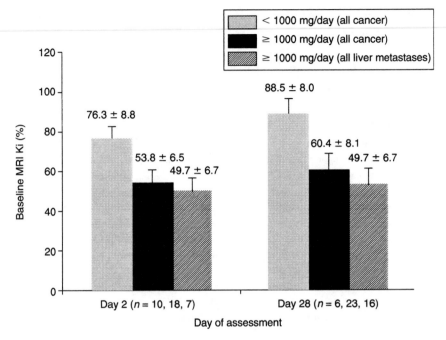

Figure 9.3 Mean (± SE) percentage of baseline magnetic resonance imaging (MRI) bidirectional transfer constant (Ki) for patients receiving <1000 mg/day and >1000 mg/day on days 2 and 28 of PTK787/ZK 222584 treatment. From Thomas *et al.* (2005) *J Clin Oncol* 23: 4162–71. Reprinted with permission from the American Society of Clinical Oncology.

comparable results, even though PET measures absolute blood flow in tumour and normal tissue, whereas DCE-MRI measures a composite of blood flow, vascular permeability, and surface area.

9.5 Summary

PK and PDs play important roles in phase I trials of anticancer agents. Both require clear protocol specifications regarding what, how, and when to collect samples or to perform other special procedures on the patient. PK and PD measures give information regarding how the drug is metabolized or cleared by the patient and what impact the drug has on normal or tumour tissues. Results from these studies may occasionally be the basis for recommending the dose at the conclusion of the phase I trial, but more often they reinforce dose recommendations. Molecular and imaging PD studies are becoming more common in phase I design and can offer useful insights into whether the drug is in fact acting on the putative molecular target (proof-of-concept).

Relationships between PK parameters and PD effects can help shape the subsequent drug development plan for a novel compound. All of these factors serve to highlight the importance of incorporating PK and PD measures in phase I studies and in investing in the necessary assay validation in preclinical models before phase I studies begin in patients.

References

1. Collins JM, Grieshaber CK, Chabner BA (1990). Pharmacologically guided phase I trials based upon preclinical development. *J Natl Cancer Inst* **82**: 1321–6.

2. Gibaldi M, Perrier D (1982). *Pharmacokinetics*, 2nd edn. Marcel Decker, New York.

3. Peng GW, Chiou WL (1990). Analysis of drugs and other toxic substances in biological samples for pharmacokinetic studies. *J Chromatogr Biomed Appl* **531**: 3–50.

4. FDA Guidance for validation of pharmacokinetic methods. May be found at: http://www.fda.gov/cder/guidance/4252fnl.htm [last accessed August 2005]

5. ICH Guideline on Good Clinical Practice (E6) may be found at the ICH web site: www.ich.org [last accessed August 2005]

6. European Union Clinical Trials Directive http://medicines.mhra.gov.uk/ourwork/licensingmeds/types/clintrialdir.htm [last accessed August 2005]

7. Good Laboratory Practice: www.accessdata.fda.gov/scripts/cdrh/cfdocs/cfcfr/CFRSearch.cfm [last accessed August 2005]

8. Stiles T, Grant V, Mawbey N (2003). Good clinical laboratory practice. A Quality System for Laboratories that undertake the Analyses of Samples from Clinical Trials. Publication available from The British Association of Research quality Assurance (web address: http://www.barqa.com/) [last accessed August 2005]

9. Banerji U, O'Donnell A, Scurr M, *et al.* (2005). Phase I pharmacokinetic and pharmacodynamic study of 17-allylamino, 17-demethoxygeldanamycin in patients with advanced malignancies. *J Clin Oncol* **23**: 4152–61.

10. Kearns CM, Gianni L, Egorin MJ. (1995). Paclitaxel pharmacokinetics and pharmacodynamics. *Semin Oncol* **22** (3 Suppl. 6): 16–23.

11. Van Kesteren C, Zandvliet AS, Karlsson MO, *et al.* (2005). Semi-physiological model describing the haematological toxicity of the anti-cancer agent indisulam. *Invest New Drugs* **23**: 225–34.

12. Beal SL, Sheiner LB (1989). *NONMEM Users Guide*. University of California, San Fransisco CA.

13. Vozeh S, Steimer JL, Rowland M, Morselli P, Mentre F, Balant LP, Aarons L (1996). The use of population pharmacokinetics in drug development. *Clin Pharmokinet* **30**: 81–93.

14. Bruno R, Hille D, Riva A, *et al.* (1998). Population pharmacokinetics/pharmacodynamics of docetaxel in phase II studies in patients with cancer. *J Clin Oncol* **16**: 187–96.

15. Ratain MJ, Vozelgang (1987). Limited sampling model for vinbastine pharmacokinetics. *Cancer Treat Rep* **71**: 935–9.

16. D'Argenio DZ (1981). Optimal sampling times for pharmacokinetic experiments. *J Pharmacokinet Biopharm* **9**: 739–56.

17. Sallas WM (1995). Development of limited sampling strategies for characteristics of a pharmacokinetic profile. *J Pharmacokinet Biopharm* **23**: 515–29.

18. Baselga J, Rischin D, Ranson M, *et al.* (2002). Phase I safety, pharmacokinetic, and pharmacodynamic trial of ZD1839, a selective oral epidermal growth factor receptor tyrosine kinase inhibitor, in patients with five selected solid tumor types. *J Clin Oncol* **20**: 4292–302.

19. Hurwitz H, Fehrenbacher L, Novotny W, *et al.* (2004). Bevacizumab plus irinotecan, fluorouracil, and leucovorin for metastatic colorectal cancer. *N Engl J Med* **350**: 2335–342.

20. Lyons JF, Wilhelm S, Hibner B, Bollag G (2001). Discovery of a novel Raf kinase inhibitor. *Endocr Relat Cancer* **8**: 219–25.

21. Wilhelm S, Carter C, Tang LY, *et al.* (2003). BAY 43–9006 exhibits broad spectrum anti-tumour activity and targets Raf/MEK/ERK pathway and receptor tyrosine kinases involved in tumour progression and angiogenesis. *Clin Cancer Res* **9**: A 78.

22. Korn EL, Arbuck SG, Pluda JM, Simon R, Kaplan RS, Christian MC (2001). Clinical trial design for cytostatic agents: are new approaches needed? *J Clin Oncol* **19**: 265–72.

23. Dowlati A, Haaga J, Remick SC, Spiro TP, *et al.* (2001). Sequential biopsies in early phase clinical trials of anticancer agents for pharmacodynamic evaluation. *Clin Cancer Res* **7**: 2971–6.

24. Hidalgo A, Tabernero J, Rojo F, Marimon I, Andreu J, Baselga J (2004). Feasibility of CT-guided serial liver biopsies to evaluate pharmacodynamic endpoints in patients with liver metastasis treated with experimental drugs. *Abdom Imaging* **30**: 65–8.

25. Tabernero J, Rojo F, Marimon I, *et al.* (2005). Phase I pharmacokinetic and pharmacodynamic study of weekly 1-hour and 24-hour infusion BMS-214662, a farnesyltransferase inhibitor, in patients with advanced solid tumors. *J Clin Oncol* **23**: 2521–31.

26. Adjei AA, Erlichman C, Davis JN, *et al.* (2000). A phase I trial of the farnesyl transferase inhibitor SCH66336: evidence for biological and clinical activity. *Cancer Res* **60**: 1871–7.

27. Stewart DJ, Donehower RC, Eisenhauer EA, *et al.* (2003). A phase I pharmacokinetic and pharmacodynamic study of the DNA methyltransferase 1 inhibitor MG98 administered twice weekly. *Ann Oncol* **14**: 766–74.

28. Plourde PV, Dyroff M, Dowsett M, Demers L, Yates R, Webster A (1995). ARIMIDEX®: a new oral, once-a-day aromatase inhibitor. *J Steroid Biochem Mol Biol* **53**: 175–9.

29. Therasse Arbuck SG, Eisenhauer EA, *et al.* (2000). New guidelines to evaluate the response to treatment in solid tumors (RECIST Guidelines). *J Natl Cancer Inst* **92**: 205–16.

30. Seddon BM, Workman P (2003). The role of functional imaging in cancer drug discovery and development. *Br J Radiol* **76**: 128–38.

31. Morgan B, Thomas AL, Drevs J, *et al.* (2003). Dynamic contrast-enhanced magnetic resonance imaging as a biomarker for the pharmacological response of PTK787/ZK222584, an inhibitor of the vascular endothelial growth factor receptor tyrosine kinases, in patients with advanced colorectal cancer and liver metastases: results from two phase I studies. *J Clin Oncol* **21**: 3955–964.

32. Leach MO, Verrill M, Glaholm J, *et al.* (1998). Measurements of human breast cancer using magnetic resonance spectroscopy: a review of clinical measurements and a report of localized 31P measurements of response to treatment. *NMR Biomed* **11**: 314–40.

33. Wolf W, Presant CA, Waluch V (2000). ^{19}F-MRS studies of fluorinated drugs in humans. *Adv Drug Deliv Res* **41**: 55–74.

34. van Oosterom AT, Judson I, Verweij J, *et al.* (2001). Safety and efficacy of imatinib (STI571) in metastatic gastrointestinal stromal tumours: a phase I study. Lancet 358:1421–3.

35. Wells P, Aboagye E, Gunn RN, *et al.* (2003). 2-[^{11}C]thymidine positron emission tomography as an indicator of thymidylate synthase inhibition in patients treated with AG337. *J Natl Cancer Inst* 95: 675–82.

36. Propper DJ, de Bono J, Saleem A, *et al.* (2003). Use of positron emission tomography in pharmacokinetic studies to investigate therapeutic advantage in a Phase I study of 120-hour intravenous infusion XR5000. *J Clin Oncol* 21: 203–10.

37. Leach MO, Brindle KM, Evelhoch JL, *et al.* (2003). Assessment of antiangiogenic and antivascular therapeutics with MRI: recommendations for appropriate methodology for clinical trials. *Br J Radiol* 76 (Spec No 1): S87–91.

38. Young H, Baum R, Cremarius U, *et al.* (1999). Measurement of clinical and sub-clinical tumour response using [18F]-fluorodeoxyglucose and positron emission tomography: review and 1999 EORTC recommendations. *Eur J Cancer* 35: 1773–82.

39. Jackson A, Haroon H, Zhu XP, Li KL, Thacker NA, Jayson G (2002). Breath-hold perfusion and permeability mapping of hepatic malignancies using magnetic resonance imaging and a first-pass leakage profile model. *NMR Biomed* 15: 164–73.

40. Galbraith SM (2003). Antivascular cancer treatments: imaging biomarkers in pharmaceutical drug development. *Br J Radiol* 76: 83–6.

41. Jayson GC, Zweit J, Jackson A, *et al.* (2002). Molecular imaging and biological evaluation of HuMV833 anti-VEGF antibody: implications for trial design of anti-angiogenic antibodies. *J Natl Cancer Inst* 94: 1484–93.

42. Aarons L, Karlsson MO, Mentre F, Rombout F, Steimer J-L, van Peer A (2001). Role of modelling and simulation in Phase I drug development. *Eur J Pharm Sci* 13: 115–22.

43. van Kesteren Ch, Mathot RA, Beijnen JH, Schellens JHM (2003). Pharmacokinetic–pharmacodynamic guided trial design in oncology. *Invest New Drugs* 21: 225–41.

44. Blesch KS, Gieschke, Tsukamoto Y, Reigner BG, Burger HU, Steimer J-L (2003). Clinical pharmacokinetic/pharmacodynamic and physiologically based pharmacokinetic modelling in new drug development: the capecitabine experience. *Invest New Drugs* 21: 195–223.

45. Kobayashi K, Jodrell DI, Ratian MJ (1993). Pharmacokinetic–pharmacodynamic relationships and therapeutic drug monitoring. *Cancer Surv* 17: 51–78.

46. Gupta E, Lestingi TM, Mick R, *et al.* (1994). Metabolic fate of irinotecan (CPT-11) in humans; correlation of glucuronidation with diarrhea. *Cancer Res* 54: 3723–5.

47. Huizing MT, Keung AC, Rosing H, *et al.* (1993). Pharmacokinetics of paclitaxel and metabolites in a randomised comparative study in platinum-pretreated ovarian cancer patients. *J Clin Oncol* 11: 2127–35.

48. Gerrits CJH, Schellens JHM, Burris H, *et al.* (1999). A comparison of clinical pharmacokinetics of different administration schedules of oral topotecan (Hycamtin). *Clin Cancer Res* 5: 69–75.

49. Schuller J, Cassidy J, Dumont E, *et al.* (2000). Preferential activation of capecitabine in tumor following oral administration to colorectal cancer patients. *Cancer Chemother Pharmacol* 45: 291–7.

50. Sarapa N, Britto MR, Speed W, *et al.* (2003). Assessment of normal and tumor tissue uptake of MAG-CPT, a polymer-bound prodrug of camptothecin, in patients undergoing elective surgery for colorectal carcinoma. *Cancer Chemother Pharmacol* **52**: 424–30.

51. Malik SN, Siu LL, Rowinsky EK, *et al.* (2003). Pharmacodynamic evaluation of the epidermal growth factor inhibitor OSI-774 in human epidermis of cancer patients. *Clin Cancer Res* **9**: 2478–86.

52. Albanell J, Rojo F, Averbuch S, *et al.* (2002). Pharmacodynamic studies of epidermal growth factor inhibitor ZD1839 in skin from cancer patients: histopathologic and molecular consequences of receptor inhibition. *J Clin Oncol* **20**: 110–24.

53. Perralba JM, de Graffenried L, Friedrichs W, *et al.* (2003). Pharmacodynamic evaluation of CCI-779, an inhibitor of mTOR, in cancer patients. *Clin Cancer Res* **9**: 2887–92.

54. Herbst RS, Mullani NA, Davis DW, *et al.* (2002). Development of biologic markers of response and assessment of antiangiogenic activity in a clinical trial of recombinant human endostatin. *J Clin Oncol* **20**: 3804–14.

55. Thomas JP, Arzoomaniam RZ, Alberti D, *et al.* (2003). Phase I pharmacokinetic and pharmacodynamic study of recombinant human endostatin in patients with advanced solid tumors. *J Clin Oncol* **21**: 223–31.

56. Dowlati A, Robertson K, Cooney M, *et al.* (2002). A phase I pharmacokinetic and translational study of the novel vascular targeting agent Combretastatin A-4 phosphate on the single-dose intravenous schedule in patients with advanced cancer. *Cancer Res* **62**: 3408–16.

57. Galbraith SM, Maxwell RJ, Lodge MA, *et al.* (2003). Combretastatin A4 phosphate has tumor antivascular activity in rat and man as demonstrated by dynamic magnetic resonance imaging. *J Clin Oncol* **21**: 2831–42.

58. Thomas AL, Morgan B, Horsfield MA, *et al.* (2005). Phase I study of the safety, tolerability, pharmacokinetics, and pharmacodynamics of PTK787/ZK 222584 administered twice daily in patients with advanced cancer. *J Clin Oncol* **23**: 4162–71.

59. Hecht JR, Trarbach T, Jaeger E, *et al.* (2005). A randomized, double-blind, placebo-controlled, phase III study in patients with metastatic adenocarcinoma of the colon or rectum receiving first-line chemotherapy with oxaliplatin/5-fluorouracil/leucovorin and PTK787/ZK222584 or placebo (CONFIRM-1). *J Clin Oncol* **23** (No 16S [June 1 Suppl.]): LBA3.

60. Anderson HL, Yap JT, Miller MP, Robbins A, Jones T, Price P (2003). Assessment of pharmacodynamic vascular response in a phase I trial of Combretastatin A4 phosphate. *J Clin Oncol* **21**: 2823–30.

Chapter 10

Running the study

Elizabeth A. Eisenhauer

10.1 Investigator and institutional responsibilities

Good Clinical Practice (GCP) outlines in detail the responsibilities of the investigator and the institution. Details of these responsibilities are found in the GCP document and are summarized in Chapter 8. In brief, some of the most important responsibilities vis-à-vis running the study are listed here:

◆ *Investigator.*

1. Qualifications: must be adequate.
2. Following the protocol: must agree to follow the protocol.
3. Designating responsibility to and supervising of study personnel.
4. Confidentiality: must maintain patient confidentiality and keep information regarding the study and agent(s) confidential as requested by the sponsor.
5. Data completeness and accuracy: must attest to accuracy and completeness of trial data.
6. Informing: must inform the patients of relevant new information and the institution Institutional Review Board/Independent Ethics Committee similarly. Must also inform the sponsor of serious events as described in the protocol.

◆ *Institutional:*

7. Ethics review and responsibility for ongoing review of trial.

8. Facilities: laboratory, radiology, medical facility, dedicated space for study materials and staff.
9. Standard operating procedures and quality control.

Chapter 8 contains more detail and documents in Appendix III provide some tools to aid in compliance with certain aspects of these responsibilities.

10.2 Identifying patients for a phase I trial

Institutions vary in their organizational structure. Many large cancer treatment facilities have subspecialist oncologists treating only one type, or only a handful, of cancers. Because phase I trials, particularly first-in-man studies, cross disease boundaries by enrolling patients with a variety of tumour types, there may be logistic challenges in arranging for the investigator or her study nurse to see or screen all potential patients for a study. There are two main approaches to addressing this, as follows.

The first is to assign several co-investigators (also called sub-investigators) to the trial team from a variety of oncology subspecialties. The disadvantage of this approach is that their practice locations and timing of outpatient clinics may not make it easy for study personnel such as research nurses to organize trial-related procedures. Furthermore, such an approach will dilute investigator experience with the drug and its effects on patients. This may mean that some subtle but real drug-related changes in patients may not be recognized as such if every patient is seen and followed by a different investigator.

The second, and preferred, approach is to organize a 'phase I clinic', or similarly titled clinic, once a week. Colleagues can refer patients who have exhausted standard curative therapeutic or palliative options to this clinic where they will be seen by the phase I investigator(s) to be screened for eligibility to any ongoing phase I trials. This organizational approach will concentrate experienced phase I personnel and resource into one place, but it will require transfer of the care of the patient from the original oncologist to the phase I investigator for the period of time they are on the trial. Concurrent care arrangements may be possible to avoid having to re-refer the patient to their original physician once the study is completed. For this to work well, a menu of several phase I trials, adequately resourced, is desirable so that referrals can be received on an ongoing basis rather than being turned on and off when trials or dose levels open and close.

10.3 Discussing the study with patients

Phase I cancer trials are unique in that the population is one of incurably ill patients, rather than healthy volunteers. Coupled with this is the fact that the trial's goals are not primarily concerned with efficacy. These factors create special challenges for disclosure and discussion. Even though a consent form may contain all the information believed to be relevant to an informed decision in a written document, the consent form itself is not a *process*: that must involve substantial discussion between the patient, members of the trial team and other caregivers if necessary. The consent process must be consistent with the principles articulated by the Nuremberg Code, the Declaration of Helsinki and the precepts of GCP. Three fundamental ethical principles are invoked in obtaining consent for research from human subjects: *respect for persons* (individuals treated as autonomous beings, capable of making informed choices), *beneficence* (maximize the possible benefits and minimize harms), and *justice* (treat research participants fairly and ensure there is a reasonable balance of risk and benefit in any experimental undertaking). These principles are reflected in the standard language required and content of consent forms (see Chapter 7) but also must be threaded through the discussions held with patients about the options to enrol in a clinical trial. Investigators and staff must be aware in discussions with patients that varying cultural backgrounds can have an impact on their, and families', willingness to have frank discussions of their prognosis or of experimental treatments. The framework for discussion of life-threatening illness that culture creates may not be well understood by caregivers (or well taught by educators) so sensitivity to the cues presented in the conversation is extremely important. See Chapter 4 for a more extensive discussion of this topic.

10.3.1 Other options for treatment

For a patient, entering a phase I trial may be one of several options at a particular time point in their illness. Thus the discussion regarding enrolment on a trial must include a conversation of other possible options for management. In combination phase I trials, it may be the case that the 'standard' regimen with which the new drug is combined is available to the patients and they do not need to be enrolled on the trial to receive it. Supportive/palliative care only is one option that is difficult but important to discuss with patients who have exhausted all forms of active therapy, as patients may feel that, if they are not enrolled on a trial, they will not have a chance to receive any care at all. It needs to be clear to patients that they will continue to receive the best medical care possible if they choose not to enrol on a trial as, if the patient believes that they will not, it may coerce them into enrolling on a trial they do not really want to join.

10.3.2 What the trial involves

To make an informed choice, not only does the patient need to know about what the other options are for managing their disease, they need to have a good understanding about what the trial itself involves: What is the goal of the study? What will treatment involve in terms of visits or tests? Are there special or genetic tests that are a mandatory part of the trial? Will there be personal costs that the patient must bear? What are expected side-effects? Expected benefits? It is clear that, despite the best process and consent form, patients will not always understand that the chances of antitumour benefit are extremely small in first-in-man phase I studies (see discussion of this topic in Chapter 4). It is the investigator's responsibility to ensure that the patient is sufficiently informed about the answers to these questions to make a truly informed decision.

10.3.3 Consent in two steps

Some studies have suggested that research subjects' understanding of informed consent is enhanced by more one-on-one interaction between the patients and investigators [1]. To accomplish this, it is recommended that the process of consenting a patient be done in two steps: in the first, the investigator (alone or with the research nurse) explains the study and determines if the patient is interested in participating. If yes, then before final consent is given, the patient is asked to think over the participation, take home, read and discuss the consent form with his/her family, family physician and/or another physician. During this interlude, any additional routine testing to ensure eligibility can be started, with the patient's agreement. Some trials require full consent to the study before even routine testing is undertaken, but others allow tests such as scans or basic haematology and biochemistry tests to be undertaken before the consent form is signed. All trials, however, require written consent before any non-standard trial-related procedures such as a fresh tumour biopsy can be done. Once the patient has had time to consider participation, a second visit is scheduled in which the investigator can review once more the major elements of the trial, ask the patient what his/her understanding is of the study's purpose and procedures (to assure the patient is adequately informed) and address any questions. If, after this is completed, the patient voluntarily agrees to proceed, the consent form can be signed and the process of trial registration and treatment begin. It is usual to give a copy of the consent form to the patient to keep.

10.3.4 During the trial: continued feedback

It is important to engage in ongoing discussion with patients (or trial subjects) during the study. As described in Chapter 4, investigators have a duty to inform patients of 'significant new findings' that arise in other patients enrolled on the same study or in experience with the drug in other studies that might have an impact on a patient's continued willingness to remain on the study. Emerging new toxicity information is an example: even before the consent form is altered to update it (if that is deemed necessary), the patient should be verbally informed about significant new toxic effects of the investigational therapy and the conversation documented in the patient's medical record. Patients may encounter symptoms or have questions that they did not think to ask about at an appointment and must have reasonable access to study personnel, such as the research nurse, to discuss these. Some research nurses make a point of telephoning patients a few days or a week after the first phase I treatment is given to see if there are any symptoms or questions; this is a good practice that should be more widely adopted. Patients can keep a diary of symptoms and questions to bring to the attention of the trial team. The use of a diary is particularly important if the trial medication is to be self-administered: the patient should record when and how much medication is taken and describe any adverse effects. The diary can be returned to the study nurse when the next scheduled visit takes place. Finally, some institutions provide the patient with a contact information card, which states he/she is on a clinical trial and provides contact numbers for the investigator, nurses, and other trial personnel for the patient or other health professional to use between scheduled visits.

10.4 Data collection and collation

All clinical trials require documentation of patient characteristics (including disease history information) at study entry, other baseline information, study treatment administration, adverse effects, various laboratory measurements (biochemistry, haematology, etc.), and radiological or clinical measures of disease over time, as appropriate. These data are then entered into a database to enable the generation of a variety of study reports and summary tables. Data collection forms, or case report forms (CRFs), are the most common approach to data collection, although some trials also utilize electronic data collection. In a trial where the information from more than one site involved in the phase I study is collected, the central site (be it an academic site, cooperative group office or pharmaceutical firm) reviews and queries the data, enters it into a database, which is created in advance using either commercial or locally designed software. Typically for single centre trials that do not have a pharmaceutical partner, those trial personnel that collect the data may also be responsible for entering the data into a local database. If the information collected is not extensive, simple electronic spreadsheets may suffice.

10.4.1 Data collection

It is vital for the credibility of results, as well as being essential for compliance with GCP principles, that the trial data are complete and accurate. As the trial CRFs are not part of the 'official' medical record, it is important that any information recorded on CRFs can be verified by examination of the official institutional patient chart or medical record. As some required information, such as patient symptoms, may not normally be recorded in the physician notes in the medical record, study nurses or data managers can create a trial-specific checklist of questions that can be appended to the patient chart to ensure information is obtained from patients at their visits and recorded in a manner that can be transferred to the CRFs. Other tools to ensure protocol compliance and facilitate complete and accurate data collection have been developed in individual cancer treatment centres, in cooperative group offices or in pharmaceutical companies.

In an individual centre, it is important that such tools and the procedures to use them are documented as part of the 'standard operating procedures' and trials staff are educated in their proper use. Undertaking this properly will not only ensure data accuracy but, if the institution undergoes an official audit, it will be clear how data are managed and collected.

10.4.2 Case report forms

Trials sponsored by industry will generally have CRF development take place within the company. It is useful for the phase I investigator and study nurses to request an opportunity to review the CRFs while they are being developed in order to ensure that all information considered important in the trial is being collected (and no extraneous information is being sought) and to be confident that the format and content of CRF is unambiguous. CRF development by an investigator or academic group should happen in collaboration between the investigator, data management, and computing/statistical staff. The CRFs must collect data required by the protocol (not more) and should be designed in such a way that the database can be easily created. Finally, the data collected for the trial must take into account what all those involved with the study can foresee will be needed in terms of reporting the trial results. A useful strategy is to imagine at the *outset* of the trial what the tables in the *final manuscript/ report* will look like. The content of the tables planned for the final report and the raw data required to populate them, tell you what the protocol must be written to collect, what goes on CRFs, and what must be put in the electronic trial database. Generally speaking, actual numbers and values should be collected on the CRFs, rather than calculated values by data managers or nurses. For example: collect actual granulocyte values, computerize them, and let a computer algorithm define the worst grade experienced, rather than have a person figure out the grade and record only the grade on the CRF. Appendix III contains a listing of the most common data elements found in phase I CRFs.

10.4.3 Database

The development of appropriate trial databases for cancer clinical trials is a topic of considerable complexity. As noted above, if the phase I trial is being conducted through pharmaceutical industry sponsorship, the database will be their responsibility. However, as described in Chapters 8 and 11, access to database information, tables, and data listings is important for the investigator to assist in the interpretation of trials results. If the trial is an academic one within a single centre or within an academic trials group, the database may be commercially purchased (e.g. Oracle Clinical) or designed by personnel in the group/institution. As phase I trials are not large in terms of sample size, some use electronic spreadsheet programs to capture data as needed. However, thought must be given as to how the clinical data in the spreadsheets will be 'merged' with special studies such as output from pharmacokinetic (PK) studies or translational research assays. Having *all* data from each patient in the *same* database facilitates analysis of the trial. Furthermore, regardless of the structure of the database, it must be possible to transform data into the format required. Examples include calculation of grades from raw values, identification of worst toxicity by patient and by dose level, the mean duration of certain toxic effects and so on.

10.5 Opening and closing dose levels

10.5.1 Who is in charge?

Each trial requires one 'co-ordinator' who takes the overall responsibility for assembling the relevant data for each dose level as the observation period ends, summarizing it, and conveying this information to colleagues for joint decisions about what the next step will be: opening the next dose level, expanding the current level, reducing to the next lower dose, etc. This may be done by the trial investigator, the main data manager or statistician at the study group or the company co-ordinating centre. This individual is responsible for making sure all relevant clinical, lab, and PK data required for decision-making is in hand.

10.5.2 Recruitment to dose levels

The rules for opening and closing dose levels should be clearly described in the design section of the protocol. Generally for the first-in-man trials for a new drug, the *first patient* at the *first dose level* should be treated and observed for a cycle (or whatever the study-designed observation period is) before others are entered on that first level (presuming that more than one patient per dose level is planned) in order to be absolutely certain that the trial starting dose is, in fact, safe. Thereafter most believe it is acceptable to enter the *required minimum* number of patients per cohort at the same time, assuming that eligible patients are available. It is also possible to continue to enrol only one patient (as for the initial dose level) and await the outcome in that individual before the remaining patients for the minimum required per cohort are enrolled. Which approach is followed can depend on the data from the previous level (e.g. was there a near dose-limiting event?), or on the nature of the drug and trial (e.g. the first ever study of an agent of a new target or class may be a situation in which a more conservative approach is warranted).

Individual patient enrolment should take place only *after* the consent form is signed for that patient and when a dose level is open for enrolment. Registration is usually done by calling, faxing, or using a web-based registration system to the central 'trial office' responsible for trial co-ordination. This may be an office in the same institution the patient is from, if the trial is being done in a single centre. As there are pauses in accrual inherent in phase I trials as one awaits the follow-up information on all patients in a previous dose level, it is highly desirable not to add to the delay by taking weeks to fill the minimum number of patient slots on a dose level. To avoid this, warning of when a new dose level is anticipated to open should be distributed about 1–2 weeks in advance to study personnel by the principal investigator or trial team member responsible for co-ordination with colleagues. In multicentre trials (some phase I trials run in more than one centre to enhance efficiency) guaranteeing a reserved slot for each institution means they can approach patient(s) for the trial without worrying that no openings will be available when they call for patient registration. In some trials it may be permissible (and if so, this should also be clearly described in the design section of the protocol) to *enrol one more patient than required* in order to ensure the specified minimum are, in fact, evaluated for the required observation period. This is a particularly useful strategy when the treatment itself is prolonged: cycles of 6–8 weeks length may not be completed by some patients if their disease rapidly progresses so having a 'back-up' patient already enrolled to replace one that drops out enhances efficiency.

10.5.3 When the dose level has completed minimum recruitment

When the dose level has completed the first stage of recruitment, the trial is put on hold and patients observed for the protocol specified period. At the end of that period *all data needed to make the end of dose level decisions must be submitted without delay* (e.g. by fax or electronically). Usually clinical data are reported in a timely fashion but there may be problems receiving PK or pharmacodynamic information expeditiously. If these latter data are critical to dose escalation decisions, then it must be clear to those concerned that 'real-time' completion of assays and analysis is essential. Once the material is received, a decision can be made by the study's co-ordinating office/investigator, in consultation with trial colleagues, regarding opening a new level, expanding the current one, or reducing the dose level.

10.5.4 When the escalation switching event is seen

As noted in Chapters 3 and 6, many protocols are designed to change the size of the dose escalation interval and/or the number of patients per dose level when a specific event is seen or criterion is met. Examples of 'switching events' include the observation of grade 2 drug-related toxicity (many protocols in which dose levels are being doubled and only one patient per level is being entered, will increase the number of patients per cohort and switch to a more conservative dose escalation scheme at that point), PK results indicated a target area under the curve of drug exposure has been achieved, or laboratory data showing that target inhibition has been accomplished. The observation of the switching event will trigger a communication from the trial co-ordinator to all concerned that from that point forward, according to protocol design, the changes in cohort size or escalation step size are in effect.

10.5.5 When a dose-limiting event is seen

If it is anticipated that toxicity will be dose-limiting, the observation of the first dose-limiting toxic effect (DLT) means the study is likely nearing the final dose level. If, at the time the first DLT is reported, only one patient has been entered on that dose level (i.e. one of one has DLT), it is wise to enrol only one (not two) more patients until the outcome of the second patient is known. If the second patient experiences DLT (that is, two of two patients), then adding a third is not necessary if the definition of maximum tolerated dose (MTD) is two of three (or six) patients with DLT. If three patients are already entered when the first DLT is seen, and only one of the three has a DLT, expansion to six is allowed. However, the same cautionary approach may apply: if patient 4 has a DLT as well, then, depending on the protocol 'rules', the MTD may have been reached without needing a total of six patients treated. Real-time inter-action between investigators and the trial co-ordinator is essential to ensure no more patients than absolutely necessary to define MTD are enrolled. If, after expansion to the maximum number of patients, no more dose-limiting events are seen, further escalation according to the scheme in the protocol can occur.

If measures other than toxicity are planned to limit dose escalation (e.g. measurement of a minimum target-related change in tumour tissue samples), then the observation of a single dose 'limiting' event need not lead to such a cautious approach to filling the dose level; the level may be filled to the maximum number planned and should then be analysed to determine if escalation can cease using the protocol-defined rules. Please note that, even when something other than toxicity is *planned* to define the upper limit of dosing in a protocol, there must be included a definition of those toxic events which, if seen, will limit further escalation regardless of whether the 'other' dose-limiting events are documented (sometimes toxicities that are unex-pected at the dose levels planned will occur).

10.6 Expecting the unexpected

10.6.1 What can go wrong?

Despite explicit and detailed design plans, not everything will go as planned in most phase I trials, particularly first-in-man studies. Table 10.1 lists some of the common problems seen during these studies and offers some practical solutions. By and large, this list is comprised of unexpected observations. Provided the protocol design section is written to allow reasonable judgement based on safety, some of the solutions proposed can be implemented without the need for a protocol amendment, which would, of course, take 2 months or so to process.

10.6.2 Conflict of trial protocol versus medical judgement

As in one of the examples in Table 10.1, sometimes what the protocol says should be done and what the investigator believes is in the best interest of the patient are in conflict. As outlined in the table, toxic effects were seen that the investigator believed needed a response, yet the protocol did not deal with this eventuality. Another circumstance where this might arise is when the protocol requires imaging studies to be done every other cycle, yet the patient's symp-toms suggest they are needed sooner. In all cases such as this, *the investigator must act in the best interests of that patient,* even if the protocol does not

Table 10.1 When the unexpected happens

If this happens.....	Consider doing this.....
Although the patient has a grade 3 toxicity (fatigue) it is not clear if this is due to drug or disease	Expand the dose level.
Two of six patients have a grade 3 event, which qualifies as DLT, but they are not the same event. (e.g. one is myelosuppression, the other is nausea)	Investigate if there are other causes for either of the events. Consider expanding the dose level further, with appropriate premedication, if applicable, if none was administered before, to see if this level is truly the MTD. Alternatively, you may declare that the MTD has been reached and decrease a dose level
Pre-clinical toxicology suggested that myelosuppression will be dose-limiting and the DLT definition is based on this. However, another grade 3 organ toxicity has been seen.	All protocol definitions of DLT should include a non-specific inclusion of 'any other ≥grade 3 organ toxicity' to cover this eventuality. If your protocol did not, this type of event should still be treated as DLT in terms of decision-making. Depending on the nature of the unexpected toxic effect, special monitoring procedures might also be advised and may need a protocol amendment (including consent form amendment to advise of new toxicity and procedures). For example, grade 3 chest pain of uncertain significance might lead to more frequent follow-up, troponin levels and ECGs in new patients.
In a weekly intravenous phase I study, the protocol calls for holding the dose if DLT criteria are met (grade 4 neutropenia for 7 days). A patient has grade 3 neutropenia on day 15: although the protocol does not require holding the dose, the investigator is uncomfortable giving treatment.	Patient *safety* concerns should take precedence over protocol direction: particularly if, as in this case, the way the protocol was written did not seem to take this type of problem into account. In weekly schedules of myelosuppressive agents it is often the case that the treatment day dose has to be reduced or held for degrees of toxicity that are less that what would be called a DLT. In fact, some would advise including as one of the definitions of DLT, the need to hold or reduce more than 1 or 2 weekly treatments per cycle because of toxic effects. In any event, the investigator should hold treatment in this case and parties to this protocol should discuss how to amend the dose reduction section.

(Continued)

Table 10.1 *Continued*

If this happens.....	Consider doing this.....
A dose level is found to meet criteria for MTD: two of three patients had DLT. The next lower dose level is expanded and no toxicity more than grade 1 is seen.	Treat a new cohort of patients at a dose level intermediate to the two dose levels described. Protocol design section should be written so as to allow this: otherwise an amendment will need to be made.
A dose level is found to produce DLT in two of six patients making it the MTD: BUT the other four patients at that dose experienced no more than grade 2 toxicity.	It may be that your drug is affecting different patient risk groups differently. Look at the entire trial database to see if there is an obvious difference in those that get toxicity versus those that do not: e.g. prior treatment, performance status, renal or hepatic function. If there is an obvious cause, consider amending the protocol to continue escalation in the low-risk group. If no obvious patient risk group is found, choices are to proceed to lower dose as per protocol *or* to cautiously add one to two more patients to the current dose level to further assess it, provided protocol language is permissive enough to allow this.

require or recommend it. The investigator's most important responsibility is to act in the best interests of the patient when matters of *safety* or *important disease management decisions* are in question. It is important, however, not to let this principle slide into areas where it is not intended; if the patient prefers, because of personal convenience, to have protocol specified blood tests drawn on Tuesday and Thursday rather than Monday, Wednesday, and Friday, then the investigator must reinforce with the patient the importance of following the protocol correctly.

Another source of conflict may arise in the interpretation of causality of an adverse event. Investigator and sponsor may disagree over whether a particular adverse event is likely to be treatment-related. It is important that investigators should not feel coerced into calling an event unrelated if their medical judgement suggests otherwise. Sometimes in the rush to move to the next dose level, it is tempting to ascribe events that might otherwise be considered dose-limiting to disease or other factors. Caution should be exercised in this; it is always better to expand a dose level to be certain that the MTD has not been reached, rather than to escalate to the next level and have serious or fatal outcomes in patients enrolled at a dose that, in retrospect, exceeded the MTD.

10.6.3 How to build in flexibility

It is useful to build into the *Design Section* of the protocol options to use *emerging data from the trial* to guide intelligent protocol decisions. Table 10.1 includes a few examples: introduction of intermediate dose levels, cautious expansion of what appears to be the MTD if interpatient variability in toxicity has been seen. Other examples include: allowing one 'extra' patient to be entered into a cohort to protect against lost time if a patient cannot complete a long cycle, allowing split dosing of oral medication if PK suggests saturable absorption, and to include in the definition of DLT missing a significant proportion of planned drug due to (even moderate) toxicity. All of these variations in the plan are permissible without protocol amendment, *provided* the protocol design section includes these options. The US Federal Regulations, as part of information supplied on Investigational New Drug Applications, states that: 'In general the protocols for Phase 1 studies may be less detailed and more flexible than protocols for Phase 2 and 3 studies' [2]. Although this document is most probably intended for phase I trials of non-cancer medications for healthy volunteer studies, it also makes the point that phase I trial design may require language that permits an appropriate response to unexpected emerging data.

10.6.4 When to stop a study

It is not problematic to stop a study when the final phase II dose recommendation is reached as per protocol design. More problematic is to stop a study for other reasons, unless these are clear and well thought through. The most common reasons for stopping a trial for unexpected scientific data are the following.

10.6.4.1 Encountering non-reversible and significant toxicity

Seeing a serious non-reversible adverse event (e.g. cardiomyopathy) in one patient may raise the question of whether this is truly due to drug effect or unrelated. If the event was predicted by animal toxicology, then observation of such an event in one patient should be enough to stop the trial and rethink what to do. If this wasn't foreseen from toxicology studies, and if there is another possible explanation for the effect (e.g. serious viral infection) then cautious enrolment of new patient(s) may be warranted. However, if a second patient experiences the same adverse effect, the trial must be stopped and the underlying mechanism investigated. Often this means taking the drug back into animal testing to see if there is a model for the toxic effect and, if so, can modifications in how the drug is administered (for example, slow infusion rather than bolus) modify the effect. If the decision is made to go back into human trials, a new protocol will need to be written, incorporating the relevant toxicology and other information that supports the new study plan.

10.6.4.2 Failing to achieve any biological effect and/or unable to achieve minimum blood levels

Sometimes doses are escalated past what was thought to be the maximum and nothing at all is seen in patients: either in terms of toxic effects or in translational lab studies. If, in addition, PK data do not show that the drug is achieving levels that are effective in animal models, there comes a point when continued study of the drug in that schedule is no longer warranted. Inadequate drug supply or the physical inability to administer the amount needed for dose escalation can also play a part in this decision. For some drugs (particularly oral agents), this situation is sometimes encountered when there is saturable absorption (or other pharmacological problem) in the drug's behaviour. Although, if written appropriately, the protocol may allow some changes in drug delivery (e.g. split dosing) to get around this, strategies like this may not solve the problem so a point of futility is reached. If, at the maximal deliverable dose, there are no signs the drug is having a biological effect and it is not achieving critical minimum blood levels, then the trial should stop. Once again, the drug should go back to the laboratory to see if there is something else that could be done in terms of formulation, for example, to rescue this.

10.7 Team meetings and communication

As is clear from the foregoing sections, running a phase I study, or in fact any type of clinical study, is the responsibility of a large team of individuals. In the institution, the investigator leads this group. The sponsor of the trial will also have a team of players working on the study. It is important therefore, to have clear lines of communication and frequent contact within the institution and between the investigator and sponsor, should they not be the same individual. While emails, phone calls, and fax contact provides some of the opportunity to communicate, it is important that face-to-face meetings occur, particularly for the investigator's team. It is in these sessions that issues about trial conduct, unusual observations, and patient recruitment can be aired. The goal is to have a smoothly running study, which is completed in a timely fashion, and from which the data generated are complete and accurate.

References

1. Flory J, Emanuel E (2004). Interventions to improve research participants' understanding in informed consent for research: a systematic review. *JAMA* **292**: 1593–601.
2. US Code of Federal Regulations, Title 21, Volume 5, Parts 300–299: Part 312: Investigational New Drug Application, Subpart B: Section 312.23 (a)(6).

Chapter 11

Reporting and interpreting results

Elizabeth A. Eisenhauer

11.1 Background

Not only is it necessary to design, conduct, and analyse phase I trials well, it is also important that the results of such trials are reported in an appropriate and timely manner. This means that the reader of a published phase I report should understand why the trial was undertaken, what the justification was for studying the agent at the doses described, what happened during the course of the study, and what the final recommendations are regarding future trials of the agent or drug combination. Despite the fact that the peer review process is designed to critique and clarify reports of trials before they are published, journals and reviewers are not consistent in what they consider to be the minimum content for a phase I report. For example, in a recent review of 57 reports of single agent phase I studies, Parulekar and Eisenhauer found that most publications did not indicate how the starting dose was justified or what was the planned dose escalation scheme [1]. Actual starting doses and dose levels were generally included, but the *plan* as described in the protocol was infrequently reported. Furthermore, some studies did not clearly state the recommended dose (RD), which was the primary purpose of the studies! The findings of this review serve to underscore the importance of a well-written phase I study report. Those who read it should be able to understand what was done and why, what the toxic and other effects of the drug(s) were, and what the authors conclude should be the RD for further study. This chapter provides a plan for generating phase I reports and some sample tables to use. As well, figures from actual phase I study publications are interspersed to illustrate how one could present certain types of data. Other formats are possible, but the one provided here is a template that covers the necessary topics. This chapter also briefly discusses what happens after phase I as new agents or combination regimens move forward into subsequent drug development steps. Readers are also encouraged to review other publications that describe standards of reporting. The CONSORT statement is the most commonly cited of these [2]; although it is targeted to publications of randomized trials, many of its recommendations apply equally to phase I or II study reports.

11.2 Contents of phase I trial report

The following pages describes the common sections with suggested content for authors to use when making a report or writing a manuscript describing the results of a phase I trial.

11.2.1 Rationale/introduction

Begin by describing briefly why the drug or regimen is of interest. This should include an outline of the key elements in preclinical and other data that justified the evaluation of the agent in a first-in-man trial. What is the drug's target or structure that makes it of interest? What preclinical efficacy and toxicology data supports its evaluation in cancer? If there are schedule and route data available that justify what will be done in the clinic, this should be referenced. If there are other agents of similar structure or target already in clinical use or development, are there any comparative data that are available that would strengthen the case for clinical study?

For phase I trials of combinations of agents, develop the rationale by describing the disease(s) for which the new combination is intended and the justification for improving on currently available therapy. The activity of the single agent investigational drug to be used in combination needs citation (if available), as does preclinical combination data justifying the expected benefits of the combination under evaluation. Combination toxicology should be summarized, if it has been done, and if not, some commentary on the probable safety of the combination in humans should be given, citing, for example, the dissimilar toxic effects in clinical studies of the standard therapy and the investigational component. Finally, for combination phase I trials, some indication of the future of the combination once doses are recommended, is advised. Thus if it is the case that a randomized trial is planned, this information is useful to include.

This section should end by a statement indicating the primary and secondary goals of the reported study. For example: 'We report here the results of a phase I trial of LTK007 given in an oral daily schedule to patients with solid tumours. The primary goal of the study was to define a recommended phase II dose for future study. Secondary goals were to describe the toxic effects, pharmacokinetic behaviour and molecular changes in cyclin dependent kinase activity in peripheral blood mononuclear cells after dosing with LTK007'.

11.2.2 Methods

The methods section is usually divided into several subsections.

11.2.2.1 Patient entry criteria

Briefly list the major inclusion and exclusion criteria. State the requirements for ethics review and informed consent.

11.2.2.2 Starting dose

State what the starting dose(s) is and justify it. For first-in-man studies, the justification will be based on animal toxicological studies. For other phase I trials, clinical data are used to set the starting dose(s).

11.2.2.3 Design

Indicate the method of dose escalation (with appropriate references), the number of patients per dose level, and the planned dose escalation steps (what actually happened appears in the results). Describe the rules for expansion, escalation or reduction of dose levels, and the basis of the decision (toxic effects or other observations). Rules for terminating escalation and declaring the RD are important to include, as are the definitions of the terms used, for example: maximum tolerated dose (MTD), maximum administered dose (MAD), dose-limiting toxicity (DLT). If intrapatient patient dose escalation was allowed, and if data from intrapatient escalation was considered in dose escalation decisions, it should be noted in this section. Sometimes the design, dose levels, or escalation approach changes mid-way through the study. If this is the case, describe briefly what occurred (details will be in the Results section) and the resulting new design.

11.2.2.4 Treatment

Describe the drug administration plan: include recommended or required premedication and postmedication. Indicate the drug route and schedule of administration and highlight the major dose adjustment criteria for adverse effects. The planned maximum treatment duration and the reasons that patients could have therapy discontinued should be detailed.

11.2.2.5 Follow-up and investigations

The standard investigations (laboratory evaluations, imaging studies) to be done before, during, and after completion of therapy are described here as well as the planned intervals at which they are repeated.

11.2.2.6 Criteria for assessing study endpoints

Describe and reference the criteria used for assessment of toxic effects, objective tumour response and other study endpoints [except for lab or imaging pharmacodynamic (PD) studies, which are described below].

11.2.2.7 Pharmacokinetics

This part of the Methods section should document the blood sampling plan, methods for measurement and analysis for pharmacokinetic assessment. Many journals permit the use of an appendix to detail the analytic methods if there is no published reference as yet available, in order to conserve space.

11.2.2.8 Special studies

Other special assays such as laboratory studies of molecular effects of the drug in normal or malignant tissue or functional imaging studies require description. The methods, frequency of repeat measurements, and analytical techniques used should be explained for each such study. If the description of the analysis or scoring method is too lengthy to describe as part of the manuscript, there is an option in many journals to use an appendix.

11.2.2.9 Statistical analysis

Phase I trials are non-randomized so no comparisons between cohorts are usually undertaken. However, there may be circumstances when more formal comparisons of measurements across dose levels are desirable. Examples might include the impact of dose on measures of target inhibition or functional imaging change, or comparison of tissue findings before and after treatment and so forth. The tests to be used for such comparisons and the methods for their application should be summarized in a special subsection of the Methods. All tests should have been described in the protocol. *Post-hoc* statistical testing of interesting observations is to be discouraged.

11.2.3 Results

Key trial results are described using both text and tabular displays of data. The following are standard subsections:

11.2.3.1 Patient entry

Describe when the trial opened and closed, how many centres participated, and how many patients were enrolled. Indicate if any were ineligible, the reasons for ineligibility and whether they received any study therapy. State how many patients were evaluable for toxicity and (if applicable) response or other secondary endpoints. As a general rule, *all eligible patients* should be included in reporting phase I trials. Some argue that reports of phase I studies should include all patients who received any drug, whether eligible or ineligible, as evaluation for toxic effects, if that is the major endpoint, need not depend on eligibility. Patient characteristics are best described in a table (see example Table 11.1).

Table 11.1 Patient characteristics: *sample*

		No. Patients
Number of patients	Entered	
	Eligible	
	Evaluable for toxicity	
	Evaluable for response	
	Evaluable for PD endpoint	
	Etc.	
Median age (range)		(years)
Performance status (ECOG)	0	
	1	
	2	
Prior Chemotherapy regimens	0	
	1	
	2	
	3	
	Etc.	
Prior taxane	(or other specific agent as appropriate)	
Prior radiation		
Primary tumour site	Lung	
	Colon	
	Breast	
	Renal	
	Melanoma	
	Gastric	
	Bladder	
	Etc.	
Sites of disease	Liver	
	Lung	
	Nodes	
	Etc.	
Measurable disease	Yes	
	No	

11.2.3.2 Drug administration and dose levels

A table of drug administration by dose level should be included. This describes how many patients were treated and how many cycles were delivered at each dose level and should include information on whether any cycles were incomplete (if treatment was given over several days or weeks). Table 11.2 gives an

Table 11.2 Dose levels and drug administration: *Sample*

Dose level	Actual dose (mg/m²) days 1, 8, 15	No. patients started at that dose	No. cycles started	No. cycles completed	No. patients escalated to that dose	No. cycles at escalated dose
1	100	1	3	2	–	–
2	200	3	8	8	1	2
3	300	8	18	15	1	1
4	400	6	15	13	2	2
Total		18	44	38	4	5

example that also shows the number of patients undergoing intrapatient dose escalation. This section should also include a brief description of what happened in dose escalation; that is, if DLT was seen at all, if so at which level(s), and how/if intermediate dose levels were created.

11.2.3.3 Toxic effects

For most phase I trials this is where the 'meat' of the report will lie. Worst grade of toxic effects by patient should be clearly described in tabular form by dose level. Some reports include columns for each grade, and some include only a column for 'any grade' and separate columns for grade 3 and 4. Usually haematological and non-haematological effects are reported in separate tables (see Tables 11.3a,b and 11.4a,b for examples). Toxic effects by cycle/by dose level may also be reported, especially if intrapatient dose escalation was common. In these circumstances patients are counted at more than one dose level and cycles are attributed to the dose level at which they were given, not to which the patient was assigned. The interval in which DLT was determined (if applicable) may also be the basis of another table (i.e. toxic effects by patient and dose level for cycle 1 only), so as to view DLT events in the window that these 'counted' as dose-limiting. In trials where toxic effects were not the major endpoint, then this tabulation doesn't add anything. Worst cycle toxicity (or worst grade by patient—the same thing) may be compared with first cycle to see if there is evidence of cumulative toxicity; if there is, first cycle data will show less frequent and severe toxic effects than worst cycle data.

The text of the report should highlight the main findings in the tables and also spend some time describing the most common and serious effects (especially DLT). This may include the description of the course of these events in individual patients. If any toxicity modifying therapies were used, this should be reported here along with an assessment of their impact.

Table 11.3a: Non-hematological Adverse Effects: Worst by patient by assigned dose level* (*Sample*)

Category	Adverse event term	100 / 1			200 / 3			300 / 8			400 / 6		
Dose level / No. patients		Any	Grade 3	Grade 4	Any	Grade 3	Grade 4	Any	Grade 3	Grade 4	Any	Grade 3	Grade 4
Gastrointestinal	Nausea	1			2			5			5	2	
	Vomiting				1			3	1		4	1	1
	Diarrhoea	1			1			3	1		5	2	
Constitutional	Fatigue	2			2			5			6	2	
Neurology	Neuropathy-sensory										2		
Etc.													

*indicate here if any of the grade 3 / 4 events were seen in patients when they were receiving an escalated dose: i.e. at one level higher than assigned and found in the table. As a way of avoiding this confusion, sometimes patients at escalated levels do not have the events ''counted'' if seen at the escalated level.

Table 11.3b: Non-hematological Adverse Effects: Worst by cycle (*Sample*)

Category	Adverse event term	100 / 3			200 / 10			300 / 19			400 / 17		
Dose level / No. cycles*		Any	Grade 3	Grade 4	Any	Grade 3	Grade 4	Any	Grade 3	Grade 4	Any	Grade 3	Grade 4
Gastrointestinal	Nausea	1			5			12			14	4	
	Vomiting				2			4	1		7	1	1
	Diarrhoea	1			1			4	1		8	2	
Constitutional	Fatigue	2			4			9			10	3	
Neurology	Neuropathy-sensory										2		
Etc.													

*this includes cycles for patients escalated to this level

Table 11.4a: Hematological Adverse Effects: Worst by Patient by Dose level (described by grade) (*Sample*)

Dose level		No. patients evaluable*	Grade 0	1	2	3	4
100	Granulocytes	1		1			
	Platelets	1	1				
	Haemoglobin	1		1			
200	Granulocytes	3		1	2		
	Platelets	3	3				
	Haemoglobin	3		1	1	1	
300	Granulocytes	8		1	2	3	3
	Platelets	8	4	2	2		
	Haemoglobin	8		1	2	3	1
400	Granulocytes	6		1	1	3	1
	Platelets	6	1	2	3		
	Haemoglobin	6		1	4	1	

*to be counted as "Evaluable" a patient must have had a baseline value and at least one follow-up determination while on study

11.2.3.4   Recommended phase II dose

This section logically follows immediately after the section reporting toxic effects, particularly if toxicity limited dose escalation. If other measures were the basis of the phase II dose recommendation, the segment on RD can be placed at the end of the Results section. Wherever it is located, it must describe if a dose is recommended for further study (and if not, why not) as well as the

Table 11.4b: Hematological Adverse Effects: Worst by Cycle by Dose level (described by grade) (*Sample*)

Dose level		No. cycles evaluable*	Grade 0	1	2	3	4
100	Granulocytes	3	1	2			
	Platelets	3	3				
	Haemoglobin	3	1	2			
200	Granulocytes	9	6	3			
	Platelets	9	9				
	Haemoglobin	9	4	4	1		
300	Granulocytes	18	6	4	5	3	
	Platelets	18	8	6	4		
	Haemoglobin	18	2	6	8	2	
400	Granulocytes	17	2	2	5	7	1
	Platelets	17	5	8	4		
	Haemoglobin	17	2	5	8	2	

*to be counted as "Evaluable" a cycle must have had at least one follow-up determination between days 8 and 22.

basis for the phase II dose recommendation. The number of patients actually treated at this level and their toxicity experience may be highlighted if it is not clear elsewhere. This information is of particular help as one moves beyond phase I into phase II single agent trials or combination phase I regimens, as knowing what the drug alone at the RD can be expected to do is important in writing future consent forms, providing patients with safety information, and in estimating starting doses for combination studies.

11.2.3.5 Pharmacokinetics

Tables showing mean [± standard deviation (SD)] pharmacokinetic parameters by dose level and overall should be included. A figure or an individual representative patient plasma × time curve is useful to illustrate general trends. If there is high interpatient variability in PK observations, having a plot of several patients treated at the same dose level makes the point very well. Figure 11.1 is an example from a study of a liposomal encapsulated topoisomerase 1 inhibitor where substantial interpatient variability was noted in C_{max} and area under the curve (AUC) (former shown) [3]. This figure also indicates which patients showed dose-limiting effects and thus makes the point that there was no obvious level at which this was to be seen.

Indicate if the PK follows a linear or non-linear pattern related to dose. If any particular circumstance appeared to have an important impact on

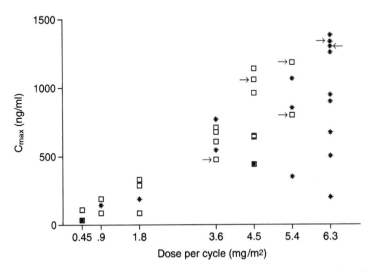

Figure 11.1 Phase I trial of OSI-211. C_{max} vs dose (dose 1 from cycle 1). □, heavily pretreated; *, minimally pretreated; →, patient with dose-limiting toxicity. From Gelmon *et al.* (2004) *Invest New Drugs* **22**: 263–75. With kind permission of Springer Science and Business Media.

expected PK observations, this can be described (e.g. if patients with high creatinine have higher AUC). These types of observations can be elaborated upon in the Discussion section and should be regarded as hypothesis generating, not conclusive.

Any relationship of PK measures with PD effects, toxicity or other correlative studies, should be explored. For example, is there a relationship between C_{max}, AUC, or steady-state levels in individual patients and the occurrence of DLT? Of grade 3 or 4 events? Of changes in surrogate markers or tumour tissue effects? A figure can tell the story very well. Interestingly, most reports seek relationships between dose and PD effect, rather than PK and PD effect, perhaps because the prescription for the patient will generally be based on dose, not PK. Figure 11.2 is an example of how both dose–PD and PK–PD effects can be effectively shown. This figure is from a phase I study report of the farnesyl transferase inhibitor BMS-214662 [4]. Measures of farnesyl transferase activity in peripheral blood mononuclear cells was incorporated into the phase I study design. The figure shows the relationship of farnesyl transferase expression over time in peripheral-blood mononuclear cells to dose in two schedules (panels A and B) and the relationship in each of those schedules between plasma levels in selected patients (panels C and D).

Other issues to address in reporting PK results: Did the trial show that the drug achieved critical minimum blood levels or some other critical measure derived from preclinical data? If so, at what dose level did this occur? Remember to factor in information about protein binding that may be at variance between species if this is important.

Finally, indicate if there is inter- or intrapatient variability seen in PK and if so, what magnitude of variability was seen.

11.2.3.6 Laboratory or imaging correlative studies

If the protocol included special tissue or blood studies designed to evaluate the impact of the treatment on the target for the drug or similar endpoint, the results of these should be included. It is preferable that these should not be published as a separate paper, otherwise the totality of the information cannot be easily digested by the reader (exceptions would be for back-to-back simultaneous publication in the same journal). The number of evaluable patients per dose level and key results by dose level should be described, not just selected cases. If there is a suggestion that there is a meaningful change in these measures, is it of the magnitude predicted/required from preclinical studies? Is there any relationship with these observations and any of toxicity, dose level, PK measure, or type of tissue? Figures are also very helpful if there are immunohistochemical or other semiquantitiative measures employed. As noted above, most such figures compare PD measures with dose, rather than with PK parameters. Figures 11.2 and 11.3 give some examples from actual phase I trials of options for displaying these data. Figure 11.2 was previously discussed. Figure 11.3(a,b) is reproduced from the publication of a phase I trial of the small molecule angiogenesis inhibitor PTK787 [5]. This agent targets

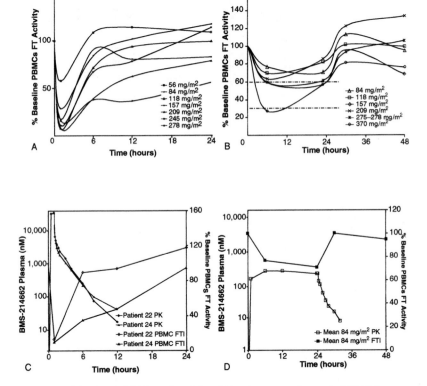

Figure 11.2 (A) Mean inhibition of peripheral-blood mononuclear cells (PBMCs) farnesyltransferase (FT) activity in the 1-hour infusion schedule; (B) mean inhibition of PBMCs FT activity in the 24-hour infusion schedule; (C) correlation between BMS-214662 PKs and PBMCs FT inhibition (FTI) in two patients at 245 mg/m^2 1-hour infusion schedule dose level; (D) correlation between BMS-214662 PKs and PBMCs FTI in patients at 84 mg/m^2 24-hour infusion schedule dose level. From Taberno *et al.* (2005) *J Clin Oncol* **23**: 2521–33. Reprinted with permission from the American Society of Clinical Oncology.

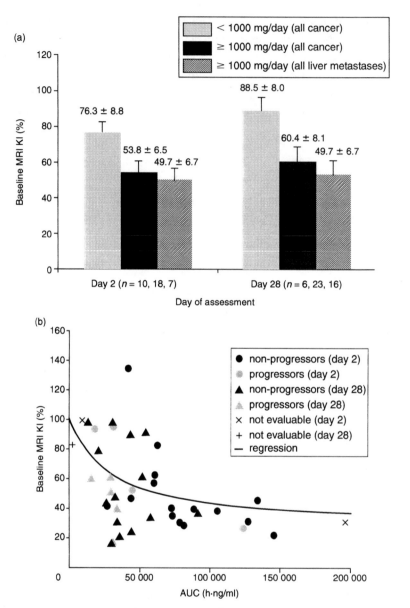

Figure 11.3 (a) Mean (± SE) percentage of baseline magnetic resonance imaging (MRI) bidirectional transfer constant (Ki) for patients receiving <1000 mg/day and >1000 mg/day on days 2 and 28 of PTK787/ZK 222584 treatment. (b) Inhibitory maximum effect (E_{max}) model fitting for percentage of baseline MRI bidirectional transfer constant (Ki) versus area under the plasma concentration curve (AUC) for patients with liver metastases. From Thomas *et al.* (2005) *J Clin Oncol* **23**: 4162–71. Reprinted with permission from the American Society of Clinical Oncology.

vascular endothelial growth factor (VEGF) receptor tyrosine kinases, including VEGFR-1/Flt-1, VEGFR-2/KDR, VEGFR-3/Flt-4, the platelet-derived growth factor receptor tyrosine kinase, and the c-kit protein tyrosine kinase. In the phase I study, dynamic contrast enhanced magnetic resonance imaging was used as a technique for studying the effect of the drug on permeability and vascularity of tumour masses measured by the bidirectional transfer constant (Ki). The results were presented in several different ways: Figure 11.3(a) shows the mean change from baseline in Ki, expressed as a percentage of baseline values, in two dose groups. The results suggest that there was a greater reduction in Ki at higher doses (>1000 mg/day) compared with lower doses (<1000 mg/day). Figure 11.3(b) shows the relationship between the effect on Ki and the plasma AUC of PTK787 in patients with liver metastases. Again results suggest that greater effects on Ki were seen at higher levels of exposure.

11.2.3.7 Antitumour effects

Phase I trials generally include a subset of patients who can be evaluated for antitumour effects using standard criteria. In this part of the Results section, indicate how many patients are evaluable for antitumour assessment (don't just select one!). Indicate if any met the criteria for objective response and if so, briefly describe the patient's story: tumour type, number of prior regimens, and disease location and extent. Some reports include several dramatic computed tomography scans as figures but this is not really necessary, and could leave the impression that activity is being overemphasized. If some other biological effects occurred that do not quite meet official response definitions it might be useful to describe them (particularly durable cases of stable disease, tumour shrinkage that is not quite sufficient to declare a response, tumour necrosis without shrinkage are a few examples). This type of information can be useful in determining in which tumour types the drug or regimen should be evaluated after phase I is complete.

11.2.4 Discussion

This section of the report pulls together the story of the trial: what was seen, how it is interpreted and what the major observations lead the authors to conclude. An opinion on the importance of the results and a review of other information on the drug in the literature should be added. In other words, how do these observations fit with other phase I trials of the compound or its analogues? Briefly reiterating the effects of the drug on toxicity and on whatever PD measures were studied is useful. This should be put in context of what was predicted by preclinical studies and the experience in other trials and of other agents with the same mechanism of action. The final dose recommendation and reasons for selecting it should be described; any particular cautions about the use of the drug in subpopulations should be emphasized. Finally, the authors should provide some indication of the future plan for the drug (or regimen). Will it proceed into phase II trials? Will more work be done defining dose–effect relationships in a phase Ib type trial? For combination phase I trials, will a randomized study follow? Tying in the observations and conclusions with the subsequent developmental plan is desirable as the report concludes.

11.3 After first-in-man phase I trials: drug development decisions

The drug development plan that is pursued after the conclusion of a first-in-man phase I trial is not usually based on only one study, but rather on the entire phase I experience with the agent given in a variety of schedules. Information on the impact of schedule on toxic effects, feasibility of delivery, effect on target (if measured), PK parameters, clinical evidence of antitumour activity, total dose of drug administered, how these findings relate back to preclinical data on the 'best' schedule, and what is happening in the clinical research realm with any similar agents, all must be considered in designing the next phases of development.

It may not be clear, in fact, which dose or schedule is best, despite various phase I trials having been completed. For example, more information on the impact of the new drug on molecular measures of target effect, on functional imaging changes, or on toxic effects may be required in order to make an informed development decision. If so, the subsequent studies should evaluate these measures as major endpoint(s) and should be designed appropriately to measure them—e.g. for studies in which tumour tissue assays are planned, all patients must be required to have biopsiable tissue; for those in which imaging changes are planned, patients must have appropriately located and sized lesions for evaluation. In these trials, sometimes referred to as phase Ib studies, larger numbers of patients are enrolled (or even randomized) at fewer dose levels (or schedules) and entry may be restricted to specific tumour type(s). Information garnered from these types of trials may assist in making more informed decisions about the dose/schedule of a new drug to carry forward.

After final decisions about RD and schedule have been made, the development path followed depends on a variety of factors: the nature and tumour expression patterns of the target (if known), the preclinical information on single agent activity, the observation of antitumour responses in phase I, and the role and efficacy of any similar agents in clinical practice, to name a few.

Agents selected for clinical development because they affect a specific molecular target may undergo phase II single agent evaluation in those tumour types in which the target is frequently expressed, move into combinations or directly into phase III trials.

Although the goals of drug development as described in Chapter 1 of this book are clear, the process and phases of development are not written in stone. Emergent data from any phase of investigation is used to shape subsequent plans and trial designs, as are data from ongoing studies with similar agents or in the target disease indications. The discussion of cancer drug development after phase I is complex and the subject of entire textbooks. Useful additional books and references on this topic are found in Appendix II.

References

1. Parulekar WR, Eisenhauer EA (2004). Phase I trials designs for solid tumor studies of targeted, non-cytotoxic agents: theory and practice. *J Natl Cancer Inst* **96**: 990–7.

2. Begg C, Cho M, Eastwood S, *et al.* (1996). Improving the quality of reporting of randomized controlled trials. The CONSORT statement. *JAMA* **276**: 637–9.

3. Gelmon K, Hirte H, Fisher B, *et al.* (2004). A phase 1 study of OSI-211 given as an intravenous infusion days 1, 2, and 3 every three weeks in patients with solid cancers. *Invest New Drugs* **22**: 263–75.

4. Tabernero J, Rojo F, Marimon I, *et al.* (2005). Phase I pharmacokinetic and pharmacodynamic study of weekly 1-hour and 24-hour infusion BMS-214662, a farnesyltransferase inhibitor, in patients with advanced solid tumors. *J Clin Oncol* **23**: 2521–33.

5. Thomas AL, Morgan B, Horsfield MA, *et al.* (2005). Phase I study of the safety, tolerability, pharmacokinetics, and pharmacodynamics of PTK787/ZK 222584 administered twice daily in patients with advanced cancer. *J Clin Oncol* **23**: 4162–71.

Appendix I: Useful web resources

The following websites provide access directly to information and documents of use in clinical trial design and development.

Submission to regulatory authorities

United States

- Chapter I—Food and Drug Administration, Department Of Health And Human Services, Part 312—Investigational New Drug Application. Available at: http://www.access.gpo.gov/nara/cfr/waisidx_00/21cfr312_00.html
- Guidance for Industry: content and format of IND applications for Phase I Studies of Drugs (etc.). Available at: http://www.fda.gov/cder/guidance/clin2.pdf
- FDA Forms Distribution Page. Available at: http://www.fda.gov/opacom/morechoices/fdaforms/cder.html

Europe

- European clinical trials database: http://eudract.emea.eu.int
- Forms for CTA process: https://eudract.emea.eu.int/eudract/index.do
- Individual member state requirements: http://eudract.emea.eu.int/docs/Detailed%20guidance%20CTA%20.pdf

Canada

- Drug Products information including application material: http://www.hc-sc.gc.ca/hpfb-dgpsa/tpd-dpt/ctdcta_ctddec_e.html

Statistical resources

- Spreadsheet-like implementation of classical design: http://biostats.upci.pitt.edu/biostats/ClinicalStudyDesign/Phase1Standard.html
- Windows implementation of CRM: http://www.cancerbiostats.onc.jhmi.edu/software.htm
- Command-line (DOS-type) implementation of CRM: http://odin.mdacc.tmc.edu/anonftp/

Good Clinical Practice

◆ E6: ICH Guideline on Good Clinical Practice: http://www.ich.org/
MediaServer.jser?@_ID=482&@_MODE=GLB

General resources

◆ International Conference on Harmonisation: ICH home page: http://
www.ich.org
◆ United States Code of Federal Regulations Title 21: Food and Drugs
(searchable data base): http://www.accessdata.fda.gov/scripts/cdrh/cfdocs/
cfcfr/CFRSearch.cfm
◆ ICH General Considerations for Clinical Trials (E8): http://www.ich.org/
MediaServer.jser?@_ID=484&@_MODE=GLB
◆ European Union Directive on Clinical Trials: http://europa.eu.int/eur-lex/
pri/en/oj/dat/2001/l_121/l_12120010501en00340044.pdf
◆ European Medicines Evaluation Agency: CPMP Note for guidance on the
pre-clinical evaluation of anticancer medicinal products. http://
www.emea.eu.int/pdfs/human/swp/099796en.pdf

Guidelines and guidance documents on preclinical safety (toxicity) testing

ICH

◆ M3: Maintenance of the ICH Guideline on Non-Clinical Safety Studies
for the Conduct of Human Clinical Trials of Pharmaceuticals: http://
www.ich.org/MediaServer.jser?@_ID=506&@_MODE=GLB
◆ S4: Single Dose Toxicity Tests: Agreement was reached, at the time of
ICH 1, in 1991, that the LD50 determination should be abandoned
for pharmaceuticals. The recommendation was published in the
Proceedings of the First International Conference on Harmonisation,
p. 184.
◆ S4A: Duration of Chronic Toxicity Testing in Animals (Rodent and
Non-Rodent Toxicity Testing) http://www.ich.org/
MediaServer.jser?@_ID=497&@_MODE=GLB
◆ S6: Preclinical Safety Evaluation of Biotechnology-Derived
Pharmaceuticals http://www.ich.org/
MediaServer.jser?@_ID=503&@_MODE=GLB
◆ S7A: Safety Pharmacology Studies for Human Pharmaceuticals (S7A)
http://www.ich.org/MediaServer.jser?@_ID=504&@_MODE=GLB

◆ S7B: The Nonclinical Evaluation of the Potential for Delayed Ventricular Repolarization (QT Interval Prolongation) By Human Pharmaceuticals http://www.ich.org/MediaServer.jser?@_ID=2192&@_MODE=GLB

FDA

◆ Guidance for single dose acute toxicity testing for pharmaceuticals: http://www.fda.gov/cder/guidance/pt1.pdf

◆ FDA Guidance on ICH S4A Chronic toxicity testing: http://www.fda.gov/cder/guidance/62599.pdf US Federal Register Vol. 64 No. 122, June 25, 1999 (FR 99–16189)

Good Manufacturing Practice

USA

◆ http://www.fda.gov/cdrh/fr1007ap.pdf

Europe

◆ http://pharmacos.eudra.org/F2/eudralex/vol-4/home.htm

Canada

◆ http://www.hc-sc.gc.ca/hpfb-dgpsa/inspectorate/gmp_guidelines_2002_entire_e.html

Good Laboratory Practice

USA

◆ http://www.fda.gov/ora/compliance_ref/bimo/glp/78fr-glpfinalrule.pdf

◆ http://www.access.gpo.gov/nara/cfr/waisidx_03/21cfr58_03.html

Europe

◆ http://europa.eu.int/comm/enterprise/chemicals/legislation/glp/index_en.htm

Endpoints criteria

Response criteria

◆ RECIST full paper reference: See Therasse et al (2000) , J Natl Cancer Inst 92: 205–16

- RECIST web resource for protocols, available at: http://ctep.cancer.gov/guidelines/recist.html

Toxicity criteria

- Common Terminology Criteria for Adverse Events (CTCAE) v. 3.0: http://ctep.cancer.gov/forms/CTCAEv3.pdf
- Medical Dictionary for Regulatory Activities (MedRA): www.medramsso.com
- ICH E2A: Clinical Safety Data Management : Definitions and Standards for Expedited Reporting: http://www.ich.org/MediaServer.jser?@_ID=436&@_MODE=GLB

Ethical guidelines

- Canadian Tri-Council Policy http://www.pre.ethics.gc.ca/english/pdf/TCPS%20June2003_E.pdf
- United States

Title 45 Code Of Federal Regulations Part 46: Protection Of Human Subjects: http://www.hhs.gov/ohrp/humansubjects/guidance/45cfr46.htm

- United Kingdom

Human Tissue Act: http://www.opsi.gov.uk/acts/acts2004/20040030.htm

- Australia

National Statement on Ethical Conduct in Research Involving Humans: http://www7.health.gov.au/nhmrc/publications/humans/contents.htm

- Europe

Ethical Aspect of Human Tissue Banking (paper): http://europa.eu.int/comm/european_group_ethics/docs/avis11_en.pdf

- Council of Europe

Convention for the Protection of Human Rights and Dignity of the Human Being with regard to the Application of Biology and Medicine: Convention on Human Rights and Biomedicine http://conventions.coe.int/Treaty/en/Treaties/Html/164.htm

Special populations

- FDA Guidance for the conduct of renal impairment studies: http://www.fda.gov/cder/guidance/1449fnl.pdf

- FDA Guidance for the conduct of hepatic impairment studies: http://www.fda.gov/cder/guidance/3625fnl.pdf
- EMEA guidance for the conduct of renal impairment studieshttp://www.emea.eu.int/pdfs/human/ewp/14701304en.pdf
- EMEA Guidance for the conduct of hepatic impairment studies: http://www.emea.eu.int/pdfs/human/ewp/063302en.pdf
- NCI Organ Dysfunction Group template for renal dysfunction studies: http://www.ctep.cancer.gov/forms/Renal_dysfunction_temp2.doc
- FDA Guideline for Industry: Studies in support of special populations. Available at: http://www.fda.gov/cder/guidance/iche7.pdf
- Note for Guidance on Studies in support of special populations: Geriatrics (CPMP/ICH/379/95) Approved by CPMP September 1993. Available at: http://www.emea.eu.int/pdfs/human/ich/037995en.pdf
- FDA Guidance for pediatric studies: http://www.fda.gov/cder/guidance/1449fnl.pdf
- EMEA Guidance for pediatric studies: http://www.emea.eu.int/pdfs/human/ewp/046295en.pdf
- FDA Guidance for pediatric oncology studies: http://www.fda.gov/cder/guidance/3765dft.htm
- FDA guidance for drug-drug interaction (1999). http://www.fda.gov/cder/guidance/2635fnl.pdf
- FDA guidance: Food effect bioavailability and fed bioequivalence studies. http://www.fda.gov/cder/guidance/5194fnl.pdf

Appendix II: Additional reading

In addition to the references found in the book chapters themselves, the following selection of articles and books are offered for further reading on specific topics.

Statistical design

Anbar D (1987). Stochastic approximation methods and their use in bioassay and Phase I clinical trials. *Communications Stat* 13: 2451–67.

Cheung YK (2002). On the use of nonparametric curves in phase I trials with low toxicity tolerance. *Biometrics* 58: 237–40.

Cheung YK, Chappell R (2000). Sequential designs for Phase I clinical trials with late-onset toxicities. *Biometrics* 56: 1177–82.

Eckhardt SG, Baker SD, Britten CD, *et al.* (2000) Phase I and pharmacokinetic study of irofulven, a novel mushroom-derived cytotoxin, administered for five consecutive days every four weeks in patients with advanced solid malignancies. *J Clin Oncol* 18: 4086–97.

Fox E, Curt GA, Balis FM (2002). Clinical trial design for target-based therapy. *Oncologist* 7: 401–9.

Gasparin M, Eisele J (2002). A curve-free method for phase I clinical trials. *Biometrics* 56: 609–15.

Gatsonis C, Greenhouse J (1992). Bayesian methods for Phase I clinical trials. *Stat Med* 11: 1377–89.

Gooley TA, Martin PJ, Fisher LD, Pettinger M (1994). Simulation as a design tool for Phase I/II clinical trials. An example from bone marrow transplantation. *Control Clin Trials* 15: 450–62.

Grossman Sa, Hochberg F, Fisher J, *et al.* (1998). Increased 9-amino camptothecin dose requirements in patients on anticonvulsants. NABIT CNS Consortium. The New Approaches to Brain Tumor Therapy. *Cancer Chemother Pharmacol* 42: 118–126.

Ishizuka N, Ohashi Y (2001). The continual reassessment method and its applications: A Bayesian methodology for phase I cancer clinical trials. *Stat Med* 20: 2661–81.

Korn EL, Midthune D, Chen TT, *et al.* (1994) A comparison of two phase I trial designs. *Stat Med* 13: 1799–806.

Legedeza AT, Ibrahim JC (2001). Heterogeneity in phase I clinical trials: Prior elucidation and computation using the continued reassessment method. *Stat Med* 20: 827–52.

Legedeza AT, Ibrahim JC (2002). Longitudinal design for phase I trials using the continual reassessment method. *Control Clin Trials* 21: 578–88.

Leung DH, Wang YG (2002). An extension of the continual reassessment method using decision theory. *Stat Med* 21: 51–63.

Mahmood I (2001). Application of preclinical data to initiate the modified continual reassessment method for maximum tolerated dose-finding trial. *J Clin Pharmacol* **41**: 19–24.

Mani S, Ratain MJ (1997). New Phase I trial methodology. *Semin Oncol* **24**: 253–61.

Mehta M, Scrimger R, Mackie R, *et al.* (2001) A new approach to dose escalation in non-small cell lung cancer. *Int J Radiat Oncol Biol Phys* **49**: 23–33.

Mick R, Ratain MJ (1993). Model-guided determination of maximum tolerated dose in Phase I clinical trials: evidence for increased precision. *J Natl Cancer Inst* **85**: 217–23.

Murphy JR, Hall DL (1997). A logistical dose-ranging method for phase I clinical investigations trials. *J Biopharm Stat* **7**: 635–47.

O'Quigley J (1990). Sequential design and analysis of dose-finding studies in patients with life threatening disease. *Fundam Clin Pharmacol* **4** (Suppl. 2): 81–91S.

O'Quigley J (1992). Estimating the probability of toxicity at the recommended dose following a phase I clinical trial in cancer. *Biometrics* **48**: 853–62.

O'Quigley J (1994). Integral evaluation for continual reassessment method. *Comput Methods Programs Biomed* **42**: 271–73.

O'Quigley J (1999). Another look at two phase I clinical trial designs. *Stat Med* **18**: 2683–90.

O'Quigley J (2002). Curve-free and model based continual reassessment method designs. *Biometrics* **58**: 245–9.

O'Quigley J, Chevret S (1991). Methods for dose finding schedules in cancer clinical trials: A review and result of a Monte Carlo study. *Stat Med* **10**: 1647–64.

O'Quigley J, Pepe M, Fisher L (1996). Continual reassessment method: a practical design for phase I trials in cancer. *Biometrics* **46**: 33–48.

O'Quigley J, Hughes MD, Fenton J (2001). Dose-finding designs for HIV studies. *Biometrics* **57**: 1018–29.

Ratain MJ, Mick R, Schilsky RL, Siegler M (1993) Statistical and ethical issues in the design and conduct of phase I and II clinical trials of new anticancer agents. *J Natl Cancer Inst* **85**: 1637–43.

Rubinstein LV, Simon RM (2003). Phase I clinical trial design. In: Budman DR, Calvert AH, Rowinsky EK, eds. *Handbook of Anticancer Drug Development*, pp. 297–308. Lippincott Williams & Wilkins, Philadelphia, PA.

Shen LZ, O'Quigley J (1996). Consistency of continual reassessment method in dose finding studies. *Biometrika* **83**: 395–406.

Smith TL, Lee JJ, Kantarjian HM, *et al.* (1996). Design and results of Phase I cancer clinical trials: three year experience at the M.D. Andersen Cancer Center. *J Clin Oncol* **14**: 287–95.

Storer BE (1993). Small-sample confidence sets for the MTD in a phase I clinical trial. *Biometrics* **49**: 1117–25.

Thall PF, Lee JJ, Tseng, CH, Estez EH (1994). Accrual strategies for phase I trials with delayed patient outcome. *Stat Med* **18**: 1155–69.

Thall P, Estey E, Sung, H (1999). A new statistical method for dose-finding based on efficacy and toxicity in early phase clinical trials. *Invest New Drugs* **17**: 155–67.

Von Hoff DD (1998). There are no bad anticancer agents, only bad clinical trial designs— Twenty-first Richard and Hinda Rosenthal Foundation Award Lecture. *Clin Cancer Res* **4**: 1079–86.

Wang O, Faries DE (2000). A low-stage dose selection strategy in phase I trials with wide dose ranges. *J Biopharm Stat* 10: 319–33.

Whitehead J (2002). Heterogeneity in phase I clinical trials: Prior elicitation and computation using the continual reassessment method. (Letter) *Stat Med* 21: 1172.

Whitehead J, Brunier H (1995). Bayesian decision procedure for dose determining experiments. *Stat Med* 14: 885–93.

Whitehead J, Williamson D (1998). Bayesian decision procedures based on logistic regression models for dose-finding studies. *J Biopharm Stat* 8: 445–67.

Whitehead J, Zhou Y, Stallard N, Todd S, Whitehead A (2001). Learning from previous response in phase I dose-escalation studies. *Br J Clin Pharmacol* 52: 1–7.

Zohar S, Chevret C (2001). The continual reassessment method: Comparison of Bayesian stopping rules for dose-ranging studies. *Stat Med* 20: 2827–43.

Ethics

American Society of Clinical Oncology Policy Statement: Oversight of Clinical Research (2003). *J Clin Oncol* 21: 2377–86.

Daughtery CK (1999). Impact of therapeutic research on informed consent and the ethics of clinical trials: a medical oncology perspective. *J Clin Oncol* 17: 1601–17.

Daugherty CK, Ratain MJ, Minami H, *et al.* (1998). Study of cohort-specific consent and patient control in phase I cancer trials. *J Clin Oncol* 16: 2305–12.

Hawkins MJ (1993). Early cancer clinical trials: safety, numbers, and consent. *J Natl Cancer Inst* 85: 1618–19.

Itoh K, Sasaki Y, Fujii H, *et al.* (1997). Patients in phase I trials of anti-cancer agents in Japan: motivation, comprehension and expectations. *Br J Cancer* 76: 107–13.

Lipsett MB (1982). On the nature and ethics of phase I clinical trials of cancer chemotherapeutics. *JAMA* 248: 941–2.

Merz JF, Leonard DGB, Miller ER (1999): IRB Review and Consent in Human Tissue Research. *Science* 283: 1647–8.

Sankar P (2004). Communication and miscommunication in informed consent to research. *Med Anthropol* 18: 429–46.

Luce JM, Cook DJ Martin TR, et al. The ethical conduct of clinical research involving critically ill patients in the United States and Canada: Principles and Recommendations (Workshop report approved by the American Thoracic Board of Directors) (2004) *Am J Respir Crit Care Med* 170: 1375–84.

Wendler D, Emanuel E (2002). The debate over research on stored biological samples: what do sources think? *Arch Intern Med* 162: 1457–62.

White MT, Gamm J (2002). Informed consent for research on stored blood and tissue samples: a survey of institutional review board practices. *Account Res* 9: 1–16.

Preclinical evaluation and targets

Kamb A (2005). What's wrong with our cancer models? *Nat Rev Drug Discov* 4: 161–5.

Newell DR, Silvester J, McDowell C, Burtles SS; Cancer Research UK (2004). The Cancer Research UK experience of pre-clinical toxicology studies to support early clinical trials with novel cancer therapies. *Eur J Cancer* 40: 899–906.

Sausville EA (2004). Target selection issues in drug discovery and development. *J Chemother* 16 (Suppl. 4): 16–18.

Shaked Y, Bertolini F, Man S, *et al.* (2005) Genetic heterogeneity of the vasculogeneic phenotype parallels angiogenesis: implications for cellular surrogate marker analysis of antiangiogenesis. *Cancer Cell* 7: 101–11.

Workman P (2003). The opportunities and challenges of personalized genome-based molecular therapies for cancer: targets, technologies, and molecular chaperones. *Cancer Chemother Pharmacol* 52 (Suppl. 1): S45–56.

Phase I trials, endpoints, and drug development

Arteaga CL, Baselga J (2003). Clinical trial design and end points for epidermal growth factor receptor-targeted therapy: implications for drug development and practice. *Clin Cancer Res* 9: 1579–89.

Blesch KS, Gieschke R, Tsukamoto Y, Reigner BG, Burger HU, Steimer JL (2003). Clinical pharmacokinetic/pharmacodynamic and physiologically based pharmacokinetic modeling in new drug development: the capecitabine experience. *Invest New Drugs* 21: 195–223.

Burczynski ME, Oestreicher JL, Cahilly MJ, *et al.* (2005). Clinical pharmacogenomics and transcriptional profiling in early phase oncology clinical trials. *Curr Mol Med* 5: 83–102.

Connors T (1996). Anticancer drug development: the way forward. *Oncologist* 1: 180–1.

Dent SF, Eisenhauer EA (1996). Phase I trial design: Are new methodologies being put into place. *Ann Oncol* 7: 561–6.

Eggermont A, Newell H (2001). Translational research in clinical trials: the only way forward. *Eur J Cancer* 37: 1965.

Eskens FA, Verweij J (2000). Clinical studies in the development of new anticancer agents exhibiting growth inhibition in models: facing the challenge of a proper study design. *Crit Rev Oncol Hematol* 34: 83–8.

Fayette J, Soria JC, Armand JP (2005). Use of angiogenesis inhibitors in tumour treatment. *Eur J Cancer* 41: 1109–16.

Fox E, Curt GA, Balis FM (2002). Clinical trial design for target-based therapy. *Oncologist* 7: 401–9.

Galbraith SM (2003). Antivascular cancer treatments: imaging biomarkers in pharmaceutical drug development. *Br J Radiol* 76 (Spec No 1): S83–6.

Gehan EA (1979). Clinical trials in cancer research. *Environ Health Perspect* 32: 31–48.

Graham MA, Kaye SB (1993). New approaches in preclinical and clinical pharmacokinetics. *Cancer Surv* 17: 27–49.

Gupta N, Price PM, Aboagye EO (2002). PET for in vivo pharmacokinetic and pharmacodynamic measurements. *Eur J Cancer* 38: 2094–107.

Hirschfeld S, Pazdur R (2002). Oncology drug development: United States Food and Drug Administration perspective. *Crit Rev Oncol Hematol* 42: 13.

Hoekstra R, Verweij J, Eskens FA (2003). Clinical trial design for target specific anticancer agents. *Invest New Drugs* 21: 243–50.

Kelloff GJ, Sigman CC (2005). New science-based endpoints to accelerate oncology drug development. *Eur J Cancer* 41: 491–501.

Miller JC, Pien HH, Sahani D, Sorensen AG, Thrall JH (2005). Imaging angiogenesis: applications and potential for drug development. *J Natl Cancer Inst* **97**: 172–87.

Morgan B, Horsfield MA, Steward WP (2004). The role of imaging in the clinical development of antiangiogenic agents. *Hematol Oncol Clin North Am* **18**: 1183–206.

Newell DR (1990). Phase I clinical studies with cytotoxic drugs: pharmacokinetic and pharmacodynamic considerations. *Br J Cancer* **61**: 189–91.

Newell DR (2003). The drug development process: from target discovery to the clinic. *Clin Med* **3**: 323–6.

Newell DR (2005). How to develop a successful cancer drug—molecules to medicines or targets to treatments? *Eur J Cancer* **41**: 676–82.

Oza AM (2002). Clinical development of P glycoprotein modulators in oncology. *Novartis Found Symp* **243**: 103–15.

Seddon BM, Workman P (2003). The role of functional and molecular imaging in cancer drug discovery and development. *Br J Radiol* **76** (Spec No 2): S128–38.

Seymour L (2002). The design of clinical trials for new molecularly targeted compounds: progress and new initiatives. *Curr Pharm Des* **8**: 2279–84.

Simon RM, Steinberg SM, Hamilton M, *et al.* (2001) Clinical trial designs for the early clinical development of therapeutic cancer vaccines. *J Clin Oncol* **19**: 1848–54.

Stadler WM, Ratain MJ (2000). Development of target-based antineoplastic agents. *Invest New Drugs* **18**: 7–16.

Tan AR, Swain SM (2001). Novel agents: clinical trial design. *Semin Oncol* **28** (5 Suppl. 16): 148–53.

Vulfovich M, Saba N (2004). Molecular biological design of novel antineoplastic therapies. *Expert Opin Investig Drugs* **13**: 577–607.

A selection of textbooks

Adjei A, Buolamwini J, eds (2005). *Novel Anticancer Agents: Strategies for Discovery and Clinical Testing.* Elsevier Science, New York NY.

Budman DR, Calvert AH, Rowinsky EK (2003). *Handbook of Anticancer Drug Development.* Lippincott, Williams & Wilkins, Philadelphia.

Girling DJ, Parmar MK, Stenning SP, Stephens RJ, Stewart LA (2003). *Clinical Trials in Cancer: Principles and Practice.* Oxford University Press, New York NY.

Schellens JHM, McLeod HL, Newell DR eds (2005). *Cancer Clinical Pharmacology.* Oxford University Press, Oxford.

Appendix III: Tools for study development

This Appendix contains a number of tools to aid in study development as follows:

Appendix IIIa: Sample phase I protocol
Appendix IIIb: Sample phase I consent form
Appendix IIIc: Sample tissue I consent form
Appendix IIId: Sample trial activation checklist
Appendix IIIe: Sample investigational agent accountability record
Appendix IIIf: Sample Standard Operating Procedures (SOP) Index
Appendix IIIg: Sample study budget
Appendix IIIh: Case report form content

Appendix IIIa: Sample master phase I protocol

Acknowledgements

This protocol template is a modified version of the master protocol utilized at the joint FECS/ AACR/ASCO workshop 'Methods in Clinical Cancer Research' (information on the workshop found at http://www.fecs.be), and is used with permission of the workshop co-chairs.

Another template that may be used is that of the US National Cancer Institute Cancer Therapy Evaluation Program. It can be found at: http://ctep.cancer.gov/guidelines/templates.html

1 Background and introduction

This section should summarize the rationale of the proposed trial including its primary and secondary endpoints, based on all background information already available, and justify its importance.

If possible, divide this section into two clear subsections, one related to the *disease* under study, and the other to the *proposed investigational therapy*.

1.1 *Background disease information*

This section should:

- Give a brief overview of the incidence, therapeutic policies and outcome of the tumour type(s) addressed in the study. For phase I trials that are *not disease specific*, general comments about the need to improve treatment of cancers should be made.
- If a *disease-oriented phase I trial*, discuss standard therapies currently available for patients to be included in the trial, as well as their expected outcome.
- For *first-in-human* phase I trials: Summarize briefly preclinical data and justification for studying agent in humans. (Note: Section 5 will include pharmaceutical and detailed drug background information.)
- Justify why an investigational therapy or approach can be studied.
- For *combination* phase I trials or single agents trials where the agent has already been studied in humans: Summarize data available for the proposed investigational treatment(s); justify selected doses and schedules and why pharmacokinetic interaction studies should (or should not, if that is

your plan) be done. (Note: Section 5 will include pharmaceutical and detailed drug background information.)

Conclude this section with one or two sentences summarizing the present status of the scientific question, to serve as a transition to the subsequent section, for instance:

- '...this study will be the first to determine the recommended dose for 'Drug X' in patients with solid tumours.'

1.2 Background therapeutic information

Summarize here the data available for the proposed investigational treatment(s); justify selected doses and schedules. For each investigational agent it is suggested the following be described.

- Name and chemical information
- Chemical structure
- Mechanism of action
- Experimental antitumour activity
- Animal toxicology (include summary statement at end to justify first-in-human starting dose if applicable)
- Phase I trials (for instances where other phase I trials have been undertaken)
- Phase II/III trials For combination phase I trials it is assumed there are data on at least one agent in phase II/III
- Animal pharmacokinetic studies
- Clinical pharmacokinetic studies (if previously conducted)
- Pharmaceutical data
  - Supplied
  - Stability
  - Storage
  - Solution preparation
  - Route of administration

When two or more drugs combined in phase I trial, include a description of each as above and at end of this section, provide a rationale/justification for the recommended starting doses in combination and consider need for pharmacokinetic interaction assessment.

2 Study objectives

This section should be reviewed with the statistician.

2.1 Primary objective

The major scientific question expected to be answered by the study that determines design and sample size. For phase I trials this is almost always to determine recommended dose(s).

Example:

♦ 'To determine the maximum tolerated dose and recommended single agent dose of drug X given in schedule Y to patients with advanced solid tumours'

2.2 Secondary objectives

Additional questions to be addressed.

Examples:

♦ To describe the nature, severity, reversibility, and dose dependence of the toxic effects of drug X given in schedule Y.
♦ To describe the pharmacokinetic behaviour of drug X given in schedule Y.
♦ In patients with measurable disease, to describe any preliminary evidence of antitumour activity by assessment of objective response.
♦ To assess any dose-related or pharmacokinetic-related pharmacodynamic effects of drug X in normal (or tumour) tissue by a number of measures.

2.3 Endpoints

Specify which primary endpoint(s) (outcome measures) will be used to address the primary objective (e.g. toxic effects, pharmacokinetic measures, etc.) and which secondary endpoints (e.g. objective response) will be studied. *The primary endpoint(s) is/are those that will address the primary objective of the trial and should be objectively measurable in all eligible patients.*

Refer to Section 7 'Criteria of evaluation' for an exact definition of the parameters used as endpoints, and the detailed method of assessment.

3 Study population: patient selection criteria

Selection criteria indicate which patients are eligible for the trial. They may be indicated as inclusion and exclusion criteria in two subsections or as inclusion criteria only.

The following items are generally used in the definition of eligibility criteria. Please include information on the test timing prior to entry if that will be considered as part of trial eligibility:

♦ Tumour type(s) (specific if restricted to one or more histologies).
♦ Extent of disease (e.g. *advanced solid tumours, incurable by standard means*) and whether entry will be restricted to those with measurable disease or if it will include measurable and non-measurable disease.

- If patients must have measurable tumour according to RECIST criteria indicate here minimum size of measurable lesions.
- Prior treatments required/allowed/not allowed and time required since discontinuation.
- Age, performance status, objectively assessable parameters of life expectancy.
- Prior and concomitant associated diseases allowed.
- Minimum required laboratory data (white blood cells, neutrophils, platelets, renal and hepatic function, etc.).
- Example:

Laboratory requirements—within 7 days prior to enrolment:

Haematology:	absolute granulocytes	$\geq 1.5 \times 10^9/l$
	platelets	$\geq 100 \times 10^9/l$
Biochemistry:	bilirubin	within normal limits
	serum creatinine	within normal limits

- Patient must be non-pregnant (if applicable) and using effective contraceptive measures.
- Other criteria related to the safety of the specific regimen to be evaluated.

The following two criteria are mandatory in all clinical trials. 'Informed consent', which is a legal requirement, is generally included as the last selection criterion to underline its importance.

- Absence of any psychological, familial, sociological, or geographical condition potentially hampering compliance with the study protocol and follow-up schedule; those conditions should be discussed with the patient before registration in the trial.
- Before patient registration, written informed consent must be given according to ICH/GCP, and national/local regulations.

4 Study design

This section should be written in cooperation with the statistician. It should specify the type of trial (phase I single agent, phase I combination, pharmacodynamic study) and if the trial is randomized. Most phase I trials will be non-randomized. For *phase I trials*, specify:

- Starting dose and rationale for selecting it.
- Whether single centre or multicentre.
- Dose escalation steps planned (table suggested for clarity: include for each dose the planned minimum number of patients to be entered). For combination phase I trials, it is recommended that only one drug be escalated at each dose level.
- Description of the number of patients to be treated at each level and how decisions about expansion or escalation will be made based on toxicity or other parameters.

- Define endpoints, specifically dose-limiting toxicity (DLT) or other measures that are intended to limit/define dose. Note that the degree of toxicity 'acceptable' varies according to whether the agent is given intermittently in 'cycles' of therapy or given continuously and the definition of limiting toxicity should reflect these differences.
- Define how maximum tolerated dose (MTD; may also be called maximum administered dose or MAD) will be determined in terms of number of patients with DLT per dose level.
- Define how recommended phase II dose (RD) will be determined with respect to the MTD or MAD and how many patients will be treated at this dose level before the study is considered complete.
- If possible include options to add 'intermediate' dose levels pending assessment of clinical effects of the regimen and also describe how RD will be determined in the absence of observation of DLT.
- Here is an example from Chapter 7 of this book:

Note: in this example DLT definition reflects that commonly used for cyclical intravenous agents. When continuous dosing daily, DLT definition should be modified appropriately and normally that would mean considering lesser degrees of toxic effects dose limiting if they were sustained.

5 Therapeutic regimens and dose modifications

5.1 Treatment plan

5.1.1 Drug administration

Indicate agent(s) dose, schedule, timing of administration, and cycle length. If special needs: e.g. tubing type, infusion rate, treatment order if more than one drug, make sure it is clear here. A pharmacist review of this section may be helpful to assure clarity.

Design section: worked example with fictional agent LTK007

Starting dose

The starting dose of LTK007 will be 100 mg p.o. b.i.d. × 5 days every 28 days. (LTH = Licensed to Kill.) This dose is based on animal toxicology (see Protocol Section XX) and represents one-tenth the mouse equivalent LD10 (MELD10) dosage in the daily oral schedule.

Dose escalation

The dose of LTK007will be escalated in increments according to the dose escalation scheme outlined in the following table.
Intermediate dose levels or further splitting of the total dose into t.i.d. or q.i.d. dosing may occur dependent on emerging safety information and/or pharmacokinetic data if available.

Dose level	Dose of LTK007 given orally, twice daily × 5 days every 28 days (total daily dose)	Minimum no. of patients
−1	75 mg b.i.d. (150 mg total)	−
1 (starting)	100 mg b.i.d. (200 mg total)	3
2	200 mg b.i.d. (400 mg total)	3
3	400 mg b.i.d. (800 mg total)	3
	Continue to double dose until grade 2 toxicity related to drug is seen at level 'n', then begin escalation as shown. Round calculated dose to nearest 50 mg	
$n + 1$	$1.4 \times n$	3
$n + 2$	$1.4 \times n + 1$	etc.
	Continue escalating at $1.4 \times$ preceding dose until MTD	

Methods

The rate of subject entry and escalation to the next dose level will depend upon assessment of the safety profile of patients entered at the previous dose level. Toxicity will be evaluated according to the NCI Common Terminology Criteria for Adverse Events (CTCAE), Version 3.0 (see Appendix ___).

A minimum of three patients will be entered on each dose level. All three will be followed for one completed cycle of therapy (28 days) and subsequent enrolment of new cohorts will be based on the toxicity assessment in that first cycle and the documentation of any dose-limiting toxicities (for definitions see below). The investigator and subinvestigators will review all the data of each cohort together by teleconference with the study sponsor before making a decision regarding the next steps to be taken.

Intrapatient dose escalation is permitted as described below.

Definitions
Maximum tolerated dose

1. *If none of three patients exhibit DLT at this dose level:*
   - dose escalation to the *next* dose level may begin in a new cohort of patients
   - patients enrolled on the *previous* dose level who are still receiving therapy may now undergo intrapatient dose escalation to *this* dose level provided they have experienced no drug-related toxicity grade 2 or more.

2. *If one of three patients exhibit DLT at this dose level:*
   - expand dose level to a total of six patients
   - if no further DLT events seen, dose escalation to the *next* dose level may begin in a *new* cohort of patients and patients enrolled on the *previous* dose level who are still receiving therapy may now undergo intrapatient escalation to *this* dose level provided they have experienced no drug-related toxicity grade 2 or more

- if one or more further DLT events are seen (i.e. two or more of six patients), this dose level will be considered the MTD.

3. *If two of three patients exhibit DLT:*
   - This dose level will be considered the MTD.

Before opening the next higher dose level all toxic effects at the preceding dose level will be reviewed and expansion or escalation will be undertaken as appropriate. Conference calls between investigators and sponsor will be organized.

Dose-limiting toxicity

Toxicity will be graded using CTCAE version 3.0 (see Appendix ___). Any DLT must be a toxicity that is considered related to study drug. DLT is defined as follows.

During cycle 1

1. *Haematological*
   - absolute granulocyte count (AGC) $< 0.5 \times 10^9/l$
   - febrile neutropenia (ANC $< 1.0 \times 10^9/l$ with fever $>38.5°C$)
   - platelets $< 25 \times 10^9/l$
   - bleeding due to thrombocytopenia

2. *Non-haematological*
   - diarrhoea $>$ grade 3 despite use of antidiarrhoeal medication
   - rash $>$ grade 3 (or grade 2 if it is medically concerning or unacceptable to the patient)
   - other grade 3 organ effects thought to be treatment related
   - missing >2 doses of treatment for toxicity reasons.

Recommended phase II dose

As described above, the MTD is that dose in which two of three or two of six patients experience DLT.

Normally *one dose level below* that dose will be considered the recommended phase II dose. If the MTD is seen at the starting dose level, then dose level '–1' will be the recommended dose.

If clinically appropriate, intermediate dose levels may be studied to assure that the recommended dose is the highest tolerable. Further, if pharmacokinetic data suggests that saturable absorption of drug is occurring on a b.i.d. oral administration level, further dose splitting to t.i.d. or q.i.d. schedules may be considered if DLT has not been seen.

Up to a total of 10 patients may be treated at the recommended dose to ensure information on the safety profile at that dose is complete.

Patient replacement

Three patients within a dose level must be observed for one cycle (28 days) before accrual to the next higher dose level may begin. If a patient is withdrawn from the study prior to completing 5 days of therapy and a further 17 days of follow-up without experiencing a DLT prior to withdrawal, an additional patient may be added to that dose level. Patients missing two or more doses due to toxicity will not be replaced as these patients will be considered to have experienced a DLT

5.1.2 Premedication

Indicate if any premedication required (for example, antiemetics).

5.1.3 Patient monitoring

Indicate if any monitoring of vital signs during or shortly after treatment is required.

Example:

♦ **Blood pressure and heart rate are to be assessed every 30 minutes during the 2-hour infusion cycle 1 and 2. If no changes are seen, then end of infusion assessment only will be required for subsequent cycles.**

5.1.4 Dose adjustments

Sample text to introduce this section:

Doses will be reduced for haematological and other adverse events. Dose adjustments are to be made according to the system showing the greatest degree of toxicity. Adverse events will be graded using the NCI Common Terminology Criteria for Adverse Events Version 3.0 (CTCAE) (see Appendix___)

Based on *(other human)* and animal studies, the major adverse effects of *Drug X/Regimen* which limit dose *is/are likely to be*: ——————————————— .

The guidelines which follow outline dose adjustments for several of these toxic effects. If a patient experiences several adverse events and there are conflicting recommendations, please use the recommended dose adjustment that reduces the dose to the lowest level.

This section must unambiguously define all modifications of doses and schedules to be applied in case of toxicity (including when therapy must be discontinued). Concomitant medications recommended to manage adverse effects should be noted.

Please note that there must be consistency between what is stated here about toxic effects that mandate dose reduction information and those events that are considered DLT events; for example, if grade 3 major organ toxicity is something requiring a dose reduction, it should also be considered part of DLT definition.

Reductions should be by dose level as described in Section 4, not by percentage dose.

Examples: see Chapter 7 for some examples of dose reduction tables.

5.1.5 Duration of therapy

Indicate expected therapy duration.

♦ Example:
  ♦ **Six cycles will be given unless disease progression (see definition Section 7) or unacceptable toxicity are encountered.**

- ◆ Or
  - ◆ Treatment cycles will be repeated until progression (see definition Section 7) unless unacceptable toxicity is encountered.
  - ◆ Patients may also discontinue protocol therapy in the following instances:
    - ◆ intercurrent illness which would in the judgment of the investigator affect patient safety, the ability to deliver treatment or the primary study endpoints
    - ◆ request by patient.

This section should unambiguously define the 'end of protocol therapy'.

5.1.6 Concomitant therapy

Indicate which concomitant therapies are permitted or not permitted and, if possible, why. Attention here should be given to haematopoietic growth factors, to agents whose metabolism might be affected.

- ◆ In general a statement should be included prohibiting other anticancer or investigational therapy while patients are on study therapy.
- ◆ A statement should be made about what radiation therapy is permitted.
- ◆ A statement should be made to indicate supportive or other palliative measures are permitted, with any exceptions as noted.

6 Clinical evaluation, laboratory tests, follow-up

6.1 Before treatment start

This section should describe all investigations (and the timelines) needed for:

- ◆ evaluating patient eligibility
- ◆ assessing baseline values of parameters used as endpoints.

6.2 During treatment

This section should describe all investigations (and their timing) needed for assessing all endpoints of the study (adverse effects, pharmacokinetic measures, protocol compliance), as well as all criteria that will be used for therapeutic decisions.

6.3 After the end of treatment (follow-up)

This section should describe all investigations (and the schedule) after protocol therapy is discontinued. In phase I studies generally follow-up is limited to one visit 4 weeks after study drug is stopped. Other data to be collected after that normally include only late toxic effects and death.

6.4 Summary table

The whole schedule should preferably be summarized as a table. Here is an example:

Required investigations	Prestudy	Indicate	frequency	on	study	here
Physical XX XX						
Haematology XX XX						
Biochemistry XX XX						
Radiology[1] XX XX						
Other investigations XX XX						
Adverse events XX						

[1]Patients with a CR or PR should have scans repeated after 4 weeks to confirm response.

7 Criteria for evaluation and study endpoints

This section should give an objective and unambiguous definition of all endpoints of the study (efficacy, toxicity ...). It should also focus on the methods to be used for assessing or measuring these criteria, if relevant, and of the time points for evaluation.

Whenever standard scales or methods of evaluation are available (i.e. NCI Common Evaluation Criteria for Adverse Events [CTCAE v 3.0], RECIST criteria for the evaluation of response ...), they should be used and described in detail here or reference made to where in protocol to find it (e.g. *CTCAE v 3.0 are found in Appendix__ or website: _____*).

For phase I protocols, toxic effects remain the most common endpoint for assessment of dose recommendations.

If response is also to be determined in the subset of enrolled patients with measurable disease, please include details on criteria and measurement here. For template for response, see: http://ctep.cancer.gov/guidelines/recist.html

8 Statistical considerations

This section should be written with the help of a statistician. Many of the design elements of the phase I trial are covered in Section 4, Trial design.

8.1 Statistical design

- Indicate type of dose escalation method (e.g. accelerated titration, modified Fibonacci, fixed dose levels, modified CRM method) and describe basic elements and assumptions for the design here along with appropriate references.
- Indicate primary endpoint and secondary endpoints.
- Indicate which endpoints will determine escalation to the next step.
- Estimate number of patients which will need to be accrued.

8.2 Statistical analysis

- Describe for each endpoint the population that will be included.
- Describe how data will be analysed (tables of frequency by dose level; by cycle or by patient) and include any information on secondary endpoints, e.g. response and pharmacokinetics and how they will be related to dose/toxicity information.
- Analysis of pharmacokinetics and pharmacodynamic studies may be included here, or in the specific protocol sections devoted to those measures.

9 Pharmacokinetics

This section should be written in cooperation with the laboratory in charge of the pharmacokinetic analysis of samples. The following aspects should be addressed:

- objectives of the pharmacokinetic study
- list of the material to be obtained for each patient, with the sampling schedule
- instructions for treating and storing samples, and sending samples to the reference laboratory
- data transfer to the data centre (parameters to be transferred, timing, etc.), if applicable
- statistical analysis of pharmacokinetics.

10 Translational research and pharmacodynamic studies

This section should be written in cooperation with the laboratory in charge of the analysis of the samples. The following aspects should be addressed:

- objectives of the translational research study
- list of the material to be obtained for each patient, with the sampling schedule

- instructions for treating and storing samples, and sending samples to the reference laboratory
- data transfer to the data centre (parameters to be transferred, timing ...) if applicable
- statistical analysis.

11 Reporting adverse events

This section should be written following discussion with relevant personnel in the data management team responsible for safety reporting, if applicable.

11.1 Definitions

Here is some sample text based on ICH GCP:

- An adverse event (AE) is defined as any untoward medical occurrence or experience in a patient or clinical investigation subject that occurs following the administration of the trial medication regardless of the dose or causal relationship. This can include any unfavourable and unintended signs (such as rash or enlarged liver), or symptoms (such as nausea or chest pain), an abnormal laboratory finding (including blood tests, X-rays or scans) or a disease temporarily associated with the use of the protocol treatment. *(ICH-GCP)*.
- An adverse drug reaction (ADR) is defined as any response to a medical product, which is noxious and/or unexpected, related to any dose. *(ICH-GCP)*.
- Response to a medicinal product (used in the above definition) means that a causal relationship between the medicinal product and the adverse event is at least a reasonable possibility, i.e. the relationship cannot be ruled out.
- An unexpected adverse drug reaction is any adverse reaction for which the nature or severity is not consistent with the applicable product information (e.g., Investigator's Brochure). *(ICH-GCP)*.
- A serious adverse event (SAE) is defined as any undesirable experience occurring to a patient, whether or not considered related to the protocol treatment. An SAE that is considered related to the protocol treatment is defined as a serious adverse drug reaction (SADR).

Adverse events and adverse drug reactions which are considered as serious are those that result in:

- death
- a life-threatening event (i.e. the patient was at immediate risk of death at the time the reaction was observed)

- hospitalization or prolongation of hospitalization
- persistent or significant disability/incapacity
- a congenital anomaly/birth defect
- any other medically important condition (i.e. important adverse reactions that are not immediately life threatening or do not result in death or hospitalization but may jeopardize the patient or may require intervention to prevent one of the other outcomes listed above).

(ICH-GCP definition)

11.2 Reporting procedure

This paragraph should describe the exact procedure implemented to ensure that SAE are handled according to GCP and national laws.

12 Data collection

This section should be written in cooperation with the data manager, if one has been selected for the trial. Otherwise, a brief outline of how data will be collected (abstracted from the medical record on to paper case report forms; captured by electronic remote data entry; etc.) and how it will be compiled (e.g. entered into a trial-specific Oracle data base; transcribed into an Excel spreadsheet etc) and how the data will be analysed (e.g. using SAS or other system).

12.1 Case report forms

If case report forms will be used (see above), this section should include the list of forms to be completed for all patients, and the expected schedule of form completion. It should be clear on who may complete forms and who is authorized to sign them. Practical details (address where forms should be sent, contact person at the data centre, etc.) should be provided.

12.2 Data flow

This section should explain how forms will be handled and who is authorized to modify them. It should describe the system in place for querying missing or inconsistent data.

13 Quality assurance
13.1 Control of data consistency

This paragraph should describe procedures implemented to check the internal consistency of collected data.

13.2 On-site monitoring and quality control

This section is intended for multicentre studies only when data are sent to a central data centre, pharmaceutical company, or similar co-ordinating centre.

If no 'on-site monitoring' is foreseen, this section does not need to be included in the protocol.

This section has to be written by the study co-ordinator/study chair, in collaboration with the person who is organizing the on-site monitoring. It should specify: (a) who will perform the monitoring; (b) what is the frequency of site visits; and (c) what are the aims of the site visits.

13.3 Audits

If audit visits are planned, a section should be included in the protocol. Here is an example:

To ensure quality of data, study integrity, and compliance with the protocol and the various applicable regulations and guidelines, the 'Sponsor' may conduct site visits to institutions participating to protocols.

The investigator, by accepting to participate to this protocol, agrees to co-operate fully with any quality assurance visit undertaken by third parties, including representatives from the 'Sponsor', national and/or foreign regulatory authorities or company supplying the product under investigation, as well as to allow direct access to documentation pertaining to the clinical trial (including CRFs, source documents, hospital patient charts and other study files) to these authorized individuals.

The investigator must inform the 'Sponsor' immediately in case a regulatory authority inspection would be scheduled.

13.4 Central review of pathology

If pathology review is planned, this section should explain the objectives of the review, describe the general review procedure, and detail the procedures to be followed by the investigators to submit material to the external reviewers.

13.5 Other central review procedures

All central review procedures (e.g. radiology) have to be addressed in this section. They should:

◆ explain the objectives of the central review
◆ detail who will be the central reviewers, and describe the general review procedure
◆ give instructions to investigators for sending appropriate material to the central reviewers.

14 Administrative considerations

This section should detail the responsibilities of all involved parties, and give their exact addresses, phone, fax, and e-mail addresses.

14.1 Trial sponsorship and financing

The name, address, telephone, and fax number of the study 'sponsor' (according to GCP definition) must be included in the protocol.

14.2 Trial insurance

European clinical trials must be covered by insurance, in accordance with GCP and most European laws and regulations (those are country dependent!). This section should specify who has subscribed the insurance, what is covered, and give the policy number (or explain how a copy of the policy may be obtained). For other jurisdictions indicate if insurance is required and, if so, who will hold it.

14.3 Investigator authorization procedure

This section should discuss the steps to be followed by the investigators to be allowed to enter patients in the trial (note: this section may be edited as appropriate for different countries. For single centre studies it may not be applicable):

- all conditions to be fulfilled by potential investigators to be allowed to participate to the trial
- documents to be provided to the data/co-ordinating centre, if applicable
- ethical committee approval
- legal requirements, submission to health authorities, etc.

14.4 Patient registration/randomization procedure

This section should explain the exact procedure to register a new patient in a trial, including:

- practical details (internet, phone, fax, mail, etc.)
- timing for registration
- if the patient eligibility is checked at the time of registration, list of information to be provided
- if the trial is randomized, details of the randomization procedure

15 Ethical considerations

The three following areas have to be addressed in the protocol. The paragraphs included hereunder are consistent with ICH GCP.

15.1 Patient protection

The responsible investigator will ensure that this study is conducted in agreement with either the Declaration of Helsinki (Tokyo, Venice, Hong Kong, Somerset West, and Edinburgh amendments) or the laws and regulations of the country, whichever provides the greatest protection of the patient.

The protocol will be approved by the local, regional, or national ethics' committees.

15.2 Subject identification

This paragraph should explain how subjects are identified in the trial database, and demonstrate how confidentiality requirements are implemented.

15.3 Informed consent

All patients will be informed of the aims of the study, the possible adverse events, the procedures and possible hazards to which he/she will be exposed, and the how treatment and dose will be determined. They will be informed as to the strict confidentiality of their patient data, but that their medical records may be reviewed for trial purposes by authorized individuals other than their treating physician. It will be emphasized that the participation is voluntary and that the patient is allowed to refuse further participation in the protocol whenever he/she wants. This will not prejudice the patient's subsequent care.

A sample of a consent form is given as an appendix, and the checklist of ICH GCP content of an informed consent document is found in Chapter 7, Table 7.10 of this book.

It is the responsibility of the individual investigator to develop the appropriate informed consent document in compliance with local and national standards. The consent form should be dated and version controlled. The informed consent form is part of the documents to be submitted to the ethics committee for approval. The competent ethics committee for each institution must validate local informed consent documents before the centre can activate the study.

16 Publication policy

Including a clear publication policy in the study protocol avoids endless discussions at the end of the trial (that can contribute to delay the publication of available results). Therefore, it is highly recommended to discuss the publication policy between the different scientists who will be involved in the conduct of the study before the trial is actually started. This policy should explain:

- when the trial results will be published
- who will be the first author, the co-authors and who will deserve acknow-ledgements
- if any restrictions apply to publication of ancillary substudies (e.g. pharmacodynamic studies) before the publication of the main results of the trial.

Appendix A: References

This appendix should include all references mentioned in the protocol, listed in a consistent way. It is recommended to use a format of 'author name(s), year' sorted alphabetically to avoid numbering errors as protocol drafts are revised.

Appendix IIIb: Sample phase I consent form for a first-in-man phase I trial

This consent form uses the language and format that is consistent with many regulations and guidelines but this is a guide only. Investigators must check with local ethics committees for specific information about content and format. Other resources to consult are the US Office for Human research Protection Informed Consent Checklist (http://www.hhs.gov/ohrp/humansubjects/assurance/consentckls.htm), the Cancer Therapy evaluation program Informed Consent Template (http://www.cancer.gov/clinicaltrials/understanding/simplification-of-informed-consent-docs/page3), and the checklist from Good Clinical Practice, found in Chapter 7 as Table 7.10.

Acknowledgements

*This document is a modified version of the generic consent form developed by the National Cancer Institute of Canada Clinical Trials Group and is used with their permission. Throughout this sample, **italicized bold text** represents examples or instructions.*

---

*Title of study (**should match final protocol title**):*_____

*Trial code number:*_____

This is a clinical trial (a type of research study). Clinical trials include only patients who choose to take part. Please take your time to make your decision. Discuss it with your friends and family.

You are being asked if you would like to take part in this study because ....

[specify here why the patient is being asked to join the study. For phase I trials, usual language is that the patient has cancer which is no longer curable by standard or available treatments, and there is a new investigational agent which they may wish to take as part of the clinical trial being proposed].

Why is this study being done?

This research is being done because *[name]* is a new drug that shows activity in animal tumours, but it has *never been tested before in cancer patients*. The first step in studying this new drug will be to determine the dose that should be given to cancer patients.

Therefore, the purpose of this study is to determine the dose of the new drug *[name]* which can be recommended for use in cancer patients. The dose will be the highest dose of the new drug *[name]* that can be given without causing very severe side-effects that are not tolerable *[or, indicate here if something other than toxic effects will determine dose]*. This is done by starting at a dose lower than the one that does not cause side-effects in animals. Patients are given *[name]* and are watched very closely to see what side-effects they have and to make sure the side-effects are not severe. If the side-effects are not severe, then more patients are asked to join the study and are given a higher dose of *[name]*. Patients joining the study later on will get higher doses of *[name]* than patients who join earlier. This will continue until a dose is found that causes severe but temporary side-effects. Doses higher than that will not be given.

How many people will take part in the study?

Up to *[number]* people will take part in this study and it will take about one year to complete.

What is involved in the study?

Please see the *[diagram or calendar]* attached to the end of this consent form.

Treatment

If you agree to take part in this study, you will be given *[name]* by needle into one of your veins. The procedure will take about 10 minutes. This will happen every 3 weeks for up to 6 months. The treatment followed by 3 weeks is called a 'cycle' of treatment. The dose may be changed or stopped if you have side-effects and the treatment may also stop if your disease grows in spite of treatment. More details on the length of treatment are found later in this form. You will not need to be hospitalized unless you have serious side-effects *[modify this section as appropriate for route and schedule of investigational drug]*.

[If applicable, prophylactic or other protocol mandated treatments (e.g. antiemetics) to be given prior to or following chemotherapy etc. should be described]

Procedures and medical tests

The following tests will be done at the *[hospital or clinic name]* to make sure that you are eligible for this study. None of these tests are experimental. They are routine.

Example:

 *   *blood tests*
 *   *physical examination*
 *   *pregnancy test*

- *chest X-ray*
- *X-rays of your bones (skeletal survey)*
- *a special X-ray to study the heart (MUGA scan)*
- *computerized scan (CT scan) of your abdomen and chest.*

Many of these tests will also be repeated during the study. Some of these tests may be done more frequently than if you were not taking part in this research study. In addition, because this will be the first time this experimental drug is given to people, *[number]* extra blood samples will be taken to find out how quickly it is removed from your circulation. *[If applicable, explain any procedures being tested or those not part of regular care.]* *[Explain any risks of procedures, e.g.]* The needles used to take blood or inject substances for body scans might be uncomfortable. You might get a bruise, or rarely, an infection at the site of the needle puncture. *[some ethical committees require explicit details on volume of blood that will be removed each cycle described in lay quantities]*

Tissue collection

[Note: some institutions prefer that the tissue consent be a separate form since this section is quite long, and a separate form facilitates tracking in the research tissue bank. If this is to be done, the following section may be replaced by a statement that the patient will be invited to undergo additional studies for tissue studies as part of the trial using a separate consent form]

Begin by stating what main purpose is and whether it is necessary or optional as follows:

When tissue studies are *optional*:

The researchers doing the study of *[drug name]* in cancer patients for the first time are interested in doing research tests on tissue samples from your cancer to see *how this new drug works inside your cancer cells, and what effects it has on your cancer cell's function.* The collection of cancer tissue samples is an optional part of this study. These tissue studies will not benefit you directly, but may help future patients. You may refuse to have your tissue samples collected and still may participate in this study.

or

When tissue studies are *mandatory*:

The researchers doing the study of *[drug name]* in cancer patients for the first time are interested in doing research tests on tissue samples from your cancer to see *how this new drug works inside your cancer cells, and what effects it has on your cancer cell's function.* These tissue studies will not benefit you directly, but may help future patients. The collection of cancer tissue samples is a necessary part of this study.

Then describe where the tissue will come from:

For *fresh* biopsies:

The collection of the tissue sample(s) will require that you undergo a biopsy *[indicate if repeated biopsies and if so timing]*. This is a type of surgical procedure which will remove *[state how much tissue is to be taken, e.g. a pea-sized piece]* of your *[type of]* cancer. It has risks such as blood loss, pain and rarely an infection at the biopsy site.

or

For *archival* tissue:

Small tissue samples will be collected from the sample of your *[type of]* cancer that has already been removed by surgery or biopsy. No further surgeries or biopsies are required of you for this purpose.

Then describe where tissue will be sent and confidentiality of the material:

Tissue samples will be sent to a research laboratory at *[institution name, place]* and studied. The only identification that will be on your tissue samples sent to the laboratory will be the code number for the trial and your patient code number which is anonymous *[add anything else that is identifier here]*. Tissue samples will be used for research to understand *[how the drug is working in your cancer cells]*.

Then describe what will happen to the tissue after this research is completed and any possibility for commercialization:

Your tissue sample will be used for research purposes only and will not be sold. The research done with your samples may or may not help develop commercial products. There are no plans to provide payment to you if this happens. Any tissue remaining after the research mentioned above is completed will be _____

[options are: kept in a research tissue bank at _____ provided you give permission for this below; returned to the hospital where you had your surgery or biopsy; destroyed. Some will allow patients the option to choose banking or not].

Then request permission for future studies on any remaining and banked tissue; the following is one approach:

If you agree to keep some of the your tissue that is leftover from the research studies described above for *future* research in a tissue bank, this tissue will be kept and may be used in research to learn more about cancer and other diseases. The research that may be done with your tissue is not designed specifically to help you. It might help people who have cancer and other diseases in the future.

Reports about research done with your tissue will not be given to you or your doctor. These reports will not be put in your health record. The research will not have an effect on your care.

If you decide now that your tissue can be kept for future research, you can change your mind at any time. Then any tissue that remains will no longer be used for research.

In order to determine what your stored tissue may be used for below, please read each statement below and consider it carefully. Put your initials beside the 'Yes' or 'No' to indicate your choice.

No matter what you decide to do, it will not affect your care.

Making your choice about tissue studies

Please read each sentence below and think about your choice. After reading each sentence, circle 'Yes' or 'No'. If you have any questions, please talk to your doctor or nurse, or the person whose name is found at the end of this consent form who is available for further questions.

[Include those of the following questions appropriate in your trial]

1. My tissue may be *[biopsied or taken from the pathology department]* and may be used to understand *[how the drug is working in your cancer cells]*. *[Indicate if this is required or optional to participate in the clinical trial, as appropriate]*

Yes   No

[Note: if the patient declines in question #1 to have biopsies done or tissue accessed from pathology, then all the remaining questions may be skipped since there will be no tissue.]

2. Any leftover tissue from the studies that will be done for this clinical trial, as described above, may be kept for use in future research to learn about, prevent, or treat cancer.

Yes   No

3. Any leftover tissue from the studies that will be done for this clinical trial, as described above, may be kept for use in research to learn about, prevent or treat other health problems (for example: diabetes, Alzheimer's disease, or heart disease).

Yes   No

4. Any leftover tissue from the studies that will be done for this clinical trial, as described above, may be kept for use may be used for genetic research (about diseases that are passed on in families).

Yes   No

5. Someone may contact me in the future to ask me to take part in more research.

Yes   No

Your signature at the end of this form will confirm your answers.

How long will I be in the study?

Study drug *[name]* will continue for *[a maximum period of 8 cycles (6 months)]* unless:

- Your cancer grows.
- You are unable to tolerate the study drug.
- New information shows that the study drug is no longer in your best interest.
- Your doctor no longer feels this is the best treatment for you.

You can choose not to take part in this study or stop taking part at any time and your doctor will continue to treat you with the best means available. If you decide to stop participating in the study, we encourage you to talk to your doctor first.

When the study drug is stopped, we would like to keep track of your health for *[insert length of time]* to look at the long-term effects of the study treatments.

What are the risks of the study?

As with any experimental drug, additional unexpected and sometimes serious side-effects are a possibility. As *[name]* is a new treatment that has never been tested in people before, all of the side-effects are not known. Long-term effects of this treatment are also unknown.

Your doctor will watch you closely to see if you have side-effects. When possible other drugs will be given to you to make side-effects less serious and uncomfortable. Many side-effects go away shortly after cancer drugs are stopped but in some cases side-effects can be serious, long-lasting or permanent. Rarely side-effects of cancer drugs can be life-threatening or fatal.

Possible risks and side-effects that may occur with *[drug name]*

Based on *[experience with other similar drugs or side-effects in animals, or effects of cancer therapy in general]* risks and side-effects related to *[drug name]* may include:

[list possible effects here. Note, some ethics committees prefer the list to be subdivided as to effects that are likely or unlikely, but as this is first-in-man study that will not be possible]

Reproductive risks

Because the effects the drug *[name]* may have on a fetus are unknown, you should not become pregnant or father a baby while on this study. An effective method of birth control should be used while you are on study treatment. *[If applicable, specify if birth control should continue for a period of time after treatment has stopped]*. Ask about counselling and more information about preventing pregnancy. You should not nurse your baby while on this study. *[Include a statement about possible sterility when appropriate]*

Are there benefits to taking part in the study?

If you agree to take part in this study, although it is unlikely there will be a direct benefit to you in terms of your cancer growth, it is still possible there might be. Overall about 5% of patients who are given experimental cancer drugs as part of studies where they are tested for the first time in people have some shrinkage of their tumour, but it is unknown if that will happen on this study. We hope the information learned from this study will help other patients with cancer in the future.

What other options are there?

If you decide not to take part in this study, your doctor will discuss other treatment options with you. These may include:

- other chemotherapy
- radiation therapy
- no therapy at this time with care to help you feel more comfortable.

Please talk to your doctor about these and other options. As with any treatment, there are possible benefits and risks. Your doctor will be able to provide you with information about any known benefits and risks of these other treatment options.

What about confidentiality?

Every effort will be made to keep your personal information confidential.

Qualified representatives of the following organizations *may inspect your medical and study records* for quality control:

- *The co-ordinating group for this trial*
- *The company which makes the drug [name] [company name]*
- *Government oversight body [name] (because they oversee the use of new drugs)*

Qualified representatives of the following organizations may receive information from your medical/study records for data analysis and quality control.

- *The co-ordinating group for this trial*
- *The company that makes the drug [name] [company name]*
- *Government oversight body [name] (because they oversee the use of new drugs)*

This information may include test results, reports of operations, X-rays, or scan reports.

The organizations listed above will keep information about you confidential, to the extent permitted by applicable laws, in the following manner:

- *you will be identified only by a trial code, a patient serial number, and initials as well as a hospital/clinic number (if permitted by your local research ethics board)*
- *identifying information will be kept behind locked doors*
- *[list others as appropriate]*

What are the costs?

The study drug, *[name]*, will be given to you free of charge as long as you receive treatment on the study. You will not be paid for taking part in this study. Taking part in this study may result in added costs to you.

In the case of research-related side-effects or injury, *[insert here relevant information about compensation]*.

What are your rights as a participant?

Taking part in this study is voluntary. You may choose not to take part or may leave the study at any time. Deciding not to take part or deciding to leave the study later will not result in any penalty or any loss of benefits to which you are entitled. Your doctor will discuss further treatments with you and continue to treat your cancer with the best means available.

[if relevant: A Data Safety Monitoring Board, an independent group of experts, will be reviewing the data from this research throughout the study.]

You will be told about new information that may affect your health, welfare, or willingness to stay in this study.

You will be given a copy of this signed and dated consent form.

Who do you call if you have questions or problems?

If you have questions about taking part in this study or if you suffer a research-related injury you can talk to your doctor. Or, you can meet with the doctor who is in charge of the study at this institution. That person is:

_____
Name Telephone

If you would like advice regarding your rights as a patient, you can talk to someone who is not involved in the study at all. That person is:

_____
Name Telephone

Signatures

My signature on this consent form means the following:

- The study has been fully explained to me and all of my questions have been answered,
- I understand the requirements and the risks of the study,
- I give permission for the tissue *[biopsies and]* studies as I have circled on this form,
- I authorize access to my medical records as explained in this consent form, and
- I agree to take part in this study.

Signature of patient   Date

Signature of investigator   Date

Obtaining informed consent

Note: The following witness signature block may not be required in some hospitals/clinics.

Signature of witness   Date

Version date and/or ethics approval date of this form: _____
Patient code no. # _____

Appendix IIIc: Sample phase I tissue consent form for a first-in-man phase I trial

This consent form assumes that tissue collected will be used for studies related to the phase I study, and possible future research. This is not a general 'tumour banking consent form, therefore.

The form uses the language and format that is consistent with many regulations and guidelines but this is a guide only. Investigators must check with local ethics committees for specific information about content and format. Other resources to consult are the US Office for Human Research Protection Informed Consent Checklist (http://www.hhs.gov/ohrp/ humansubjects/assurance/consentckls.htm), the Cancer Therapy evaluation program Informed Consent Template (http://www.cancer.gov/clinicaltrials/understanding/simplifi-cation-of-informed-consent-docs/page3) and the checklist from Good Clinical Practice, found in Chapter 7 as Table 7.10.

Acknowledgements

This document is a modified version of the generic tissue consent form developed by the National Cancer Institute of Canada Clinical Trials Group and is used with their permission.

Throughout this sample, ***italicized and bold text*** represents examples or instructions

---

*Title of study (**should match final protocol title**): _____*

Trial code number: _____

Tissue collection

Begin by stating what main purpose is and whether it is necessary or optional as follows:

When tissue studies are *optional:*
The researchers doing the study of *[drug name]* in cancer patients for the first time are interested in doing research tests on tissue samples from your cancer to see ***how this new drug works inside your cancer cells, and what effects it has on your cancer cell's***

function. The collection of cancer tissue samples is an optional part of this study. You may refuse to have your tissue samples collected and still may participate in this study. These tissue studies will not benefit you directly, but may help future patients.

or

When tissue studies are *mandatory*:
The researchers doing the study of *[drug name]* in cancer patients for the first time are interested in doing research tests on tissue samples from your cancer to see *how this new drug works inside your cancer cells, and what effects it has on your cancer cell's function.* The collection of cancer tissue samples is a necessary part of this study, so if you choose not to take part in this aspect of the study, you will not be able to join the rest of the study. These tissue studies will not benefit you directly, but may help future patients. [*note: some would argue that mandatory tissue collection should be included in the main study consent form, not a separate document, so that the patient understands all the aspects of what the study involves before consenting to it*]

Then describe where the tissue will come from:
For *fresh* biopsies:

The collection of the tissue sample(s) will require that you undergo a biopsy *[indicate if repeated biopsies and if so timing]*. This is a type of surgical procedure that will remove *[state how much tissue is to be taken, e.g. a pea-sized piece]* of your *[type of]* cancer. It has risks such as blood loss, pain, and rarely an infection at the biopsy site.

or

For *archival* tissue

Small tissue samples will be collected from the sample of your *[type of]* cancer that has already been removed by surgery or biopsy. No further surgeries or biopsies are required of you for this purpose.

Then describe where tissue will be sent and confidentiality of the material:

Tissue samples will be sent to a research laboratory at *[institution name, place]* and studied. The only identification that will be on your tissue samples sent to the laboratory will be the code number for the trial and your patient code number, which is anonymous *[add anything else that is identifier here]*. Tissue samples will be used for research to understand *[how the drug is working in your cancer cells]*.

Then describe what will happen to the tissue after this research is completed and any possibility for commercialization.

Your tissue sample will be used for research purposes only and will not be sold. The research done with your samples may or may not help develop commercial products. There are no plans to provide payment to you if this happens. Any tissue remaining after the research mentioned above is completed will be *[options are: kept in a research tissue bank at _____ provided you give permission for this below; returned to the hospital where you had your surgery or biopsy; destroyed. Some will allow patients the option to choose banking or not].*

Then request permission for future studies on any remaining and banked tissue; the following is one approach.

If you agree to keep some of the your tissue that is leftover from the research studies described above for future research in a tissue bank, this tissue will be kept and may be used in research to learn more about cancer and other diseases. The research that may be done with your tissue is not designed specifically to help you. It might help people who have cancer and other diseases in the future.

Reports about research done with your tissue will not be given to you or your doctor. These reports will not be put in your health record. The research will not have an effect on your care.

If you decide now that your tissue can be kept for future research, you can change your mind at any time. Then any tissue that remains will no longer be used for research.

In order to determine what your stored tissue may be used for below, please read each statement below and consider it carefully. Put your initials beside the 'Yes' or 'No' to indicate your choice.

No matter what you decide to do, it will not affect your care.

What are the risks?

The risks to you include *[the risk of biopsy… list consequences if appropriate]* and a potential risk to your privacy. As noted, your tissue sample will not have personal information attached and will be identified only by a code number, so you name will not known to the laboratory researchers doing the tissue studies *[add anything else here that will be done to assure confidentiality]*.

What are the benefits?

Although participating in this research will not be of direct benefit to you, what is learned may be of help to future patients, by *[explain]*.

Making your choice about tissue studies:

Please read each sentence below and think about your choice. After reading each sentence, circle 'Yes' or 'No'. If you have any questions, please talk to your doctor or nurse, or the person whose name is found at the end of this consent form who is available for further questions. *[Include those of the following questions appropriate in your trial]*

1. My tissue may be **[biopsied or taken from the pathology department]** and may be used to understand **[how the drug is working in your cancer cells]**. *[Indicate if this is required or optional to participate in the clinical trial, as appropriate]*

        Yes   No

[Note: if the patient declines in question 1 to have biopsies done or tissue accessed from pathology, then all the remaining questions may be skipped since there will be no tissue.]

2. Any leftover tissue from the studies that will be done for this clinical trial, as described above, may be kept for use in future research to learn about, prevent, or treat cancer.

Yes   No

3. Any leftover tissue from the studies that will be done for this clinical trial, as described above, may be kept for use in research to learn about, prevent or treat other health problems (for example: diabetes, Alzheimer's disease, or heart disease).

Yes   No

4. Any leftover tissue from the studies that will be done for this clinical trial, as described above, may be kept for use may be used for genetic research (about diseases that are passed on in families).

Yes   No

5. Someone may contact me in the future to ask me to take part in more research.

Yes   No

Signatures

My signature on this consent form means the following:

- The tissue research study has been fully explained to me and all of my questions have been answered,
- I understand the requirements and the risks of the study
- I agree to take part in this tissue study, with the conditions as indicated on future research as indicated by my answers to the YES/NO questions above.

Signature of patient	Date
Signature of investigator	Date

Obtaining informed consent

Note: The following witness signature block may not be required in some hospitals/clinics.

Signature of witness	Date

Appendix IIId
Sample Trial Activation Checklist for a Phase I First-in-man Oncology Study

Not all items need to be done in sequence. In fact, wherever possible, simultaneous action on the checklist items is encouraged to make the process of trial activation more efficient.

Acknowledgment: This document is a modified version of a similar checklist used at the National Cancer Institute of Canada Clinical Trials Group and is used with their permission.

TRIAL ACTIVATION CHECKLIST			
Trial Code:			
Full Title:			
Principle Investigator (Study Chair):		Statistician:	
Data Manager		Other personnel:	
Pharmacist Contact:	Industry Sponsor (if applicable):		Industry Contact(s) (if applicable):
PROTOCOL DEVELOPMENT			**DATE**
Concept sheet to sponsor (if applicable)			
Circulate draft protocol for comments to:			
Members of protocol committee			
Industry Sponsor, if applicable			
Data manager			
Pharmacist			
Contacts for tumour banking, other special studies			
Statistician			
Revise protocol. FINAL Protocol with appropriate covering letters to:			
Protocol/ trial committee			
Scientific/protocol review committee (if appropriate)			
Other: specify (note: there may be other documents required depending on trial)			
FINAL Protocol to your internal regulatory office to begin to prepare submission to Health Authorities, if applicable			
CONSENT FORM			
Drafted by Study Chair/ Study Coordinator according to 'generic' format			
Once final, to go for translation if necessary (note: should be done in time to be included with 'final' protocol in distribution for Ethical committee approval)			
CASE REPORT FORMS/DATA COLLECTION FORMS (INCLUDING SAE FORM)			
Forms design initiated by Study chair/Study coordinator or clinical trials office staff			
Draft to Data manager			
Draft to Industry Sponsor, if applicable			
Draft to Study Chair/Study coordinator			
Draft to Statistician for review			
Research Nurse Guidebook, if applicable			
Patient Diary, if applicable (Patient Diary for translation, if necessary)			
Other: specify			
TRIAL INSURANCE			
Trial insurance in place			
Other (specify)			
CONTRACT			
Contract drafted *(including elements noted in Table 8.4, Chapter 8 of this book)*			
Contract finalized			
Contract signed			
INVESTIGATOR DRUG BROCHURE			
Investigator Drug Brochure received			

	DATE
GOVERNMENT/REGULATORY AND OTHER APPROVALS	
Government regulatory submission done on FINAL approved protocol	
Government approval received	
Industry submission (if applicable)	
Industry approval Received (if applicable)	
Other submission (specify)	
ETHICAL REVIEW AND APPROVAL	
Prepare submission of FINAL protocol for ethical committee, submit protocol and all required papers	
Submission completed	
Submission reviewed	
Final Approval received	
DRUG SUPPLY AND ACCOUNTABILITY	
Establish with pharmaceutical company (if applicable) or other provider procedure for drug distribution............	
Arrange with Director of Pharmacy storage of drug	
Drug accountability logs developed, if applicable	
Other (e.g. training in administration procedures): specify	
REVIEW MECHANISMS (ESTABLISH, AS APPLICABLE)	
Pathology review (procedures and form)	
Radiology review (procedures and form)	
Central laboratory (procedures and form)	
Other: specify	
PHARMACOKINETIC STUDIES	
Supplies (tubes, labels, packaging) received. Ensure proper equipment available (e.g. centrifuge)	
Education of study personnel on sample timing, acquisition, processing and storage	
Shipping instructions and materials received	
TRANSLATIONAL RESEARCH STUDIES (IF APPLICABLE)	
Supplies (tubes, labels, packaging) received	
Education of study personnel on sample timing, acquisition, processing and storage. This should include meeting of study personnel with relevant scientist colleagues.	
Identification and agreement of any consultant specialists (e.g. surgeon, radiologist, pathologist) required	
Shipping instructions and materials received.	
OTHER SPECIAL RESEARCH STUDIES (IF APPLICABLE)	
Establish procedures, training for other special research studies (e.g. EKG monitoring, special radiology)	
FILES AND RECORDS	
Authorization list (names of participating centres, investigators, research nurses, data managers, pharmacists, etc.)	
Trial files (create trial related files)	
Registration or randomization Log Books	
Other: specify	
COMPUTERIZATION AND DATABASES	
Verify randomization/registration mechanism	
Meetings with computing/analysis team to review data entry plans and screens	
Meet with statistician to confirm data entry plans/screens once drafted	
Finalize computing/data entry procedures, programs and screens	
Other: specify	
FINANCE OFFICE	
Notify financial officer of new trial and establish per case funding amount (if applicable)	
Other: specify	
EDUCATION	
Education session for nurses, data managers and other team members re study conduct and procedures	
Other: specify	
STUDY ACTIVATION	
Activation package (includes protocol, forms, registration log, etc) to institution(s) once regulatory authorization completed, ethics approval received, contract in place and drug/study supplies ready.	
Drug supply shipped to centre with drug accountability logs, if applicable	
Other: specify	

Appendix IIIe: Investigational Agent Accountability Record

Appendix IIIe

EXAMPLE: INVESTIGATIONAL AGENT ACCOUNTABILITY RECORD
Main Record ☐   Satellite Record ☐   Page No. _____

Name of Institution:		Protocol No:		Investigator:
Agent Name:		Strength: Dosage Form: Manufacturer:		Dispensing Area:
Protocol Title				

Line No.	Date	Patient Initials	Patient Study ID	Dose	Received (+)	Dispense/ Destroyed (–)	Balance	Lot #	Expiry Date	Recorder Initials	Date of Return	Quantity Returned	Recorder Initials
1.													
2.													
3.													
4.													
5.													
6.													
7.													
8.													
9.													
10.													
11.													
12.													

1 – If multiple dose(s) or strength(s) of the drug are used, then logs for each dose/strength must be used as per regulatory requirements.
2 – Columns not required to be completed for IV drugs.

Acknowledgment: This document is a modified version of the drug accountability form developed by the National Cancer Institute of Canada Clinical Trials Group and is used with their permission.

Appendix IIIf: *Sample*: Standard Operating Procedures (SOPs) Index

Acknowledgement: This list of SOPs is a modification of the SOP topic list of the Ontario Cancer Research Network, found at http://www.ocrn.on.ca/pdf/CTNSOPIndex16Jul04.pdf. We acknowledge and thank colleagues at the OCRN for allowing us to use this material.

Appendix IIIg:
Sample Phase I Budget:

This budget assumes that trial management, PK assay, and sponsorship will all be undertaken by the clinical centre that is enrolling patients on the study. *It does not include funding for nested translational research or functional imaging studies.* Make sure appropriate overhead (indirect costs) is included in each item.

Clinical Data: Per Patient Costs	Baseline	Cycle 1, 2 etc (separate column for each cycle Estimate total number of cycles for Totals)	Follow-up visits	Total
Research nurse or Clinical Research Associate or Data manager *(see note below about cost calculation for personnel)*				
Special investigations (e.g. MUGA scan)				
Routine Laboratory studies				
PK sampling	███████			
PK supplies (collection)				
Radiology				
Pharmacy dispensing fee	███████			
(Physician fee)				
Supplies				
Mailing/Faxing				
Other				
Pharmacokinetic assay	Per sample costs	Number of samples per patient	Number of patients	Total
Pharmacokinetic assay development and validation	████████████████████████████			
Pharmacokinetic supplies				
Pharmacokinetic assay				
Shipping				
Computing				
Administrative costs				Total
Ethics committee (IRB, IEC or REB) fee for initial review	██████████████████████████████			
Initial pharmacy review fee				
Regulatory submission				
Adverse event reports (per report)				
Other (specify)				
Central Study Management	%FTE	Costs (including indirect costs)		Total
Data manager				
Statistician				
Regulatory specialist				
Secretarial and data entry				
Equipment: (Specify)				Total
Other Central Costs (Specify)				Total
Travel				
Publication				
Other				
GRAND TOTAL				

* Costs based on hourly wage for each professional. Time spent in patient contact, telephone calls, forms completion etc. should be accounted for. Include indirect costs (overhead) for institution and benefits in calculation. Costs for this aspect are sometimes also calculated using % FTE.

Appendix IIIh:
Case Report Form Content:
Baseline and On-Study forms

Although each case report form will have format defined by users, it is useful to consider what variables should be collected at baseline, during study drug administration, and after therapy is complete. The following lists are reasonably standard compilations of the data required for the *baseline* and *on treatment periods* of a phase I study.

FORM	Item number	Data element	*Comment*
Eligibility checklist			
	1	Include all items found in inclusion and exclusion criteria	*May have yes/no answers or require actual numbers/dates to check eligibility*
	2	Dose level	*Dose level assigned and calculated starting dose to be completed at time of patient entry.*
Baseline (Pre-Study)			
	1	Patient identification (coded) Institution and investigator	*Due to privacy concerns, it should not be possible to identify an individual patient on the basis of what is included on the CRF.*
	2	Disease History: Date of cancer diagnosis Primary site Histology	*Optional: stage/grade at diagnosis Optional: date of first relapse Optional: hormonal status of tumour*
	3	Previous chemotherapy. Date of first and last doses	*Start date, stop date, total dose for each agent or regimen may be collected*
	4	Previous radiation	*Dates, sites, total dose*
	5	Previous surgery	*Dates and procedures relevant to study disease*
	6	Other major medical problems	*Include name of problem and date of diagnosis along with relevant details*
	7	Sites of disease	*Include measurements for lesions that are measurable. Divide date form into Target and Non-Target lesions if using RECIST criteria*
	8	Symptoms/adverse events	*Use standard criteria (e.g. CTCAE v. 3.0) Include symptoms of disease and from previous therapy*
	9	Concomitant measures and medications	*Details variable but this may be an important list for phase I trials to assess eligibility (if any medications are prohibited) and to look for explanations for inter-patient variability in symptoms*
	10	Physical exam	*Performance status, height, weight vital signs (all with dates)*
	11	Lab studies (hematology, chemistry, coagulation etc.)	*Date, absolute values, units, normal range (latter may be collected separately).*
	12	Imaging studies	*Check list of studies performed, date and whether normal or abnormal*
	13	Urinalysis	*Date and results*
	14	Other studies	*e.g. MUGA scan, EKG. Date and results*
	15	Research procedures	*e.g. tumour biopsy, baseline normal tissue collection*
	16	Signature of person completing form	*Must be authorized person*

FORM	Item number	Data element	Comment
On Treatment			
Captures data from day 1 cycle 1 to end of that cycle. In phase I trials usually one form for each "cycle" of therapy.	1	Patient identification, institution, investigator	*As for baseline*
	2	Cycle or visit number and assigned dose level	
	3	Study drug administration	*Collect actual dose and units. Start date/time and stop date/time for each dose of treatment. If continuous infusion, capture beginning and end. Identify if drug interrupted, held, or dose reduced and reason*
	4	Radiation therapy this cycle	*To document concurrent radiation site, dose and reason*
	5	Surgical procedures this cycle	*To document any procedures (major or minor such as paracentesis)*
	6	New major medical problems	*Normally these will also be documented in adverse events page*
	7	Sites of disease	*As for baseline. Normally disease is followed every 2nd or third cycle. May include a section for investigator response assessment here.*
	8	Adverse events	*Capture all events, assign proper term name, (worst) grade, relationship to study drug (investigator opinion). Normally in phase I start and stop dates are also collected. Must specify criteria to be used in grading and naming events (e.g. CTCAE v. 3.0)*
	9	Concomitant measures	*New or changed concomitant measures are most important to capture.*
	10	Physical Exam	*Record as for baseline; Expected frequency as per protocol*
	11	Lab studies	*Record as for baseline; Expected frequency as per protocol*
	12	Imaging studies	*Record as for baseline; Expected frequency as per protocol.*
	13	Urinalysis	*Record as for baseline; Expected frequency as per protocol*
	14	Other studies	*Record as for baseline; Expected frequency as per protocol*
	15	Research Procedures	*Record as for baseline; Expected frequency as per protocol*
	16	Pharmacokinetics	*May be collected on separate specialized form. Record date, time of sampling, and volume sampled*
	17	Signature of person completing form	*Must be authorized person*

Appendix IV: List of courses

Courses and workshops on cancer clinical trials

The following are a sampling of educational workshops and courses available in North America, Europe, Australia and Asia-Pacific regions.

North America

A workshop on *Methods in Clinical Cancer Research* is held each summer in Vail, Colorado and is co-sponsored by the American Society of Clinical Oncology (ASCO) and the American Association of Cancer Research (AACR). Information and application forms available at http://www.asco.org and http://www.aacr.org

Other workshops on specific research methodology topics are periodically developed by both ASCO and AACR. Details are available at their websites.

Europe

A workshop on *Methods in Clinical Cancer Research* is held each summer in Flims, Switzerland and is co-sponsored by the Federation of European Cancer Societies, the American Society of Clinical Oncology (ASCO) and the American Association of Cancer Research (AACR). Information and application forms available at http://www.fecs.be, http://www.asco.org, and http://www.aacr.org

An annual course on *Clinical Trial Statistics for Non-Statisticians* is sponsored by the Education Department of the European Organization for Research and Treatment of Cancer (EORTC). EORTC also organizes a course on *Cancer Clinical Trials: Methods and Practice* that is held every other year. Information on these courses and other is found in the education section of the EORTC website: http://www.eortc.be/Seminar/Educationpgm/Programs/prog2005.htm

Australia and Asia-Pacific

Australia and Asia Pacific Clinical Oncology Research Development Workshop: A Workshop in Effective Clinical Trials Design is planned for every other year and is co-sponsored by ASCO, AACR, the Medical Oncology Group of Australia and the Clinical Oncology Society of Australia. Information and application details are found at http://www.acordworkshop.org.au

Index